MW01031302

DROP ACID

ALSO BY DAVID PERLMUTTER, MD

―――――

*Brain Wash: Detox Your Mind for Clearer Thinking,
Deeper Relationships, and Lasting Happiness*

*The Grain Brain Whole Life Plan: Boost Brain Performance,
Lose Weight, and Achieve Optimal Health*

*Brain Maker: The Power of Gut Microbes to Heal and
Protect Your Brain—for Life*

*The Grain Brain Cookbook: More Than 150 Life-Changing
Gluten-Free Recipes to Transform Your Health*

*Grain Brain: The Surprising Truth About Wheat, Carbs, and
Sugar—Your Brain's Silent Killers*

*Raise a Smarter Child by Kindergarten: Build a
Better Brain and Increase IQ Up to 30 Points*

*The Better Brain Book: The Best Tool for Improving Memory and
Sharpness and Preventing Aging of the Brain*

Power Up Your Brain: The Neuroscience of Enlightenment

Brainrecovery.com: Powerful Therapy for Challenging Brain Disorders

DROP ACID

The Surprising New Science of Uric Acid — The Key to Losing Weight, Controlling Blood Sugar, and Achieving Extraordinary Health

Featuring the LUV Diet™

DAVID PERLMUTTER, MD

WITH KRISTIN LOBERG

Little, Brown Spark
New York   Boston   London

Little, Brown Spark
Hachette Book Group
1290 Avenue of the Americas, New York, NY 10104
littlebrownspark.com

First Edition: February 2022

Little, Brown Spark is an imprint of Little, Brown and Company, a division of Hachette Book Group, Inc. The Little, Brown Spark name and logo are trademarks of Hachette Book Group, Inc.

The LUV Diet is a trademark of David Perlmutter, MD.

The publisher is not responsible for websites (or their content) that are not owned by the publisher.

The Hachette Speakers Bureau provides a wide range of authors for speaking events. To find out more, go to hachettespeakersbureau.com or call (866) 376-6591.

ISBN 9780316315395
LCCN 2021919579

Printing 1, 2021

LSC-C

Printed in the United States of America

This book is dedicated to the ever-increasing numbers of people who desperately seek to understand the true underlying causes of their metabolic issues.

And to Dr. Richard Johnson, whose careful and compassionate uric acid research over the past twenty years has provided all of us with powerful new tools aimed at resolving these health challenges. I am deeply grateful for his guidance in the creation of this book.

Contents

INTRODUCTION   The Acid Test   3

PART I

THE BASICS OF URIC ACID

CHAPTER 1   U Defined
The Hidden Connection Linking Our
Modern Ailments, from Diabetes to Dementia   23

CHAPTER 2   Survival of the Fattest
How Prehistoric Apes Hardwired Us
with the Fat Gene   50

CHAPTER 3   The Fallacy of Fructose
How Uric Acid Amplifies the Threat   72

CHAPTER 4   The U-Bomb in Your Brain
The Emerging Role of Uric Acid in
Brain Decline   97

CHAPTER 5   Acid Rain
How Sleep, Salt, Psoriasis, Seafood,
and Sitting Connect with Uric Acid   112

CHAPTER 6   New Habits to LUV
The Acid-Dropping Power of Five Key
Supplements, CGM Technology, and
Time-Restricted Eating   137

Contents

PART II

U-TURN: THE LUV PLAN OF ACTION

CHAPTER 7   Prelude to LUV
Start Your Engines   163

CHAPTER 8   Week 1: Dietary Edits to Lower Uric Values
*How to Make Over Your Metabolism on
the LUV Diet*   173

CHAPTER 9   Week 2: Companions to LUV
*Sleep, Movement, Nature, and an
Eating Window*   201

CHAPTER 10   Week 3: A Sweet Opportunity
Learn to LUV and Live High   218

CHAPTER 11   Recipes to LUV
Breakfast   232
Lunch   242
Dinner   251
Snacks   265
Drinks   269

EPILOGUE   273

ACKNOWLEDGMENTS   279

NOTES   281

INDEX   313

Perfect health is above gold; a sound body before riches.

— Ecclesiasticus 30:15

DROP ACID

Introduction

The Acid Test

YOU ARE HEREBY EMPOWERED::::::::::::

— TOM WOLFE, *THE ELECTRIC KOOL-AID ACID TEST*

IF YOU WERE LOOKING FOR Tom Wolfe's follow-up to his counterculture classic from the 1960s about adventures in psychedelic drug use, you've come to the wrong place. The acid we're talking about in this book is of an entirely different type, one that has everything to do with being in control of your health and feeling empowered to live a full, long, and vibrant life with a fit body and sharp mind to the very end. You may have never heard of *uric acid* before or put any serious thought into this metabolic compound aside from perhaps its role in gout and kidney stones. And if that's the case, there is no fault on your part, because this has been the messaging for years. Get ready: I'm going to give the term *drop acid* a whole new meaning. Your body and brain will thank you for it.

In the fall of 2020, as the COVID-19 pandemic continued to rage across the world, I was on a run outside listening to one of my favorite podcasts: Dr. Peter Attia's *The Drive*.[1] I always get a lot done while running; it's as much exercise for my mind as it is for my body and brain. On this particular day, Dr. Attia's guest had a deep impact on me. Dr. Richard (Rick) Johnson, a professor of nephrology at the University of Colorado, was basically providing a master class on uric acid, revealing the stunning connection between this little-known, underestimated metabolite in the body and overall metabolic health—as well as its downstream biological effects, which can influence virtually every condition and ailment you can imagine. Uric acid is often described as a harmless inert "waste product" of metabolism that is normally excreted in urine (and in stool, though to a lesser extent). It is cast as a trivial, incidental by-product of our normal biology. But it is anything but meaningless or unworthy of our attention. It sits at the heart of regulatory mechanisms involved in our most fundamental processes of metabolism. And it is these processes that, when they go awry, end up manifesting themselves as the most pervasive health issues of our time—from obesity and insulin resistance to diabetes, elevated blood fats, hypertension, cardiovascular disease, and even cognitive decline and dementias.

The following day, I listened to the podcast again. The message and the data behind it were so compelling that I immediately started to take notes and do my own deep dive into the scientific literature. That's when I fell down the proverbial rabbit hole, albeit a satisfying and illuminating one. Dr. Johnson is one of many scientists around the world researching the role of uric acid in our lives—especially in light of modern diets riddled with uric acid–stimulating ingredients. My own research led me to pose a simple question that has an eye-opening answer.

Q: What do obesity, insulin resistance, diabetes, nonalcoholic fatty liver disease, hypertension, coronary artery disease, stroke, neurological disorders including Alzheimer's disease, and premature death have in common?

A: High uric acid levels.

My exploration into the science of uric acid finally answered many questions that had remained in my mind for years. Yes, we know that sugar can threaten health, but *how?* Why do so many people stick to stringent diets and yet still have problems controlling their weight and blood sugar and go on to develop serious illnesses? Why are rates of high blood pressure going up, even in adolescents and in people who maintain an ideal weight (a staggering one in three adults has hypertension and one in ten youths between the ages of twelve and nineteen has elevated blood pressure)?[2] What is the connection between the sugars added to approximately 74 percent of the foods and beverages sold in America's grocery stores and the ever-increasing rates of chronic degenerative diseases, including those that rob people of their mental faculties?[3]

You're about to find out.

If you've tried everything to gain control of your health but still feel like you can't reach your goals, I think you'll appreciate what I have to say. When you discover what I've learned down this rabbit hole, you'll be immediately empowered. This book, part personal journey and part medical investigative reporting, is the culmination of my efforts. I don't want the science screaming from the literature to take decades to reach everyone in their doctors' offices (as it usually does, to the tune of nearly twenty years). I have taken this new knowledge seriously and adjusted my own habits to ensure that I maintain my uric acid level within a healthful range. It's not that difficult and will be incredibly beneficial to your vibrancy and longevity. For an apt analogy, think about the story of smoking and the ills of even secondhand smoke. Until enough people convincingly proved the link between tobacco and cancer, we were tolerant of the habit. Even those of us who never smoked didn't become overly concerned when the air filled with fumes in bars, restaurants, and airplanes. But now look at how we perceive smoking.

Managing uric acid levels to achieve radiant health is a strategy that's been validated by science for decades. But it remains a blind spot in general medicine today. I'm about to equip you with a new pair of glasses that will give you a totally new perspective about what it means to be in — and to achieve — robust health.

HIDDEN HISTORY

More than a century ago, Scottish physician Alexander Haig sounded
the alarm about the connection between uric acid levels in the body and
conditions as diverse as migraine, depression, epilepsy, diabetes, obesity,
liver disease, high blood pressure, cardiovascular disease, stroke, cancer,
dementia, and rheumatism. His revolutionary findings, which culmi-
nated in a book published in 1892 and a subsequent review of the fourth
edition in 1898 in the *Journal of the American Medical Association,* did
not travel far into the next century.[4] Although prescient, they were too
forward-thinking for the era. Thereafter, uric acid continued to be dismissed as an inert waste product of cellular metabolism that at high levels could cause kidney stones and a form of arthritis called gout. But for
most people who never develop gout or kidney problems, uric acid was
thought to be an innocuous biological compound undeserving of any
scrutiny.

Although gout has been described for centuries, dating back to the
ancient Egyptians, an English Dominican monk by the name Randolphus of Bocking first used the term *gout* around 1200 CE to describe
podagra (which literally means "foot trap" in Greek).[5] The word *gout*
comes from the Latin word *gutta,* meaning "a drop" (of liquid), and
owes its origins to humorism, which is an ancient system of medicine
based on the role of bodily fluids, or humors, in the development of
disease.[6] In this case, gout was defined as the "dropping" of bad,
disease-causing material from the blood to the joints. But the relationship between gout and other ailments had long been known.
Galen, a Roman physician of the second century, described the
association between gout, which he called a disease caused by
"debauchery and intemperance," and cardiovascular diseases.[7]

In gout, which is considered a metabolic disease, excess uric acid erodes bone tissues and forms sharp, needlelike mineral crystals (urate) in the joints, which causes inflammation and pain, sometimes severe. Gout notoriously strikes the bunion joint in the big toe. From kings and queens to poets, scientists, and explorers, history is home to many famous gout sufferers, including Alexander the Great, Charlemagne, Henry VIII, Christopher Columbus, Leonardo da Vinci, Isaac Newton, John Milton, Queen Anne of Great Britain, Benjamin Franklin, and Alfred, Lord Tennyson. Although gout is more common in men, the rate evens out a little more after women hit menopause.

From the 1960s to the 1990s, the number of gout patients more than doubled in the United States, and it has continued to rise—affecting nearly ten million people.[8] It's one of the most common inflammatory and immune-system diseases of our era.[9] And how interesting that the prevalence of obesity and metabolic syndrome has also increased in lockstep with gout. These surges parallel the upswing in the consumption of the very ingredients that cause *hyperuricemia* (elevated uric acid) and gout: sugar-sweetened foods and drinks, including soda pop and fruit juice (and, yes, the much-beloved orange and apple juices).

But again, this conversation about uric acid isn't just about gout. An estimated 21 percent of the population in the United States lives with hyperuricemia, putting them at risk for a host of health challenges.[10] That's roughly one in every five individuals. And the vast majority of these people don't know it because they don't have gout or kidney issues. (While a test for uric acid levels is commonly included in the general blood work many of us have done as part of an annual physical, it's safe to say that patients and their physicians rarely pay attention to the result.) In fact, there is a term I'll discuss at length called *asymptomatic hyperuricemia*—high uric acid levels with no adverse symptoms to show for it. It's important to note that the *only* adverse symptoms included in this medical definition are gout and kidney stones. But asymptomatic hyperuricemia is far from innocent or just an early signal of gout or kidney problems. As you will soon learn, long before any symptoms develop, asymptomatic hyperuricemia may well be fomenting an unending, irreversible storm and subtly stoking biological processes that ultimately result in elevated blood sugar and blood pressure, bad cholesterol, excess body fat, and systemic inflammation, which opens the door for any number of chronic degenerative conditions. Put simply, hyperuricemia *precedes* these debilitating ailments that become difficult to manage once they take root. And, incredibly, in our distant evolutionary past, elevated uric acid served as a survival mechanism, as I will soon explain.

Only in the past two decades have research scientists revisited Dr. Haig's discoveries and confirmed that he had indeed identified what has turned out to be a central mechanism in many preventable maladies. Today's medical literature is exploding with evidence that elevated uric acid levels are the bellwether of many ills, such as type 2 diabetes, excess weight and obesity, and hypertension, to name just a few. What's more, some clinicians are now specifically treating elevated uric acid with pharmaceuticals as a way of bringing these conditions under control. But as you will learn, we have the ability to lower our levels of uric acid with simple, straightforward lifestyle adjustments, almost always without having to resort to drug interventions.

For years now I've repeatedly turned to the best medical literature from around the world to figure out why our rates of these diseases have continued to skyrocket. Sure, our diets and lifestyles have changed, but I felt there was a missing piece to the puzzle. And what finally leaped out from the pages of the most leading-edge journals is undeniable evidence that these challenging conditions are the end product of the connection between our modern lifestyle choices and uric acid. Uric acid is a key central player that we need to understand. Much as we learned in the twentieth century that C-reactive protein tells us about the body's level of systemic inflammation, which is linked to many of the diseases that afflict us today, we are discovering in the twenty-first century that uric acid levels are associated with dysfunction and disease in the long term. We all need to keep weight, blood sugar, and blood pressure in check, and the same goes for uric acid. Uric acid is not a minor idle character in the story of our body's chemistry. It's a perpetrator of ill health when it's not well managed.

Unfortunately, most physicians are not yet attuned to this new knowledge — knowledge that tells us, according to one landmark scientific paper published by the American College of Rheumatology, that elevated uric acid is responsible for 16 percent of all-cause mortality and an astounding 39 percent of total cardiovascular disease.[11] (All-cause mortality refers to death from any cause.) In a compelling review published in 2017, investigators wrote: "An elevated serum uric acid [level of uric acid in the blood] is also one of the best independent predictors of diabetes and commonly precedes the development of both insulin resistance and diabetes type 2, as it was discovered that one quarter of diabetes cases can be attributed to a high serum uric acid level and elevated serum uric acid levels were found to be closely associated with insulin resistance and diabetes mellitus type 2."[12] They went on to write that "serum uric acid is a strong and independent risk factor for diabetes in middle-aged and older people."[13] *Independent risk factor* is a term you will hear repeatedly. It's a phrase that research scientists use to define a certain circumstance or measurement, in this case uric acid level, that *on its own* corresponds to harm or injury to the body. As I'll explain, a person with a heightened uric acid level who has no other risk factor for type 2 diabetes (e.g., obesity) can indeed develop diabetes at a healthful weight because of uric acid's sneaky shenanigans.

Without a doubt, the overwhelming contributor to elevation of uric acid in our modern world is the cheapest, most abundant ingredient around — it's the kind of sugar we've been told is relatively "safe" because it doesn't directly raise blood sugar: fructose.[14] And I'm not vilifying fructose from fresh whole fruits. I'm talking about the refined, highly processed fructose that finds its way into many of our daily provisions, including our beloved salad dressings, sauces, condiments, baked goods, snack and energy bars, packaged foods, beverages, and foods you wouldn't even think contain sugar. You probably have a general sense that high-fructose corn syrup isn't good for you, but you don't realize how pervasive this ingredient has become and that you can consume too much fructose by eating other forms of sugar. The science showing fructose's true colors has only been elucidated in the medical journals over the past decade or so—and it doesn't concern what your grandmother knew as fructose. Although the prestigious medical journal *The Lancet* reported on fructose-induced hyperuricemia in 1970,[15] in the years since then we've come to understand the full range of fructose's adverse effects.

It's not news that sugar-rich diets are linked to all kinds of health problems. But we haven't been told the *why* and *how* of sugar's devastating blow to our bodies, especially as it relates to fructose from nonnatural sources. We now understand fructose's biological mechanisms and its veiled relationship with uric acid, both of which help explain the root causes of these intractable conditions—and this is not merely a flimsy association. In fact, evidence from human and animal studies indicates that the connection between dietary sugars and obesity is probably driven primarily by the metabolic effects of fructose.[16] The way the body handles fructose involves uric acid and directly favors the development of obesity.

The other main culprit that leads to elevated uric acid levels is a class of chemicals called *purines*, which are found in all living cells and contribute to healthy physiology but, like body fat, are problematic in excess. Purines are organic compounds that cells use to make the building blocks of DNA and RNA, and when purines are naturally broken down by the body, uric acid is formed. Because purines—two of which, adenine and guanine—provide the backbones, or nucleotides, for DNA and RNA formation, anything that has to do with tissue (cellular) breakdown will raise uric acid levels. As damaged, dying, and dead cells are degraded, purines are released and turned into uric acid during the process. Purines are also constituents of other important biomolecules, such as the energy giant ATP (adenosine triphosphate) and the coenzymes we need for the biochemical reactions that sustain life.

Purines are more common than people realize. In addition to being naturally produced by the body during cellular turnover, they are abundant in a wide array of foods, including certain seafoods, meats, multigrain breads, beer, and even some legumes and vegetables. As these external sources of purines are processed by the body, uric acid is synthesized mainly in the liver, intestines, and inner cellular lining of blood vessels (what's called the *vascular endothelium*). Their prevalence in what we view as rich, lavish fare fit for the wealthy is why gout has long been known as the "king of diseases and the disease of kings."[17] But purines also lurk in many foods touted as healthful in popular diets. During the last decade, large epidemiological surveys have revealed an association between the intake of purine-rich food and the blood concentration of uric acid. Let's not blame vegetables, however, because as we shall see, despite the fact that certain vegetables (e.g., cauliflower, spinach, and mushrooms) might be rich in purines, they may not trigger an increase in uric acid.[18]

For half a century, low-purine diets have been prescribed for people prone to gout and kidney stones. But this dietary protocol is increasingly recommended for anyone looking to control uric acid and rein in the body's metabolism. Just because you don't develop gout or kidney stones, conditions that can have genetic origins as well, doesn't mean you won't suffer from the consequences of chronic high uric acid.[19] Our understanding of this compound we all have coursing through us provides vital clues to unlocking the mystery of optimum human health.

For people who have gone on every "doctor-approved" diet to little or no avail, targeting uric acid fills in a giant blank in the equation. If you don't factor in the uric acid component, going low-carb, vegan, keto, paleo, pescatarian, lectin-free, or even Mediterranean might not be enough to help you permanently drop excess weight or easily manage both blood sugar and blood pressure. Moreover, this new science calls for a revision of the way we reference the glycemic index and consume certain so-called healthful foods. Uric acid levels can generally be brought into balance by (1) implementing simple dietary tweaks, (2) getting quality sleep and adequate exercise, (3) minimizing the intake of uric acid–increasing drugs, and (4) consuming acid-reducing gems such as tart cherries, coffee, vitamin C, and quercetin (the last two are found in many foods and can be taken in supplement form). Nurturing the microbiome is also vital to controlling uric acid; studies reveal correlations between elevation in uric acid and significant increases in the types of bad bacteria in the gut that are associated with inflammation. I call the protocol outlined in this book the LUV Diet—using an acronym for "lower uric values." In this book, you will learn how to both lower uric acid levels and maintain ideal levels once you've achieved them.

My research taught me things my medical education decades ago—and my experience in all the years since, working as a neurologist treating patients—never did. One important reason I became a physician to begin with was my own curiosity. Curiosity plays a key role in why I do what I do. I like to live on the edge of wonder, continually asking: Why do patients develop the problems they do? And once we unravel these mysteries, how might we change what we do as physicians so we can better serve our patients? For me, it has never been enough to simply treat the symptoms of a problem—for example, using a drug to lower blood pressure or balance blood sugar. I want to understand the root of these problems and so many others, then address the causes, not just the manifestations. As I have been fond of saying for many years, I'm really interested in focusing on the fire, not just the smoke.

THE NEW BELLWETHER OF HEALTH

Despite the publication of Dr. Haig's work more than a century ago, only since 2005 or so has uric acid finally been viewed as anything more than a risk marker for gout and kidney stones. Scientists around the world are confirming, in study after study, the fact that uric acid factors into our health. In Japan, controlling uric acid has already entered the mainstream practice of medicine quite apart from solely treating gout. I've learned a wealth of surprising and empowering information in my quest to understand the role of uric acid in our lives. For example, elevated uric acid levels directly lead to increased fat storage, and there's a reason for that, dating back millions of years, which you'll soon come to grasp (and appreciate). Our primate ancestors needed high levels of uric acid in order to build fat stores that would ensure their survival during times of environmental challenges, such as food and water scarcity.

But we all know that food scarcity is not a modern reality for most people living in developed nations. In the pages that follow, I will explore the idea that we humans have acquired genetic mutations that cause us to experience elevations in our uric acid far in excess of those in our ancestral primates, who did not carry these genetic mutations. (Our uric acid levels far exceed those in other mammals, too.) By making early humans increasingly fat and insulin-resistant, uric acid proved life-sustaining. I will examine how this powerful survival mechanism led to passing on these genes to future generations as they allowed us the ability to persevere and procreate. We will then see how environment and evolution butt heads today, when we live in a time of caloric abundance, and how these genetic mutations are now proving so devastating to our health. It's a fascinating story that ultimately empowers us to rein in our insulin sensitivity, blood pressure, fat production, and even our waistlines and risk for all manner of illnesses.

When the original research on the role of uric acid in diseases other than gout and kidney stones began to appear, as expected, mainstream medicine cast it off as folly. We have now reached a point where this thesis has gained considerable traction and is being explored globally because of its potential to affect the major health issues of our time, including obesity, diabetes, cardiovascular disease, hypertension, and other chronic inflammatory, degenerative conditions. This message is one we all need to hear if we're to live longer, fitter, and healthier lives and avoid life-crushing conditions that are wholly preventable.

SELF-ASSESSMENT: HOW TO SPOT THE U-BOMB IN YOUR LIFE

Don't know what your uric acid (UA) levels are? You've surely been tested routinely in the past and can actually test yourself at home, just as you would check your blood sugar, weight, or temperature. Even if you have a sense of your UA level, which is of course a dynamic number that changes throughout the day, it's important to know generally what factors into that level—from what you consume to which medications you take and even how well you sleep and how much you physically move. Before we delve into all the dazzling science behind uric acid's role in your life, let's start with a simple questionnaire that reveals what habits could be silently harming you right now.

Respond to these statements as honestly as possible. Don't think about the connections to sickness implied by the statements; just respond truthfully. In the following chapters you'll begin to understand why I used these particular statements and where you stand in your risk factors. Note that if you feel like you're in between yes and no, or if "sometimes" or "rarely" feels like your knee-jerk response, then answer yes for now.

1. I drink fruit juices (any kind).

2. I drink sugar-sweetened beverages such as soda pop, flavored teas, and sports drinks.

3. I eat sugary foods, including cereals, baked goods, dried fruits, and candies.

4. I use xylitol as an artificial sweetener or consume products that contain it.

5. I take diuretics (also known as water pills) or low-dose aspirin.

6. I drink beer and liquor.

7. I have an underactive thyroid.

8. I take immune-suppressant drugs (e.g., cyclosporine) and/or a beta-blocker.

9. I am overweight or obese (body mass index of 30 or above).

10. I have been diagnosed with high blood pressure.

11. I love wild game meats (e.g., venison, veal, moose, elk, buffalo).

12. I eat organ meats such as liver, kidney, and sweetbreads.

13. I eat red meat (beef, lamb, pork, ham) three or more times a week.

14. I eat lots of high-purine seafoods such as sardines, anchovies, mackerel, mussels, scallops, herring, and haddock.

15. I eat deli or processed meats, including bacon.

16. I have psoriasis and/or joint injuries.

17. I have a metabolic disorder (e.g., insulin resistance, type 2 diabetes).

18. My family has a history of gout and/or kidney conditions (e.g., renal insufficiency).

19. I'm a poor sleeper.

20. I am not an active, regular exerciser.

The more yeses you tallied up, the greater your health risks. But don't panic. Once you gain the knowledge and know-how to rethink your habits, you'll soon lower your risks dramatically.

Interestingly, a sudden infection, dehydration, excessive exercise, fasting, and crash diets can also elevate uric acid levels in the body. I left these risk factors out of the questionnaire because they typically relate to temporary rises in uric acid and do not reflect the main cause of most people's chronic problems with it. Nevertheless, I'll explore all these factors, and for those of you who have been infected by the virus that causes COVID-19, I'll address your issues directly in the first chapter, given that you may carry unknown risks to your future health that require special attention. Later in the book, I'll teach you how to understand your UA values and offer target numbers that totally redefine the reference range—the way doctors determine the difference between normal and abnormal.

Being in the normal range is no longer good enough. It's time we talk about being in the optimal range. You deserve it. You also deserve to know how to rethink other values in your health equation, such as your blood sugar and A1c levels. A test for the latter measures your average blood sugar levels over the previous three months (and is also known as the hemoglobin A1c, or HbA1c, blood test). It's a commonly used way to diagnose prediabetes and diabetes. But the target numbers your doctor may recommend are not the same ones I'll prescribe. News flash: brain degeneration begins at a hemoglobin A1c of 5.5 percent, which doctors deem a normal value.[20] Even a blood glucose level of 105 mg/dL (milligrams per deciliter), which your doctor might say is fine, is significantly associated with the development of dementia.[21] No matter what health issues you worry about or currently manage, two fundamental goals to achieve are metabolic health and controlled levels of systemic inflammation. If you don't know what I mean by these goals, you soon will. And uric acid control helps you find your way to these goals. It's a gateway to vibrant health.

As this book will show, uric acid is far from a by-product or inert waste product. It's time to change the dogmatic narrative about this compound, which orchestrates and instigates many reactions in the body. With all due respect to other physicians, I must warn you that your doctor may have dismissed an abnormally high level of uric acid in your routine tests if you don't have gout or kidney issues. He or she may have said, "Don't worry about it." Nothing could be further from the truth. He or she may scoff at the idea that lowering uric acid is an important health goal. Remember, people tend to be down on what they are not up on.

As I've stated in the past, we can choose to live our lives, come what may, and hope that modern medical science will provide a remedy for the ills that inevitably develop. But this is a model destined for failure. One has only to look at Alzheimer's disease, for example, to see that there is no medical treatment for it of any merit whatsoever. Such a treatment would be welcomed beyond measure. But right now we have the science that clearly reveals how making the right lifestyle choices can go a long way toward *preventing* this untreatable condition. Treating the symptoms of disease — such as lowering blood pressure with medication, reducing blood sugar with medication, and taking drugs designed to help the heart beat more forcefully — doesn't address the causes of the underlying disease process. Again, this means treating the smoke while the fire is ignored. The goal of this book is to keep you healthy. It is written to equip you with a new, state-of-the-art, deeply validated tool that will soon become a central player among the other implements in your toolbox.

Ready? Let's get to it!

PART I

THE BASICS OF URIC ACID

IF THE THOUGHT OF *NOT* KNOWING this secret to gaining control of your health—including your weight—makes you mad, prepare to become a happy, informed individual.

We all know that our nutritional choices and factors such as exercise, sleep, and stress reduction are key to overall wellness. But sometimes knowing exactly *what* to eat, *how* to exercise and achieve restful sleep, and the best ways to unwind can seem difficult when we're bombarded daily with directives to do this, not that. And when we don't know *why* these goals are important, motivation can wane. It's time to learn the hidden difference between health and sickness within the context of uric acid. It's time to gain a radical new perspective that will show you the way toward radiant health and vitality. I've spoken with the world's experts on this subject, devoured all the scientific literature, and done all the homework for you. As I mentioned, like many nuggets of wisdom in medicine, knowledge that can help us all live better, longer lives can often get siloed in medical literature for years before it lands in clinical settings. The translation from laboratory to clinical medicine (i.e., your doctor's office) has its own natural timeline for a variety of reasons. Luckily, uric acid is finally having its moment. Ask the people who study this fascinating new area of research, and they will tell you that a revolution is afoot.

In part 1, we'll do a deep dive into the surprising and truly fascinating biology of uric acid. This will involve some history, a little science and physiology, and a lot of LUV notes of wisdom that you'll then put into practice in part 2. Reducing uric acid and managing healthful levels is not nearly as hard as you might think. And it won't require an impossible overhaul of your life or an elimination of all things sweet and delicious. I promise to use validated strategies to make this effortless to understand and easy to execute. Subtle tweaks to your daily habits are all you need. But before we get to those details, it's helpful to have a complete, 360-degree panoramic view of this chemical compound that has a profound impact on your current and future well-being. By the end of part 1, you'll have a new appreciation for your bodily processes, which want to run as optimally as possible.

You have the power to protect your body from premature decline, prevent the deterioration of your mental faculties, and even influence the way your genetic code behaves thanks to the magic of *epigenetics*, a topic we'll explore. Some fun facts to lure you in from the get-go:

• Uric acid comes from only three sources: fructose, alcohol, and purines (organic molecules found in DNA and RNA that are also found in foods, some beverages, and the body's own tissues).

• Uric acid triggers fat production — from thickening your waistline to filling your liver with dangerous fat even if you're not overweight or obese.

• High levels of uric acid are strongly related to being overweight or obese as well as to the risk of cardiovascular problems and hypertension, cognitive decline, abnormal blood fats, and death from *any cause.*

I don't know about you, but for me, reducing the risk of death from any cause is a top priority. And if it means paying attention to uric acid levels in addition to other factors that contribute to longevity, then I'm all in. Join me.

CHAPTER 1

U Defined

The Hidden Connection Linking Our Modern Ailments, from Diabetes to Dementia

But not only is the pulse affected in this way by the uric acid, but it in turn affects the circulation in, and the function of, several important organs in a way, and to an extent which leads little doubt as to the real existence of the cause and effect of which I have been speaking.

— ALEXANDER HAIG, URIC ACID AS A
FACTOR IN THE CAUSATION OF DISEASE, 1892

WHEN YOU THINK ABOUT the laws of nature we've all come to accept and live by, such as the effects of gravity, the principles of time and space, and even the importance of food and water to human survival, you probably think of some old philosophers whose legacies are preserved in paintings and busts in museums today. Even if you've never studied physics, chemistry, or medicine, a few names likely come to mind: Hippocrates, Aristotle, Plato, Newton, and perhaps the Greek physician Galen, who — before the fall of the Roman Empire — was the first to describe the blood in our arteries and cranial nerves. In more recent history, we've had the great Louis Pasteur, who introduced us to the world of microorganisms; Edward Jenner, who created the first functional vaccine; Ignaz Semmelweis, who taught us the importance of hand washing, especially in health-care settings; Albert Einstein, with his theory of relativity; and Sir William Osler, who revolutionized the practice of medicine in the twentieth century, teaching doctors the importance of clinic-based learning rather than exclusive reliance on textbooks. But you probably have not heard of the nineteenth-century doctor from Scotland whom I introduced a few pages ago by the name of Alexander Haig.

Like other doctors who have achieved medical breakthroughs, Dr. Haig experimented on himself first. He documented tremendous health improvements after he went on a diet designed to drop his uric acid level. In the late 1800s, he eliminated meat in a bid to snuff out the migraines he'd suffered from for years, and it worked. Meat, as you'll soon learn, contains ingredients that raise uric acid levels in the body (purines; see the box on page 25 for details). He then suggested that excess uric acid may cause not only headaches and migraines but also depression and epilepsy. He ultimately came to the conclusion that a vast array of common diseases was related to elevated uric acid, including cardiovascular disease, cancer, dementia, gout, hypertension, and stroke. Haig in fact is credited for being one of the first physicians to link a surfeit of uric acid to hypertension as he painstakingly explored the relationship of uric acid to blood pressure and blood flow. In his seminal 1892 book *Uric Acid as a Factor in the Causation of Disease,* he wrote:

> If my premises are good, and my deductions are sound, and if uric acid really influences the circulation to the extent which I have been led to believe that it does, it follows that uric acid really dominates the function, nutrition, and structure of the human body to an extent which has never yet been dreamed of in our philosophy, and in place of affecting the structure of a few comparatively insignificant fibrous tissues in which it is found after

death, it may really direct the development, life history, and final decay and dissolution of every tissue, from the most important nurse centres and the most active glands, to the matrix of the nails and the structure of the skin and hair.[1]

Although Dr. Haig's book went through seven editions and was translated into several languages, and although he consulted with patients around the world and as far away as India and China, his work was only whispered about during the twentieth century. But then, in the twenty-first century, the evidence supporting uric acid's role in Western society's health challenges became too voluminous to be ignored. It was time to revisit this "physiologic alarm signal," as Dr. Richard Johnson calls it.[2]

PURINES AND URIC ACID: WHAT'S THE CONNECTION?

Purines are natural organic substances found in the body, where they serve important functions and help form our body's core genetic material—both DNA and RNA. Purines, in fact, belong to a family of nitrogen-containing molecules known as nitrogenous bases; they help build certain nucleotide base pairs (backbones) in both DNA and RNA. Picture the classic image of the helical, twisted, ladderlike structure of DNA: its rungs include purine molecules. Which means when genetic material is broken down, purines are released.

Purines are truly building blocks of life: along with pyrimidines, which are also nitrogenous bases, purines help build the genetic material in every living organism. They also serve important roles when they connect with certain cells via special receptors on those cells, initiating far-reaching repercussions—affecting blood flow, heart function, inflammatory and immune responses, the experience of pain, digestive function, and the absorption of nutrients. Some purines even act as neurotransmitters and antioxidants.

Around two-thirds of purines in the body are *endogenous* — they are produced naturally by the body and found inside cells. Your body's cells are in a perpetual state of death and renewal, and the endogenous purines from damaged, dying, or dead cells must be processed. Purines are also found in many foods such as liver, certain seafoods and meats, and alcohol. These are the *exogenous* purines that enter the body through our diets and are metabolized as part of the digestive process. So your body's total *purine pool* is a combination of both endogenous and exogenous purines, and when these are processed by the body, the final end product of their metabolism is uric acid. Purines themselves are not necessarily harmful, but if the amount of purines becomes excessive and the body cannot keep up with processing them, too much uric acid builds up in the bloodstream. Most of the excess uric acid produced dissolves in the blood, passes through the kidneys, and leaves the body in urine. But many things can prevent proper elimination of uric acid, which can build to high levels in the blood and cause adverse effects on metabolism that have a domino effect throughout the body and brain.

THE FAT SWITCH

Getting to the root of high blood pressure and heart disease — driving forces in mortality — has been a vexing endeavor for decades among scientists worldwide. A game-changing study that began in the middle of the last century and continues today has sparked new insights, leading to a refresher course on uric acid in modern medicine. Let me explain.

One of the most prized and respected studies ever done in America, the famous Framingham Heart Study, added volumes of data to our understanding of certain risk factors for disease, especially for the leading killer of all: heart disease.[3] It commenced in 1948 with the recruitment of 5,209 men and women between the ages of thirty and sixty-two from the town of Framingham, Massachusetts, none of whom had yet suffered a heart attack or stroke or even had symptoms of cardiovascular disease. Since then, the study has added several generations stemming from the original group to the pool, which has allowed scientists to carefully monitor these populations and gather clues to physiological conditions within the context of myriad factors—age, sex, psychosocial issues, physical traits, and genetic patterns. Although it was originally focused on heart disease, the study has provided extraordinary and, frankly, irresistible opportunities to examine the processes of other diseases, from diabetes to dementia.

In 1999, the study's authors reported that elevated uric acid did not by itself cause heart disease, arguing instead that high blood pressure elevated the risk of the disease and happened to raise uric acid levels at the same time.[4] This conclusion, however, did not sit well with Dr. Rick Johnson, because the researchers had not tested their hypothesis on laboratory animals. It was an incomplete conclusion. Johnson, then at the University of Florida College of Medicine, had been studying the underlying causes of obesity, diabetes, hypertension, and kidney disease for decades and had authored hundreds of research articles about his findings.[5] He led his own study to see if raising uric acid levels with a drug would also raise blood pressure or harm kidney function.[6] Just a few years previously, he'd shown that subtle kidney injuries in rats could cause high blood pressure, a finding that had stunned him and his colleagues.[7] The experiment led them to conduct a series of further studies, revealing that elevated uric acid levels in rats caused high blood pressure in two ways.[8]

First, high uric acid sets off a cascade of biochemical reactions collectively called *oxidative stress,* which constricts blood vessels. In turn, blood pressure rises as the heart is forced to pump harder to circulate blood. But lowering uric acid reverses this effect. Second, when there's an unrelenting surplus of uric acid, lasting injury and inflammation in the kidneys can occur, which makes them less able to do their job and excrete salt. This salt retention further contributes to rising blood pressure, as that extra salt in the bloodstream pulls water into your blood vessels, increasing the total amount (volume) of blood inside them. And with more blood flowing through your blood vessels, the pressure inside them increases, just as it does in a garden hose when it's turned on high.

When Johnson and his team studied humans to see if they responded similarly to elevated levels of uric acid, he measured the acid in obese adolescents who'd been recently diagnosed with hypertension.[9] To his astonishment, fully 90 percent of them had elevated uric acid. He and his team then proceeded to treat thirty of the patients with *allopurinol*, a drug that lowers uric acid by blocking an enzyme in the body that's needed to produce the acid. It's important to note that the drug restored blood pressure to normal in 85 percent of the adolescents simply by lowering their uric acid. This enlightening study landed in the prestigious *Journal of the American Medical Association* back in 2008, and the results have since been replicated numerous times by other researchers around the world, including in studies focused on adults. In fact, studies done on adults with asymptomatic hyperuricemia show that administering allopurinol to lower uric acid improves many factors involved in cardiovascular and cerebral functioning, from blood pressure and blood fats to inflammatory markers.[10] But it would take scientists time to fully elucidate the cause-and-effect connections in such eye-opening findings — time for them to notice and catch up on all the accruing evidence about uric acid.[11]

A provocative question that Johnson sought to answer: Which comes first, obesity or high blood pressure? Could uric acid, he wondered, be the trigger not only for high blood pressure but also for obesity itself? He then thought about our evolution and the concept of "survival of the fattest": we are hardwired, like other primates, to store fat when calories are abundant in preparation for times of food shortage. We are very efficient at storing energy when food is plentiful. We are also programmed to become insulin-resistant under certain circumstances in order to save precious glucose in the blood for the brain, so it can remain fully functional and quick-witted—a survival mechanism that allows us to find food and water. Johnson called this special programming the "fat switch" and went so far as to explain that it resulted from a series of genetic mutations that took place over millions of years in our ancestral great apes before we *Homo sapiens* emerged. As you'll see in the next chapter, at the heart of this biology in the animal kingdom is an enzyme called *uricase*, which converts uric acid into other substances that can be easily expelled by the kidneys. Uricase is found in most species of fish and amphibians, some other mammals, and even bacteria—but not in birds, most reptiles, or mammals of the hominoid family, which includes our fossil ancestors, the anthropoid apes, and us.

What exactly happened to our uricase? Did Mother Nature make a horrendous mistake? No: over the course of evolution, and for the sake of their own survival, our ancestral apes disabled the genes needed for making uricase, turning them into "pseudogenes," or the biological version of corrupted computer files.[12] Put simply, the genes that encode uricase developed mutations that stopped our distant ancestors, and us, from making the enzyme at all. In order to develop the fat switch, we had to increase our uric acid levels by deactivating the various genes holding the instructions to produce uricase. Less uricase equals more uric acid, enabling the fat switch to turn on.

It was a dicey evolutionary compromise: cut the function of the uricase genes to allow for more efficient energy storage, less risk of starvation, and ultimately better chances of survival. Our defunct uricase genes are the reason why our blood contains three to ten times more uric acid than that of other mammals, predisposing us to certain health conditions. Indeed, we simply have not evolved the physiology to handle the many calories that are available to us around the clock year-round. Fructose is particularly offensive because, as you'll see later on, it's been shown to be incredibly effective at flipping that switch and causing the body to hoard fat and raise both blood sugar and blood pressure levels—directly through the actions of uric acid. Briefly, fructose generates uric acid as the body metabolizes it, and without uricase to break all that uric acid down easily, the fat switch stays in the On mode and that fructose gets turned into fat. "Fruit-to-fat" physiology saved ancient primates from dying during long fruitless winters. But circumstances have changed, although our genetics—and, therefore, our physiology—have not.

Making matters worse, uric acid buildup amplifies fructose's effects. It's a double whammy. Researchers have shown that mice fed a high-fructose diet ate more and moved less than mice on a more healthful diet.[13] The mice also accumulated more fat: this increase in body weight happens in part because fructose silences the hormone leptin, which we need to tell us to stop eating. Even moderate consumption of fructose can have monumental effects on liver health, fat metabolism, insulin resistance, and eating behavior.[14] I'll get to all this biochemistry in more detail soon, but for now know that while we may be genetically doomed to be fat in a world of calories galore, we get to consciously choose those calories, and they are not all created equal. We also get to decide how to leverage the body's preferred support staff: sleep, exercise, and time-restricted eating.

In the title of a 2016 paper, a group of researchers in Turkey and Japan put it bluntly: "Uric Acid in Metabolic Syndrome: From an Innocent Bystander to a Central Player," stating that uric acid has officially been "incriminated in a number of chronic disease states, including hypertension, metabolic syndrome, diabetes, non-alcoholic fatty liver disease, and chronic kidney disease."[15] Their conclusion is informative: "While uric acid was once the lonely dinner conversation for those suffering from gout or kidney stones, it is now being evaluated as a potential master conductor in the worldwide symphony of obesity, diabetes, and cardiorenal disease." (Cardiorenal disease refers to a spectrum of disorders involving both the heart and kidneys.) I'd italicize *master conductor* because it says so much.

In a larger study conducted in Japan in 2020, which followed more than half a million people between the ages of forty and seventy-four over the course of seven years, researchers looked at the association between uric acid in the blood and both cardiovascular and all-cause mortality.[16] They found that "A significant increase in the hazard ratio for all-cause mortality was noted with serum uric acid levels ≥ [greater than or equal to] 7 mg/dL in men and ≥ 5 mg/dL in women. A similar trend was observed for cardiovascular mortality." The study disclosed that even a *slight* increase in blood levels of uric acid was an independent risk factor for death in both men and women. Moreover, the threshold values of uric acid for mortality might be different for men and women. I know I haven't covered these values yet, but as a prelude to information later in the book, I'll say that you want to keep your uric acid level at or below 5.5 mg/dL whether you're a man, woman, or child. This recommendation is a more rigorous goal than established medical guidelines deem normal, but remember we're aiming for optimal—a loftier bar. Although men generally have higher uric acid levels than women (and bear a higher overall risk for hyperuricemia and gout), that does not mean that maintaining a level below 5.5 mg/dL is impossible. It may mean that some men will have to work harder at dropping their acid than women will, but that's all the more reason for them to follow this program.

We can't forget the seminal study I briefly highlighted in the introduction, which found, over an eight-year period, a 16 percent increase in the risk of death from any cause among people with elevated uric acid as well as a nearly 40 percent increase in the risk of death from cardiovascular disease and a 35 percent increase in the risk of death from ischemic stroke, which is caused by a blocked artery that supplies blood to the brain.[17] Moreover, the researchers discovered a snowball effect—an 8 to 13 percent increase in the risk of death with every milligram per deciliter of uric acid in the blood above 7 mg/dL. This was no small study, as it involved more than forty thousand men and nearly fifty thousand women thirty-five years of age and older who were tracked over those years. What I find truly remarkable is that research now shows that the risk of death from having elevated uric acid is higher than it would be even if you had a history of coronary heart disease! Something else that struck me in my deep dive into the research: you may not have high blood pressure; you may not be obese or diabetic or even a cigarette smoker; nonetheless, having elevated uric acid—*even minimally*—increases your risk of premature death.

A good question: Why haven't we heard of this before? Well, historically, as I've mentioned, we've only heard about elevated uric acid in the context of gout and kidney stones. But now we are finally documenting the silent killer: asymptomatic hyperuricemia. Uric acid levels on the high side do harm the body, but you don't know it's happening because you don't experience symptoms and you don't suffer from gout or kidney issues. Yet asymptomatic hyperuricemia can *predict* the development of high blood pressure, obesity, diabetes, chronic kidney disease, and nonalcoholic fatty liver disease. Nonalcoholic fatty liver disease, or NAFLD, happens to be one of the most common chronic liver diseases and has been called an "emerging driver of hypertension."[18] The prevalence of NAFLD has doubled during last twenty years, ranging from 24 to 42 percent in Western countries and 5 to 30 percent in Asian countries.[19] And once again, uric acid plays a prominent role, directly increasing the production of fat in the liver cells, which ultimately leads to NAFLD.

Fatty livers are commonly seen among alcoholics, whose overconsumption triggers an excessive amount of fat in the liver. But many people who don't drink much or even *any* alcohol can wind up with the same problem thanks to the same process—disruption in the body's metabolism causes the buildup of fat in the liver, crippling its function and potentially leading to irreversible scarring and cirrhosis. The well-known primary causes of NAFLD are obesity, diabetes, abnormal blood fats (dyslipidemia), and insulin resistance. High blood pressure and high uric acid levels are also implicated, and new research reveals that, contrary to received wisdom, you don't have to be overweight or obese to have NAFLD.[20] Plenty of people are walking around today at an ideal weight but carrying a heavy fatty liver on the road to failure. In fact, some doctors have slowed the progression of NAFLD just by reducing levels of uric acid with drugs and lifestyle strategies.[21] That speaks volumes.

One of the underlying forces connecting all these conditions is inflammation. Elevated uric acid and elevated systemic inflammation go hand in hand, as high uric acid amplifies and stokes inflammation.[22] Many people have gotten the memo that chronic inflammation is a fundamental cause of serious health challenges and death; it's associated with coronary artery disease, cancer, diabetes, Alzheimer's disease, and virtually every other chronic disease you can imagine. Nobody debates this fact now, but it wasn't long ago that we couldn't fathom a connection between stubbing a toe (and experiencing acute redness and swelling— the clear and obvious signs of inflammation) and developing Alzheimer's disease (whose central mechanism is invisible and imperceptible inflammation). That doesn't mean that stubbing your toe causes Alzheimer's, but both problems share the same underlying phenomenon: inflammation. Similarly, heart disease and cancer are two different diseases with a single common denominator: inflammation.

On February 23, 2004, the cover of *Time* magazine pictured a silhouette of a human seemingly on fire with the bold headline: THE SECRET KILLER.[23] The feature story was about the "surprising link between inflammation and heart attacks, cancer, Alzheimer's, and other diseases."[24] The concept was merely a "theory" then, with most of the evidence "circumstantial" but "starting to look pretty good" as doctors began to note dramatic improvements across the board when patients with various conditions benefited from anti-inflammatory drugs.[25] In retrospect, it's astonishing to think that fewer than twenty years ago we were just beginning to grasp a fundamental cause of chronic diseases. It's also astonishing to think that the same inflammatory strategies our bodies have used for millennia to ward off microbial invaders and help heal open wounds could slip beyond our control and leave us chronically inflamed: it's as if, from an evolutionary perspective, we've become victims of our own success.

Rather than a transitory and helpful immunological defense mechanism, inflammation has become persistent and harmful — ultimately preventing us from reaching a ripe old age.

I love borrowing the analogy that my good friend and colleague Dr. David Ludwig, a nutrition researcher, physician, and professor at Harvard Medical School, uses to describe the fires within: "Imagine rubbing the underside of your arm with sandpaper. Before long, the area would become red, swollen, and tender — the hallmarks of acute inflammation. Now imagine that this inflammatory process took place over many years within your body, affecting all the vital organs as a result of poor diet, stress, sleep deprivation, lack of enough exercise, and other exposures. Chronic inflammation may not be immediately painful, but it silently underlies the greatest killers of our era."[26] Now we need to factor in uric acid as an important part of the story — another way we've become victims of our own success from an evolutionary standpoint. Studies are under way that chart parallel rises in both uric acid levels and chronic inflammation, which is often measured by the amount of C-reactive protein in the blood.

Some of you may already know that C-reactive protein (CRP) is a common marker of inflammation in the body that's easily tested through blood work. Ideal levels are 3 mg/L (milligrams per liter) or below; elevations above that are linked to all manner of ills. Many factors are associated with increased CRP, including extra weight, diabetes, hypertension, cigarette smoking, estrogen replacement therapy, high cholesterol, and even some genetic predispositions. High CRP is a common denominator in physical dysfunction and disease and is associated with a wide spectrum of inflammatory conditions, such as rheumatoid arthritis, coronary heart disease, age-related macular degeneration, Parkinson's disease, hemorrhagic stroke, and type 2 diabetes. In my world, high CRP is a huge risk factor for brain damage, cognitive decline, depression, and dementias, including Alzheimer's disease. And now we know that uric acid levels and CRP share a relationship: elevated uric acid directly correlates with the presence of elevated CRP as well as other inflammatory chemicals (cytokines). In one study, for example, which involved a collaborative effort between Italian researchers and the National Institutes of Health's National Institute on Aging, increases in uric acid directly predicted increases in CRP over a three-year period among a large group of men and women between the ages of twenty-one and ninety-eight.[27]

In another rather alarming study that attempted to determine the connection between uric acid and inflammatory chemicals, including CRP, a team of German researchers found that elevated uric acid in a group of more than a thousand high-risk patients between the ages of thirty and seventy, all of whom had stable coronary artery disease, was a better predictor of future adverse cardiovascular disease (CVD) events than either CRP or IL-6 (interleuken-6), another marker of inflammation in the body.[28] In their conclusions, they stated that the relationship between elevated uric acid and increased risk for future CVD events was "statistically significant," even when they adjusted for other risk factors. And they suggested that elevated uric acid *alone* could be causing these adverse episodes—a connection not seen between the inflammatory markers and CVD events. The most troubling finding in this study is that it showed an increased risk for CVD events from elevations in uric acid still within the normal range.

It bears reiterating: the risk increase was clearly evident at levels considered normal. Other studies have confirmed these findings, showing that uric acid levels mirror levels of systemic inflammation and can actually serve not only as a surrogate marker of inflammation but also as an *amplifier* of that inflammation. Which means that uric acid levels are directly tied to every malady under the inflammatory sun. This is what places high uric acid at the heart of any conversation about risk of disease.

The lesson is clear: unchecked uric acid could be a death knell. I should add that this is not just about adults and senior citizens who misguidedly assume they will struggle with chronic conditions stemming from age and the natural wear and tear on the body. This message has important implications for children, too, who are increasingly diagnosed with problems previously only seen in adults—insulin resistance, diabetes (cases of type 2 diabetes more than doubled among children during the coronavirus pandemic), hypertension, obesity, NAFLD, early signs of cardiovascular disease, and, yes, elevated uric acid.[29] It's now been established in the medical literature through large studies spanning more than a decade that elevations in uric acid in childhood play a key role in— and can in fact predict—the development of high blood pressure and kidney disease in adulthood.[30] Clearly, the manifestations of illness start in youth simply with hyperuricemia, much of which goes unnoticed. And, intriguingly, uric acid levels in teenagers' saliva can even predict their body fat accumulation in later life.[31] This could mean that we have a new noninvasive way to detect early changes in an adolescent's physiology that could lead to unwanted outcomes with regard to weight and metabolism.

THE HIGHS AND LOWS: KNOW YOUR NUMBERS

When we get to the programmatic instructions in part 2, I'll recommend that you test your uric acid level first thing in the morning at least weekly, before eating or exercising. Testing for uric acid affords you a window into the health and function of your metabolism that has everything to do with your total health and risk of decline. Uric acid tends to increase during sleep and reaches its highest point at around 5:00 a.m., which is, interestingly, about the same time of day that heart attacks peak.

In addition, I'll encourage you to test your blood glucose regularly, ideally with a continuous glucose monitor so you know exactly where you are at any given time and how your daily choices are affecting your biology. You can track how your body responds to food, meal timing, exercise, stress, and sleep in real time. The combination of routinely testing your uric acid and blood glucose is among the most powerful strategies for managing your health and knowing when to take action through interventions such as reducing your intake of certain foods and timing your workouts to streamline your metabolism. Self-testing, however, will not be a requirement on the LUV Diet. If you follow the program, even without the testing, I trust you'll experience positive changes that will keep you going strong and progressing toward optimal health. But at that point, you'll probably want to see your numbers!

URIC ACID: FROM YOUR METABOLISM TO YOUR IMMUNITY

For years doctors have known that obese people and people with heart disease and unhealthful levels of blood fats have higher uric acid levels than their lean, fit counterparts who have normal levels of blood fats. But they didn't pay much attention to those uric acid levels or realize that these levels were playing a big role in the connection between obesity and blood fats — until now.

The prevalence of obesity and obesity-related diseases in the United States and worldwide is increasing rapidly: an astounding 73.6 percent of the US population over the age of twenty is considered overweight or obese.[32] That's roughly three out of four adults. In the obesity category alone, 42.5 percent of adults over twenty are obese.[33] And, as noted by scientists in a 2019 paper published in the *International Journal of Obesity*, it is estimated that fully half of adults in the United States will be classified as obese by 2030.[34] That's breathtaking. Even more breathtaking is the fact that diabetes, the condition most associated with obesity, now afflicts a little more than 10 percent of the US population. And kids are not spared: more than 20 percent of adolescents between the ages of twelve and nineteen, and children between the ages of six and eleven, are obese.[35] In the two-to-five age group, the percentage of obese kids hovers just above 13 percent.[36]

Obesity is just one of many metabolic diseases that fall under the umbrella term *metabolic syndrome* (also known as MetS or syndrome X), which poses the greatest public health threat in the twenty-first century. To be clear, metabolic syndrome refers to a cluster of conditions that increase the risk of heart disease, stroke, diabetes, sleep apnea, liver and kidney disease, cancer, and Alzheimer's disease. And it even immensely raises the risk of dying from an infection such as COVID-19 (see the box on page 40) or at least the risk of suffering from long-term symptoms that don't abate after the acute infection has cleared.

Metabolic syndrome comprises five key characteristics—you only need to check three of the boxes below to receive the diagnosis:

☐   high blood pressure;

☐   elevated blood sugar;

☐   excess body fat around the waist (greater than forty inches in men or thirty-five inches in women);

☐   elevated triglycerides in the blood (a type of blood fat); and

☐   abnormal cholesterol levels (notably, low HDL, or low "good" cholesterol).

Most of the characteristics of metabolic syndrome aren't obvious unless you're looking for them. Many medical experts say that metabolic syndrome may be the most common and serious condition *you've never heard of.* And yet it's on the rise. The condition is now known to affect nearly 35 percent of adults, a percentage that increases to around 50 among people at least sixty years old.[37] Although metabolic syndrome is less common among normal-weight individuals than among overweight and obese people, it does occur in the former group. As the CDC said in

2020, in the wake of a study by researchers at New York University, people who are of normal weight and have metabolic syndrome have a 70 percent higher risk of dying than people who do not have the condition.[38] Moreover, the mortality rate was found to be even higher in the group of people of normal weight with metabolic syndrome compared to people in the overweight or obese group without the syndrome. The authors of the study stressed the importance of finding those individuals with metabolic syndrome who defy the stereotype of being overweight or obese as well. When you're at a normal weight but can check off three of those boxes, then you've got a lot going on behind the scenes, and that surely involves uric acid, especially its role in creating and storing fat. In fact, creating and storing fat is so central to all the components of metabolic syndrome that researchers are now looking at giving metabolic syndrome a new name: "fat storage condition."[39]

Many people don't think metabolic diseases are all that harmful, or that they can factor so enormously into the risk of contracting very disparate illnesses, deadly infections included. After all, the thinking goes, people with elevated blood sugar, hypertension, and/or high cholesterol can manage and control their conditions with drugs and lifestyle strategies. But metabolic disorders are scourges. They significantly raise the risk not only of developing diabetes, cardiovascular disease, and chronic kidney disease but also of developing many degenerative diseases in later life—dementias and Alzheimer's disease included. In fact, as I've written extensively in the past, diabetes and brain disease are this country's costliest and most pernicious diseases, yet they are largely preventable and are uniquely tied together: having type 2 diabetes at least doubles one's risk for Alzheimer's and may increase a vulnerable person's risk for the disease as much as *fourfold*.[40] Specifically, contracting type 2 diabetes before age sixty doubles dementia risk, and for every five years a person lives with diabetes, his or her dementia risk increases by 24 percent.[41] Research also has shown that the road to serious cognitive decline from consuming too many sugary foods doesn't even have to involve diabetes.[42] In other words, the higher the blood sugar, the faster the cognitive decline — regardless of whether a person is diabetic or not. This relationship holds true with uric acid, too, as you'll see: the higher the uric acid level, the faster the cognitive decline, even in the absence of gout or kidney disease. Scientists have already documented a direct correlation between elevated uric acid and brain shrinkage with declining cognitive performance. (So much for hyperuricemia being "asymptomatic"!) What's more, you'll see how "cerebral fructose metabolism" is now considered a potential major driver of Alzheimer's disease.[43] The way fructose behaves in the brain, and how it's metabolized, can be deleterious to the brain's energy dynamics and, ultimately, its health and functionality.

A NOTE ABOUT COVID

The connection between the risk of dying from an infection such as COVID-19 and having metabolic dysfunction may not seem obvious at first, but it's profound and relates to the entire premise of this book. To grasp the elusive link, look no further than the high mortality rate among people with metabolic syndrome who suffered from COVID-19. By mid-January of 2021, researchers had declared metabolic syndrome a striking forecaster for severe disease outcomes in COVID-19 patients.[44] The numbers are stunning: patients with metabolic syndrome have a 40 percent increase in all-cause mortality, a 68 percent increase in the need for critical-care services, and a 90 percent increase in the need for mechanical ventilation compared to patients without metabolic syndrome. And studies on the relationship between uric acid and COVID-19 are beginning to appear in the literature, showing that people who are admitted to a hospital with the infection and elevated levels of uric acid are 2.6 times more likely to end up in the ICU on a ventilator, or dying, than patients whose levels are normal.[45]

It's no wonder that the stage was already set for a health catastrophe when COVID-19 hitched a ride across the world on boats, planes, trains, and automobiles.

There's a lot we still don't know about this virus and its long-term effects in people who've been exposed to it. In my field, doctors and researchers are furiously trying to figure out what kind of long-term complications a COVID-19 infection may have on brain function and the risk of neurodegeneration, including Alzheimer's disease, later on. COVID-19 is at first a respiratory infection, but we know it's also an inflammatory vascular disease that has far-reaching, ricocheting effects throughout the body, with damage to virtually all tissues, including those of the cardiovascular and neurological systems. When it became obvious that the virus caused neurological deficits, from minor ones such as temporary loss of taste and smell to more serious problems such as stroke, seizures, and delirium—not to mention psychiatric disorders such as anxiety and depression—people woke up to the fact that this is not just a bad flu. By one large study's calculation, a third of patients diagnosed with COVID-19 experience a psychiatric or neurological illness within six months.[46] That places COVID-19 in its own unique box.

Once this pandemic subsides, we will still live in a long aftermath during which tens of millions of people who've been infected may be managing COVID-related symptoms indefinitely—the so-called long-haulers. The two main drivers of long-haul COVID-19 seem to be organ and blood vessel damage as well as immune overreaction. Whether an individual becomes a long-hauler is likely the result of a complex interplay of genetic, epigenetic, and environmental factors. My hope is that patterns in the accumulating data will help us better predict who is more likely to have a prolonged illness and learn how best to treat those individuals. Long-haul recovery programs are appearing throughout the country, including at places like Mount Sinai Hospital in New York City, where a post-COVID clinic has been established. If you're among the long-haulers, I recommend participating in one of these programs and staying as close to the cutting edge of new treatments as possible.

We may not have a lot of control over factors that can threaten immune regulation, such as cancer and chemotherapy, but when it comes to problems such as diabetes, coronary artery disease, and obesity, our lifestyle choices turn out to be highly influential. Among the common conditions that separate people who either suffered immensely or died from COVID-19 from those who did not is obesity. In a study published in *Obesity Reviews,* researchers at several universities and the World Bank performed a meta-analysis of seventy-five studies that looked at the relationship of obesity to the spectrum of COVID-19 events—from the risk of contracting it to death as a result of it.[47] The findings of this report are telling. In comparing obese to nonobese individuals, obesity was associated with a 46 percent higher risk of being COVID-positive, a 113 percent higher risk of hospitalization, a 74 percent higher risk of ICU admission, and a 48 percent higher risk of death from the virus. The authors made it quite clear that mechanistically, one of the main reasons for these metrics related to obesity centers on disruption of immune function, stating, "The immunological impairments from individuals with obesity demonstrate the convergence of chronic and infectious disease risks. They expose a large portion of the world population with overweight/obesity status to greater risk of pulmonary viral infections like COVID-19."

We hopefully await the development of global herd immunity as well as more effective treatment protocols for the virus's impact in the people who contract it. But it's important to embrace the fact that we are not powerless when it comes to both our infection risk and outcomes. Our lifestyle choices in areas such as diet, sleep, exercise, and dealing with stress all factor into our immune competence and may well deny this coronavirus the chance to take additional advantage of us and spread itself even further.

Another way to look at the pandemic is to appreciate the opportunities it affords us to become more aware and proactive in our daily lives in pursuit of optimal health. And as this book shows, if uric acid levels, like a road sign on our journey, can help us predict future health challenges, we had best pay attention. We had best open our eyes to this new perspective and strategy in our toolbox.

A LURID AFFAIR

The relationship between uric acid and metabolic syndrome is among the hottest areas of study today, and fructose is public enemy number one because of its role in fueling ever-increasing levels of uric acid and aggravating metabolic syndrome. In a large, carefully conducted meta-analysis covering fifteen studies worldwide, a team of Iranian researchers showed that consumption of fructose in industrialized foods, such as sweetened beverages, is one of the chief causes of metabolic syndrome in otherwise healthy adults.[48] Although the researchers did not look specifically at uric acid, we know it's a prominent downstream product of fructose metabolism, and plenty of other studies have established a causal role for it in fructose-induced metabolic syndrome—so much so that hyperuricemia is now considered a "new marker for metabolic syndrome."[49]

Highlights of these recent findings prove that we can no longer ignore uric acid or cast this metabolite aside as an innocent bystander. Uric acid must be prioritized right alongside other biomarkers such as blood glucose, body weight, blood pressure, and LDL (the bad kind of cholesterol). I'd go further, however, and agree with the many researchers who are now declaring uric acid a *contributory causal factor* in elevating these measurements.[50] This is the central thesis of *Drop Acid*—you're going to learn how uric acid worsens the very biomarkers that healthcare providers have been focused on for decades. And this is precisely why it's been conclusively shown that high uric acid precedes and *predicts* the development of many cardiometabolic and kidney diseases.[51]

Uric acid belongs with other commonly measured biomarkers of health, such as blood glucose, body weight, blood pressure, triglycerides, and the ratio of good to bad cholesterol.

The underlying connections among all these conditions from a biological standpoint — and within the context of uric acid — are complex, but I'll be offering them to you throughout the book in digestible bites. And truthfully, it's incredibly interesting from so many perspectives. For example, one of the explanations for the relationship between elevated uric acid and insulin resistance, which is a core factor in type 2 diabetes and obesity, seems to be damage to the lining of the blood vessels — the endothelium.[52] Here's how this works.

First, it helps to know that *nitric oxide* (NO) is produced naturally by your body, and it's important for many aspects of your health. Perhaps its most vital function is vasodilation, meaning it relaxes the inner muscles of the blood vessels, causing them to widen and increase circulation. As such, NO is considered one of the most powerful regulatory molecules of the cardiovascular system. But it's also important in insulin function, because another important role of blood vessels is to facilitate insulin's move from the bloodstream into the cells, primarily the muscle cells, where it allows glucose to enter and make glycogen (the stored form of glucose).[53]

Uric acid undermines NO activity in two ways: (1) by compromising its production and (2) by jeopardizing the way it does its job.[54] So if there's a lack of NO and a damper on the way NO works, both insulin function and overall cardiovascular health are compromised. Which is why a deficiency of NO and damaged NO functionality are associated with heart disease, diabetes, and even erectile dysfunction (see the box on page 46). Scientists who study NO's effects in the body have long documented the fact that reducing NO levels is a mechanism for inducing insulin resistance. When they experiment with NO-deficient mice, the rodents display the features of metabolic syndrome. And the biological reason for this is that a roadblock of sorts has been erected between insulin and glucose. Insulin is supposed to stimulate the uptake of glucose in skeletal muscle by increasing blood flow to these tissues through a pathway that depends upon nitric oxide. So without adequate NO, insulin cannot do its job—the insulin-glucose correspondence, or activity, is disrupted. Loss of nitric oxide also triggers hypertension and a loss of vascular compliance, which refers to the ability of blood vessels to respond appropriately to changes in blood pressure.

The Uric Acid–Nitric Oxide Connection

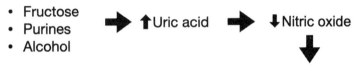

- Fructose
- Purines
- Alcohol

➡ ↑Uric acid ➡ ↓Nitric oxide
↓

- Insulin resistance
- Hypertension
- Reduced blood flow to organs

Let me mention one more study that showed the striking difference, in terms of uric acid, between people newly diagnosed with type 2 diabetes and their healthy counterparts.[55] It involved people between the ages of forty and sixty-five in whom the researchers measured fasting blood glucose, insulin, A1c, and uric acid—charting higher values across the board for people diagnosed with type 2 diabetes. Studies like this and many others expose the ways in which elevated uric acid induces diabetes. There are a few pathways: one is the simple activation of inflammation brought on by elevated uric acid, which causes insulin resistance. And uric acid is a powerful generator, as I noted, of oxidative stress, which damages tissues and DNA and reduces nitric oxide function (thereby causing endothelial function damage), all of which further incite inflammation. The cumulative inflammatory effect alone could injure cells in the pancreas and even cause problems with the expression of the *insulin gene*, which causes a decrease in insulin secretion. Once the insulin-signaling system is impaired, metabolic trouble looms large.

SEX ED: URIC ACID AND ED — WHAT'S THE CONNECTION?

Although I'm a neurologist, and as I've written about previously, I've treated a fair share of men who suffer from sexual dysfunction and are either impotent or have some level of erectile dysfunction. Many of them rely on drugs like Viagra to help them out. These patients didn't come to me for erectile dysfunction specifically, but it was a noted issue when I asked them about that part of their lives in addition to the neurological concerns I was addressing. Had I been attuned to the uric acid connection, however, I could have added that topic to the conversation.

Erectile dysfunction, or ED, has long been associated with blood-vessel problems and cardiovascular disease. The condition is a marker of vascular dysfunction and correlates strongly with coronary artery disease. Men with a history of cardiovascular conditions such as hypertension and small vessel disease are at high risk for ED; and now elevated uric acid *alone* is an independent risk factor as well — even when there is no hypertension.[56] How so?

We know that uric acid damages the inside lining of blood vessels, the endothelium, via inflammation and oxidative stress. This reduces the activity of nitric oxide, which is necessary for erectile function. In fact, ED drugs like Viagra and Cialis may work by increasing nitric oxide. In several recent studies, high levels of uric acid have been associated with a 36 percent increase in the risk of ED. The overconsumption of soft drinks has even been implicated in the "slow and asymptomatic progression of ED," which eventually results in full manifestation of ED.[57] So for men who are not concerned about high blood pressure, diabetes, and obesity but are concerned about their sexual health, these findings will likely speak to them.

If you didn't follow all that science, rest assured that you'll grasp it soon. You'll also learn how this vital biological process relates to problems as disparate as an underactive thyroid and immune dysfunction. Given the experience of COVID-19, we all have a heightened awareness of immunity. We seek the secrets to building immune resilience, including resilience against autoimmune diseases, and this quest most definitely involves an understanding of uric acid.[58] There's even a process in the body called autophagy, which has a starring role not only in your immunity but also in your longevity.

Autophagy (which literally means "self-eating" in Greek) is a form of cellular housecleaning that enables cells to act in a youthful manner. Fundamentally, it's how the body removes or recycles dangerous, damaged cellular parts, including troublemaking dead "zombie cells" and pathogens. In the process, the immune system gets a boost, and this may have an impact on the risk of developing cancer, heart disease, autoimmune diseases, and neurological disorders. And here's the critical point: uric acid suppresses autophagy and diminishes the anti-inflammatory capacity of cells. Put another way, uric acid prevents your cells from clearing out dangerous clutter and calming down inflammatory reactions.

THE SWEET SPOT: MIDDLE OF THE U

In astrobiology, a field of astronomy that studies life on earth and beyond, the phrase "the Goldilocks zone" refers to the range of distances between a planet's orbit and its star within which the planet's temperatures are ideal for generating liquid water. (To be sure, the phrase can be applied across many disciplines to describe phenomena that only happen within certain "just right" constraints.) The Goldilocks zone is the place where a planet can sustain life because its temperatures remain stable in the "middle"—not too hot and not too cold. Earth is a prime example of a planet in the Goldilocks zone. Medical biologists often borrow the term to describe the ideal quantities of things the body needs for health-promoting effects. Exercise too much or too little, and the result can be damaging. Same goes for sleeping too much or too little, eating too much or too little, having dangerously low or high blood sugar, and taking too much or too little of a necessary drug. You get my point. Obviously, the terminology is based on the fairy tale "Goldilocks and the Three Bears," in which Goldilocks tastes three different bowls of porridge and finds she prefers porridge that is neither too hot nor too cold but just right.

When it comes to uric acid, finding the Goldilocks zone is essential.[59] Although it's rare these days to suffer from dangerously low uric acid, I should point out that there are some health issues that could be associated with extremely low uric acid over time (defined as below 2.5 mg/dL for men and 1.5 mg/dL for women), and they include a *potentially* higher risk of certain neurological disorders, cardiovascular disease, cancer, and a very rare kidney disease called Fanconi syndrome. But these associations have not been fully validated, and other factors could be at play that have nothing to do with low uric acid. While you might hear that uric acid is an antioxidant and hence has benefits, it's the ultimate two-faced character: it may have some antioxidant properties in plasma outside cells, but inside cells it's a pro-oxidant offender. I'm honestly not worried about people having persistently super-low uric acid levels, because that is simply not the reality for the vast majority of people. Yes, the highs and lows of body fat are hazardous, but overweight and obese people far outnumber underweight people. Same goes for the highs and lows of uric acid. People who live with chronically low uric acid likely have genetic underpinnings to the condition and are anomalies—one in several million.

Another way to think about the ideal zone is to picture the letter U—you don't want to be out on a limb with sky-high uric acid at the tops of the U. You want to be in the sweet-spot middle. And of course I'll show you how to do just that.

The dramatic rise in uric acid levels since the mid-1970s has clear origins that I'll delve into shortly. I have no doubt that our dietary changes are significantly responsible. Our DNA has not evolved fast enough to handle our current caloric load, in particular the dark force of fructose in our daily fare. You will be stunned to learn the science behind fructose and how pervasive it is in our lives. In fact, test it out yourself: spend a day making note of all the sources of fructose in your foods and beverages. Read your labels. Ask questions where you buy your groceries. It's no wonder we are documenting rising levels of uric acid as well as a rising prevalence of degenerative conditions across all segments of society.

The laws of nature that govern and regulate every aspect of our physiology have been written in our code of life for millennia. Some of that encoding has led to the precarious situation we find ourselves in today. Let's travel back in time.

CHAPTER 2

Survival of the Fattest

How Prehistoric Apes Hardwired Us with the Fat Gene

Nothing in biology makes sense except in the light of evolution.

— THEODOSIUS DOBZHANSKY, 1973

SUE WAS NOT A HAPPY DINOSAUR.* We all know that T. rexes were among the fiercest and most famous of the reptilian giants that roamed the planet some sixty-six to sixty-eight million years ago. They were carnivorous animals, and cannibalism was not beneath them. Like other T. rexes, Sue had short forelimbs and probably a short temper, too, and she was maybe a bit edgier and moodier than her fellow dinosaurs. She had good reason to be extra grumpy, because studies of her bones (and she may have been a male, for we don't know her sex) have resulted in an extraordinary diagnosis: gout.[1] Even though reptiles today lack uricase,

---

* Sue, a tyrannosaur skeleton, was unearthed in 1990 in South Dakota. The story of her discovery and her subsequent acquisition is a dramatic tale all on its own, complete with the jailing of a fossil dealer, a seizure by the FBI and National Guard troops, and an auction in which she sold for $8.3 million. Sue Hendrickson, after whom the dinosaur is named, found her protruding from a butte; she has become one of the largest and most complete preserved tyrannosaur skeletons in the world. She now resides in all her fossilized glory in Chicago's Field Museum of Natural History.

this condition was probably not common among dinosaurs (and tyrannosaurs in particular), but it raises questions such as why this ailment goes back so far in time.

While we'll never manage to blast to the past or spy on Sue and her Cretaceous prey, astrophysicists tell us that we may be able to travel into the future at some point. I can't help but wonder: What does the future human look like? How long can we push the limits of longevity? Where will our genome take us? Obviously, I don't have the answers, but if history tells us anything, it is that we must learn to respect our genome—its powers as well as its weaknesses. In fact, that is the most important lesson of all. Unfortunately, we've arrived at a critical moment in our evolution that demands we pay special attention to this lesson if we're to carry on as a species and thrive. Many of us do not respect our genome and have plenty of chronic diseases to show for it. The disconnect between our genome, established long ago, and our environment in the twenty-first century is what scientists call an *evolutionary/environmental mismatch*. Let me explain.

Despite the wonders and technological marvels of modernity, we still have a hunter-gatherer genome; it's "thrifty" in the sense that it's programmed to make us fat during times of abundance. The thrifty-gene hypothesis was first proposed by University of Michigan geneticist James Neel in 1962 to help explain why type 2 diabetes has a strong genetic basis and results in the negative effects favored by natural selection (his scientific paper's title says it all: "Diabetes Mellitus: A 'Thrifty' Genotype Rendered Detrimental by 'Progress'?").[2] Why, he wondered, would evolution support a gene that caused debilitating symptoms, even during one's prime reproductive years, from blindness and heart disease to kidney failure and premature death? That doesn't seem, at least on the surface, to be a good omen for the future of our species. He also wondered what changes in the environment were responsible for the increase in cases of type 2 diabetes. Well, according to his theory, which is now established, the genes that predispose a person to diabetes—thrifty genes—were historically advantageous. They are what turned on the fat switch to help one fatten up quickly when food was available, since long stretches of food scarcity were an inevitable part of life. But once modern society transformed our access to food, the thrifty genes, while still active, were no longer needed—essentially preparing us for a famine that these days never materializes.

Human evolution has its own timeline. We don't yet know how to speed it up. It takes between forty thousand and seventy thousand years for any significant changes to take place in our collective human genome—changes that could accommodate drastic shifts in our diet. Our innate thrifty genes are not trained to ignore the instruction to store fat. Most of the genome that defines us as human comprises genes selected during the Paleolithic era in Africa, a period that lasted from roughly three million years ago to roughly eleven thousand years ago, when the agricultural revolution took hold. (These numbers are a moving target: archeologists continue to find new clues to the chronology of our evolution. The agricultural revolution occurred between ten and twelve thousand years ago, so eleven thousand years is close enough for my purposes.) And eleven thousand years comprise approximately 366 human generations, which in turn comprise only 0.5 percent of the history of the genus *Homo*. Moreover, the Industrial Revolution and the modern age, which mark the beginning of the Western lifestyle, comprise only seven and four human generations respectively. This period of just a few hundred years was marked by rapid and radical changes in lifestyle and diet that are still ongoing and that caused unprecedented modifications in people's habits—habits that naturally led to rises in uric acid levels. The Industrial Revolution introduced the widespread use of refined vegetable oils, refined cereal grains, and refined sugar, while the modern age gave us the junk food industry.

Our dietary habits took a particularly devastating turn for the worse between 1970 and 1990, when the consumption of high-fructose corn syrup ballooned more than 1,000 percent—an increase that far exceeded the changes in intake of any other ingredient or food group. This surge has paralleled the rise in obesity and other conditions aggravated by high uric acid. Today in the United States, dairy products, cereal grains (especially the refined form), refined sugars, refined vegetable oils, and alcohol make up a little more than 72 percent of the total energy consumed daily.[3] These types of foods would have contributed little or no energy to the typical preagricultural hominid diet. In fact, the food industry that provides us processed food has only been around for a scant 0.005 percent of the time that humans have been on this planet! We have not genetically adapted yet to thrive on our Western diet and lifestyles.

While some of us like to believe we're saddled with genes that promote fat growth and retention, thus making weight loss and maintenance hard, the truth is that we *all* carry thrifty genes that turn on the fat switch. It's part of our human constitution, and for the majority of our existence on this planet, it has kept us alive. But this evolutionary mismatch between our ancient physiology and the Western diet and lifestyle underlies many so-called diseases of civilization, including coronary heart disease, obesity, hypertension, type 2 diabetes, cell cancers, autoimmune diseases, and osteoporosis, which are rare or virtually absent in hunter-gatherers and other non-Westernized populations (more on this below).[4] We'll see later the cascading effects of this modern lifestyle, from fanning the flames of inflammation to changing our microbiome, which has everything to do with metabolism and immunity. We even have new evidence that adverse changes to the gut microbiome directly relate to uric acid metabolism and the consequences of its accumulation in the body—even in the absence of gout or kidney issues.

The idea that *Homo sapiens* is best adapted to an ancestral environment is reinforced by data showing that the hunter-gatherers living today and other populations minimally affected by modern habits exhibit superior health markers, body composition, and physical fitness compared to industrialized populations whose diets are high in refined sugars and unhealthful fats.[5] These markers include:

- healthfully low blood pressure;

- lack of association between blood pressure and age (a common association in the rest of us);

- excellent insulin sensitivity, even among middle-aged and older individuals;

- lower fasting insulin concentrations;

- lower fasting leptin levels (which control hunger signals);

- lower body mass indexes;

- lower waist-to-height ratio (meaning less abdominal fat);

- lower triceps skin-fold measurements (another marker of body fat);

- greater maximum oxygen consumption, or VO_2 max (a marker of cardiopulmonary functionality);

- better visual acuity; and

- better bone health markers and lower fracture rates.

So unlike these non-Westernized populations, we're trying to force our bodies to speak a language it never learned — our desire to operate in a new 2.0 world with 1.0 technology is working against us. That's not to say that our genome is stupid or primitive. It's a remarkable piece of machinery that can do a lot for us when we learn how to work with it.

ONCE UPON A TIME

Our story begins sometime between fifteen and seventeen million years ago, during the early to middle Miocene epoch, when the world looked a little different from the way it looks today. Two major ecosystems — the kelp forests and grasslands—were just getting started here on earth as the continents continued to drift toward their present positions. Antarctica became isolated; Mount Everest rose high in East Asia as mountain building took place in western North America and Europe; and the African-Arabian plate joined to Asia, closing the seaway that had previously separated Africa from Asia. Animals of the Miocene were fairly modern, as mammals and birds were well established and apes arose and diversified. The earliest apes evolved from a common ancestor with monkeys, probably in East Africa around twenty-six million years ago.[6] Those apes walked on all fours and, like monkeys, lived in trees, but they had big bodies, no tails, and larger skulls and brains. This was when Africa was full of deciduous and tropical rain forests—a paradise of sorts where the apes feasted primarily on fruit.[7]

But the earth would undergo a progressive decline in temperatures during this epoch, taking a sharp drop around fourteen million years ago. This led to an ice age that helped form the land bridge between Africa and Europe. As we all learned in high school science class, this facilitated the migration of our distant primate ancestors into Asia and Europe. The cooling continued and eventually became a powerful environmental pressure, favoring survival among those who were able to sustain significant periods of caloric scarcity. This "weeding out" process was slow, taking place over several million years and honing animals' genetics along the way. A certain group of primates pulled through the challenges and would become our ancestors. These ancestors ultimately migrated back to Africa, sowing the seeds for future humans.

Their secret to survival? They had a unique ability to generate high levels of body fat as well as to preserve and store that body fat, creating a reservoir for caloric energy during long stretches of food insecurity.[8] Indeed, it was a matter of survival of the fattest. Now, that's not to say they were necessarily overweight or obese, but they had become genetically hardwired to pack away those "just-in-case" calories to survive at normal weight and hold on to every bit of extra energy they could.

Among the mutations that occurred to equip our ancestors with this gene-based survival skill were three that practically deleted the gene for coding a functional uricase enzyme.[9] As I mentioned in the previous chapter, uricase is the enzyme that breaks down uric acid. It's a liver enzyme that converts uric acid into allantoin, which is more easily excreted by the kidneys because of its water-soluble characteristics. I should reiterate that the mutations that deactivated the uricase genes were ones that served us in advantageous ways millions of years ago, but they also took something away from us: the ability to eliminate uric acid from the body and avoid the side effects that result from too much of the substance circulating through our bloodstreams.

For modern humans, these mutations are mucking up the quest for fitness. And by fitness, I'm talking about all forms of fitness, from healthful weight and other physical markers of wellness to the absence of disease and metabolic disorders. We are, as it were, evolutionarily mismatched with our current environment. It took perhaps fifty million years for our

The Uricase Mutation—Then and Now

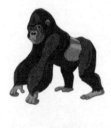
Increased uric acid
(Food scarcity)
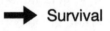
Survival

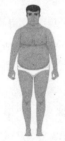
Increased uric acid
(Food abundance)
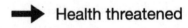
Health threatened

uricase genes to mutate through various iterations and achieve our genome's current state, but we haven't yet had the benefits of another fifty million years of evolution to force new mutations to correct for our modern environment.

This mismatch between our environment and evolution, which is also the central premise of the so-called Paleo movement, has been an interest of mine for most of my life. In fact, on March 26, 1971, when I was sixteen years old, the following letter was published in the *Miami Herald* as the "feature letter" of the day. It was my first publication.

To the Editor:

After spending three days and two nights at the Sebring car races, I found myself to be in question: "Can we adapt ourselves to this future environment?"

Perhaps our bodies are more suited to the lush forest bed or soft sandy beaches where former humans lived in duration.

I don't believe that the two weeks in the mountains or a Saturday at the beach will be enough to keep this body, which has evolved under less strenuous conditions, content.

Perhaps the human will change rapidly in the next centuries to adapt himself to beer cans, concrete, and shattering noise. Our generations are each contributing to the evolution of pollution-resistant lungs. But what about the people of today who are stuck with the outdated machinery?

In the decades since that publication, we have seen what happens when humans can't adapt fast enough to match our endless desire for "beer cans, concrete, and shattering noise." We are fat, addicted to being indoors and sedentary, and suffer from the adverse effects of a very noisy modern and largely urban lifestyle that aggravates our stress levels and mucks up our sleep habits.

OUR ORIGIN STORY IS STILL BEING WRITTEN

Our understanding of the human origin story and our evolution is a work in progress. Much of the story has shifted since I first learned about early humans in my own formal education. What we didn't realize until the twenty-first century, when new fossil evidence was discovered, is that there were at least two migrations out of Africa, if not more, as soon as a series of land bridges began connecting Africa to Europe and Asia (Eurasia) some twenty-one million years ago. Which means that the pressures to modify the mother-ship genes for the uricase enzyme could have occurred outside Africa, especially since fossil evidence suggests that some European apes journeyed to Asia and became the ancestors of gibbons and orangutans, whereas others returned to Africa and evolved into African apes and humans. By seven million years ago, there were no longer any apes in Europe.

The uricase defect benefited our ancestors not only because it padded their bones with much-needed fat for survival but also because the increase in blood pressure that occurred with elevated uric acid further helped them endure periods of dehydration and salt scarcity. Salt, as you probably know, can lead to high blood pressure because it stops the kidneys from removing water from the body efficiently.* Salt is nature's way of helping us retain precious water. But when there's a drought, and no salt to help, the body needs another way to survive.[10]

Our ancestors turned fruit sugar into fat and, through the actions of uric acid, simultaneously bumped up blood pressure to keep it normalized (not too low). In fact, the metabolism of fructose also drives the production of *vasopressin*, the very hormone the body uses to boost blood pressure and help the kidneys retain water. As summed up nicely in the

---

* Note that the words *salt* and *sodium* are often used interchangeably; technically, however, *sodium* refers to a mineral—it's one of the two chemical elements found in salt, or sodium chloride, which is the crystal-like compound we shake onto foods and into recipes. Semantics aside, it doesn't matter whether we're talking about sodium or table salt, because both are the same for my purposes. Sodium is the ingredient in salt that has effects in the body.

Journal of Internal Medicine in 2020: "Thus, one of the primary functions of fructose is to conserve water by stimulating vasopressin which reduces water loss via the kidney while also stimulating fat and glycogen production as a source of metabolic water."[11] What's more, consuming fructose may also increase thirst, which acts as yet another mechanism to stimulate an increase in precious water content.

You can likely see where I'm going with this line of reasoning. There's no shortage of fructose, especially the refined kind, or salt in our sustenance today. But we're missing the uricase genes to keep us lean and fit in our world of abundance. The plethora of sugar- and salt-rich calories in our diets over the past century in particular is why researchers have tracked a dramatic rise in hyperuricemia-related disorders, from gout to cardiometabolic conditions that set us up for other problems, including cancer and dementia. And the number one dietary culprit that screams from the scientific literature is fructose.[12] Fructose may have been the ticket to fitness eons ago, but it's the body's license to kill when its intake is not under control.

FROM FRUCTOSE TO FITNESS

While it's common knowledge that consuming too much sugar of any kind can fatten us up as those extra calories get packed away in adipose (fatty) tissue, what's not commonly understood is the fact that excess fructose is particularly harmful because of its impact on our mitochondria, the tiny organelles in our cells that generate chemical energy in the form of ATP (adenosine triphosphate). Too much fructose impairs energy production in the mitochondria, and this alone leads to energy storage. Translation: more fat.

Fructose is nature's sweetener, found exclusively in fruit and honey: it's the sweetest of all naturally occurring carbohydrates, which probably explains why we love it so much (and why scientists can attribute the prevalence of diabetes to our love affair with sugar).[13] Most of the fructose we consume, however, is not in its natural form of whole-fruit sugar. The average American consumes seventeen teaspoons (71.14 grams) every day of added sugar. (The term *added sugar* refers to any sugar added to foods and beverages during preparation or processing that those foods and beverages would not otherwise contain. Added sugar can come from sucrose, dextrose, table sugar, syrup, honey, and fruit or vegetable juice concentrates.) That translates into around fifty-seven *pounds* of added sugar each year, per person—much of which comes from the highly processed form of fructose derived from high-fructose corn syrup.[14] High-fructose corn syrup, which is what we find in our sodas, juices, and many tremendously palatable processed foods, is yet another combination of molecules dominated by fructose—it's around 55 percent fructose, 42 percent glucose, and 3 percent other carbohydrates. I use the word *around* because some studies have shown that high-fructose corn syrup can contain much more fructose than other formulations—one concoction of high-fructose corn syrup comes in at 90 percent fructose (though you won't see the percentage breakdown on the label).[15]

High-fructose corn syrup, or HFCS, gained popularity in the late 1970s, when the price of regular sugar was high while corn prices were low because of government subsidies (HFCS is usually made from the starch of genetically modified corn). Hailed as a "case history of innovation" early on, it's been a case history of ruination in health ever since.[16] We'll get into the details of fructose biology and its relationship to uric acid levels later, but I want to prime you now for that part of the book.

Fructose is often touted as the "safe" or "safer" sugar because it has the lowest glycemic index of all the natural sugars, meaning that it does not directly trigger a rise in blood sugar with the reflexive release of insulin from the pancreas. Unlike other types of sugar, which immediately go into circulation and raise blood sugar levels, fructose is handled exclusively by the liver. If it's combined with other forms of sugar, as it is in high-fructose corn syrup, the glucose ends up in general circulation and raises blood sugar levels while the fructose is metabolized by the liver. While fructose does not have an immediate effect on blood sugar or insulin levels, make no mistake: its long-term dangerous effects on these measurements and so many other markers of metabolic health are profound.[17]

The facts I'll lay out in the next chapter are well documented: consuming fructose is associated with impaired glucose tolerance, insulin resistance, high blood fats, and hypertension. And because fructose does not trigger the production of insulin and leptin, two key hormones in regulating our metabolism, diets that contain high amounts of it lead to obesity and its metabolic repercussions. Indeed, our fructose consumption is increasingly being implicated in the development of the obesity epidemic in the United States, and fructose is edging out other forms of sugar as the culprit at the top of the list.

A look at the geographical areas where obesity rates soar will give you a vivid picture of the evolutionary mismatch of the modern era. And they're not the places you might think. The most overweight and obese humans on the planet live in Polynesia, an expansive region made up of more than one thousand islands scattered over the central and southern Pacific Ocean. Travel magazines may advertise this exotic destination as a vacationer's paradise, but it's ground zero for people living with hypertension, obesity, and diabetes.[18] Polynesians also have an unusually high prevalence of hyperuricemia and gout. Nowhere in the world has the evolutionary mismatch been more striking.

According to the World Health Organization, more than half the residents of the Cook Islands, for example, are obese; percentages of obesity range from 35 to more than 50 throughout the Polynesian islands.[19] And diabetes is rampant: 47 percent of the inhabitants of the Marshall Islands carry this diagnosis. According to Professor Jonathan Shaw of the Baker Heart and Diabetes Institute, in Australia, "This is a population with a genetic predisposition and when exposed to Western lifestyles results in high rates of diabetes... [This is] undoubtedly caused by high rates of obesity."[20] And nearly a quarter of Polynesians have hyperuricemia today.

Historically, the Polynesians are a hardy group who endured long voyages at sea. But genetically, they carry those same thrifty genes that enabled them to survive seafaring migrations but make living difficult in the twenty-first century, when they have access to cheap, highly caloric, processed, sugar-rich foods. Interestingly, in Polynesian countries such as Fiji, where there is a mixed ethnicity (just over half the people are indigenous, and most of the rest are of Indian origin), the rate of obesity is significantly less, at 36.4 percent. Fully 40 percent of the Polynesian population of nearly ten million people has been diagnosed with a noncommunicable disease — e.g., diabetes, cardiovascular disease, and hypertension — which can be tied to both chronic blood-sugar chaos and elevated uric acid. In fact, these diseases alone account for three-quarters of all deaths in this area and 40 to 60 percent of total health-care expenditures.[21]

Concerns about the health of Pacific Islanders date back decades. In 1960, doctors from what was then called the Queen Elizabeth Hospital for Rheumatic Diseases, in New Zealand, began publishing papers about the stark rise in metabolic diseases and elevated uric acid levels among the country's Maori people.[22] When Westerners first encountered the Maori people of New Zealand, there was virtually no evidence of gout or even obesity in the native population, even at a time when gout was highly prevalent in northern European areas. By the middle of the twentieth century, however, gout had made its appearance among many inhabitants of the Pacific basin. One 1975 study noted that "half the Polynesian population of New Zealand, Rarotonga, Puka Puka, and the Tokelau Islands proved to be hyperuricemic by accepted European and North American standards, the associated gout rate reaching 10.2% in Maori males aged 20 and over." The researchers went on to write: "The trends towards hyperuricemia and gout, on the one hand, and towards obesity, diabetes mellitus, hypertension, and associated degenerative vascular disorders, on the other hand, which manifest themselves separately in some Polynesian Pacific Islanders, run together in the Maori and Samoan people, presenting a combined problem of considerable importance to the public health."[23]

More recently, scientists from the University of California at San Francisco, the University of Southern California, and the University of Pittsburgh have documented the same concerns among native Hawaiians with Polynesian ancestry, whose risk for obesity, type 2 diabetes, cardiovascular diseases, and several common cancers is much higher than it is for European Americans or Asian Americans living in the Hawaiian Islands.[24] And the reason for it is the same: strong thrifty genes that predispose people to elevated uric acid and its downstream effects in the face of a Western lifestyle rich in calories. After studying the DNA of four thousand native Hawaiians, this consortium of epidemiologists determined that for every 10 percent increase in the amount of DNA that indicated Polynesian genetic ancestry, there was an 8.6 percent increase in the risk of diabetes and an 11 percent increase in the risk of heart failure. As Dr. Veronica Hackethal, writing for *Medscape Medical News*, observed, "Three thousand years of cross-ocean migration in Polynesia may have provided a selective advantage for a genetic variant favoring obesity."[25] And clearly, this offers up a compelling explanation as to why this population has such a prevalence of hyperuricemia.

In addition to strong thrifty-gene predispositions to hyperuricemia and gout among this unique group of people, other genetic variants have been discovered that further increase that predisposition. Evolutionary protections, for example, against the mosquito-borne infection malaria could have led to genetic changes thousands of years ago that now predispose these populations to more hyperuricemia and gout. (To be sure, monosodium urate, which is formed from uric acid, triggers a strong inflammatory response. During the infection process caused by the malaria parasite, urate is released.) In other words, high uric acid levels could have been "selected for" by evolutionary changes to enhance the survival rates of humans who had this variation in their genetic makeup in regions where malaria was endemic.[26] Again, these were compromises made under survival pressures.

The genetic underpinnings of obesity and other metabolic disorders are not often discussed in medicine, or at least they are downplayed. In most obese people, for example, no single genetic cause can be identified, and there have not been a lot of genes found to be directly related to obesity. In studies that have identified parts of our genome associated with obesity, their total contribution to variation in BMI (body mass index) and body weight is estimated to be less than 2 percent, suggesting that environmental influences are more important than genetic factors. Exceedingly rare genetically driven obesity conditions do exist, such as Prader-Willi syndrome. Not only does the syndrome involve hormonal disruptions that delay puberty and trigger constant, insatiable hunger, it also entails behavior problems, intellectual disability, and short stature.

Highly unusual conditions such as Prader-Willi syndrome aside, the dramatic shift in health trends among Pacific Islanders in the past half century shows that genetic variations can indeed pave the way for metabolic problems that are not in any way related to a genetic "defect." It was a survival mechanism established long ago that ran up against the twentieth- and twenty-first-century lifestyle with dreadful consequences. When scientists probe further into this disturbing trend, they find that, for these Polynesians, being encumbered with commanding thrifty genes and modern diets high in purines and fructose is akin to "dietary genocide."[27]

Pacific hyperuricemia is now a standard term in medical literature. And I think it's safe to say that we're all now suffering to some degree from Pacific hyperuricemia. The medical literature tags both Pacific Islanders and Caucasians as being the peoples most susceptible to hyperuricemia and gout. Even if you have no Pacific Island ancestry, you're likely harboring genes fit for a forager, not a gorger. And your uric acid levels can help tell the story. Now, this does not mean that high uric acid alone is causing obesity, but it's an important part of an intricate metabolic picture that must be taken into account. Below are graphics adapted from recent studies showing the parallels between rising levels of uric acid and rising BMI and waist circumference.[28]

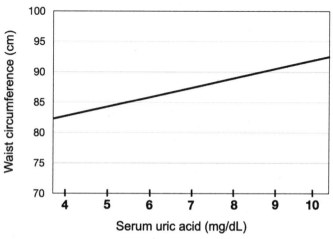

How Uric Acid Relates to BMI

Adapted from Nurshad Ali et al., *PLOS ONE,* November 1, 2018

How Uric Acid Relates to Waist Circumference

Adapted from Nurshad Ali et al., *PLOS ONE,* November 1, 2018

STORING FAT VERSUS BURNING FAT

Most of us are attracted to things that will help us burn excess fat, from metabolism-revving workouts and ideal meal timing to simply getting a good night's sleep (and if you don't how sleep burns calories, wait until chapter 5). But it's probably not common knowledge that there are mechanisms within our physiology that determine, from moment to moment, whether we need to make and store fat or burn fat—that is, use it as an energy source. And empowering research over the past several years has revealed that we have control over the way our metabolism deals with fat.

The study of fat metabolism could fill a book all on its own, but here I want to highlight a few aspects of human physiology that are central to this book's theme. In particular, let's home in on one molecule in the body you've likely never heard of: AMPK, short for "adenosine monophosphate–activated protein kinase." This gem not only plays a role in determining whether we store fat or burn fat, it also has a big say in how we age. You got that right: AMPK acts as the body's Swiss Army knife. It's an all-purpose tool that helps us get important tasks done — tasks that can either lead us to become old and fat or stay young and lean.

Biologists consider AMPK an antiaging enzyme that, when activated, promotes and helps the body's cellular housecleaning as well as its energy balance, whether you're burning or storing fat. I don't want to get too deeply into the weeds, but AMPK, when activated, basically tells your body that "the hunting is good," meaning that food is abundant and therefore there's no need to make and store fat or increase the production of blood sugar. Your metabolism shifts from storing fat to burning it, creating a lean, streamlined hunting machine. And when food is abundant, AMPK helps the body reduce its production of glucose. Metformin, the popular diabetes drug, takes full advantage of this mechanism by the direct stimulation of AMPK, bringing blood sugar levels down. This activation explains why people taking this drug—or stimulating AMPK by exercising or taking berberine—often experience the "side effect" of reduced abdominal fat stores.

As you'll read later in the book, several strategies can help activate AMPK that don't require drugs—notably, certain foods and supplements, exercise, and even intermittent fasting (also called time-restricted eating). And while it is certainly desirable to keep AMPK activity going strong, what you don't want is to activate too much of AMPK's evil twin: AMPD2, short for adenosine monophosphate deaminase 2. This is also an enzyme but has an opposing effect—reducing the burning of fat and increasing its storage. Essentially, the way in which our bodies deal with fat is regulated by these two enzymes, and to a significant degree, it is uric acid that determines which one is activated. High levels of uric acid push activation of AMPD2 and reduce or silence AMPK.

In a 2015 study done on hibernating animals who develop fatty livers when they're active in summertime and undergo a switch to fat-burning mode during their sleep-filled winters, researchers found that fat accumulation in liver cells was attributable to the activation of AMPD2 and reduced AMPK activity.[29] Animals that hibernate switch between activating AMPD2 to store fat when they are preparing to hibernate and activating AMPK to burn fat when they are hibernating. And uric acid flips this switch.

In a similar study, these same researchers found that when rats were given sucrose, a source of fructose, the animals developed fatty liver, as one might expect.[30] But if AMPK was activated by giving the rats the drug metformin, fat accumulation in the liver did not occur. Again, uric acid determines which pathway is taken, either for producing fat or burning fat. Specifically, when the body breaks down purines and fructose, among the many molecules produced in a long chain of reactions is AMP (adenosine monophosphate), which goes on to trigger uric acid production—the final product of this metabolism. AMP production means that energy is being consumed, and this system tells our bodies that we need to conserve energy—to make and store fat. This is how the environment (not enough food) runs the show. And, as this particular study revealed for the first time, uric acid at the end of that biological sequence directly inhibits AMPK while turning on AMPD2. The study further singles out fructose as being especially culpable in driving the AMPD2 actions.

In the next chapter, we'll take this knowledge one step further as I show you how and why fructose is so damaging. For now, keep in mind that fructose consumption and the resulting levels of uric acid have everything to do with whether your body is activating AMPK or AMPD2. The level of uric acid acts as a kind of traffic signal at a major intersection, telling your body to either store or burn fat. In a very real sense, our empowerment over our metabolism begins and ends with our understanding of uric acid. Because uric acid plays a pivotal role in determining whether or not we pack away pounds for a winter that never comes, we must learn to control our levels of it and finally achieve so many of our health-related goals.

SHARING THE PLANET: URIC ACID AND GUT HEALTH

For millennia, humans and other living things have shared more than a unique evolution from prehistoric ancestors. We've also coevolved with colonies of microbes that now collectively make up our microbiome. In my book *Brain Maker*, I covered the science of the microbiome in depth, and I encourage you to read it to learn more. The LUV program is designed to cultivate a healthy microbiome, and this has everything to do with controlling uric acid, too. But before we get to that connection, I want to present some basic information about your microbiome.

Gut bacteria are key to our survival. They exist in what we call an intestinal microbiome, and they play a role in many physiological functions: they manufacture neurotransmitters and vitamins that we couldn't otherwise produce, promote normal gastrointestinal function, provide protection from infection, regulate metabolism and the absorption of food, and help control blood sugar. They even affect whether we are overweight or lean, hungry or satiated. Your microbiome as a whole, which encompasses microbes that live in many places in and on your body (think skin), is unique to you. Although patterns do exist in the microbiomes of people living in similar environments, individual microbiomes are like personal fingerprints—no two are exactly alike.

Because the health of your microbiome factors into your immune-system function and inflammation levels, those microbes may ultimately factor into your risk for illnesses as varied as depression, obesity, bowel disorders, diabetes, multiple sclerosis, asthma, autism, Alzheimer's disease, Parkinson's disease, and even cancer. These microbes also help control gut permeability—the integrity of your intestinal wall, which acts as a gatekeeper between you and an outside world that's filled with potential threats to health. A break in the intestinal wall (called a leaky gut) allows food toxins and pathogens to pass into the bloodstream, triggering an aggressive and often prolonged immune response. Components of bacteria such as lipopolysaccharide, or LPS, can also pass through a leaky gut and ignite inflammation. Many strains of good gut bacteria need LPS for protection and to maintain their structure, but LPS should not traverse over into the bloodstream; it's a harmful endotoxin (LPS is classically used in laboratory experiments to instantly create inflammation in animals, humans included). In fact, measuring LPS in the blood is one way to detect leaky gut, because it's not supposed to be there. In my field, LPS is now being looked upon as playing a central role in neurodegenerative diseases. And surprise: uric acid is connected with gut health and whether or not LPS lands in your bloodstream.

Any breach in the gut lining affects the health and function not only of the gut but also of other organs and tissues, including the skeletal system, the skin, the kidneys, the pancreas, the liver, and the brain. How does uric acid play a part? Turns out that uric acid in the body is excreted to a significant degree by the intestines. As such, our intestines are exposed to uric acid, and elevations in the acid can change the composition of gut bacteria, favoring pro-inflammatory strains. Elevations also promote the decay of the intestinal lining, further paving the path toward systemic inflammation. It's no wonder that researchers are now documenting a strong association between hyperuricemia, intestinal barrier dysfunction, and immune disorders.[31]

In cutting-edge studies that have leveraged the power of CRISPR technology, which allows scientists to "edit" mice DNA so they have abnormally high levels of uric acid, the mice routinely develop sick microbiomes, with pro-inflammatory bacteria dominating and clear signs of a compromised intestinal lining. The relationship between elevated uric acid and changes in the gut bacteria is so profound that researchers are now performing fecal microbial transplants (FMT) in research settings to see whether they might constitute a treatment for both acute and recurrent gout. Fecal microbial transplants involve taking a sample of the microbiome of a physically healthy donor via his or her stool and giving it to an ill patient after it's been filtered. Experiments so far in humans have revealed that FMT leads to a significant reduction of uric acid immediately after the treatment and decreases the frequency and duration of acute gout attacks. Interestingly, after the FMT treatment, measurements of the endotoxin LPS decreased.

What I find even more intriguing are studies that refer to the bad bacteria related to high uric acid as "gout bacteria." In one of the first explorations of its kind, researchers identified seventeen gout-associated bacteria and were able to predict diagnoses of gout with close to 90 percent accuracy simply by looking at the gut bacteria.[32] And not surprisingly, they found that the bacteria in the guts of gout patients were quite similar to those found in people with type 2 diabetes and other features of metabolic syndrome.

All these conditions have underlying commonalities, and uric acid is but one strong thread in the tapestry of our biology that we can no longer neglect. The sooner we can drop acid to healthful levels and support the strength and function of our guts' microbiomes, the sooner we can usher in better health. I'll help you do that in part 2. For now, let's get up close and personal with the sugar that's had a hidden agenda for far too long.

CHAPTER 3

The Fallacy of Fructose

How Uric Acid Amplifies the Threat

Whoever is careless with the truth in small matters cannot be trusted in important affairs.

— Albert Einstein

When Joanna turned fifty, she treated herself to a visit to a medical spa equipped with state-of-the-art technology and on-site physicians who specialize in helping people create custom plans for optimizing their health and, presumably, their longevity. After years of struggling to gain control of nagging health conditions, including high blood pressure, prediabetes, and an extra sixty pounds, she had reached the point where she said to herself, *Enough is enough.* None of her regular doctors offered any useful advice other than the canned, "Just watch what you eat and try to exercise more." And nobody had ever discussed metabolic syndrome with her, a condition she surely suffered from but had never been officially diagnosed with.

Despite her primary care physician's urging that she try pharmaceuticals to manage her blood sugar and hypertension, Joanna resisted taking any medications, hoping to achieve her goals through lifestyle hacks. But no matter what she tried, from popular diets to torturous exercise boot camps, nothing worked. That is, until she met a prescient doctor at the spa who diagnosed her with metabolic syndrome and asked a simple question: How much fructose are you consuming?

Joanna didn't know how to answer the question. Her mind immediately went to fruit, which she admitted she probably didn't eat enough of. Then she thought about her love of soda pop and other sweetened beverages made with high-fructose corn syrup. Sugary drinks were the main weakness in her diet, which was otherwise pretty good. When the doctor ran a few basic tests to confirm his suspicion — that she could check off at least three of the five boxes on the metabolic-syndrome list of symptoms (page 38) — he discovered that she met all five criteria for the condition. Even her blood fats, both her triglycerides and cholesterol levels, pointed to concerning issues with her metabolism. Crucially, he also noticed that her uric acid level was high. In addition, the tests revealed that her thyroid was underactive, which she later learned may have exacerbated the elevated uric acid. Because thyroid hormones help regulate metabolism and kidney function, when there's an imbalance in those hormones, uric acid is not properly excreted by the kidneys and builds up in the blood. Joanna's C-reactive protein value, a measure of systemic inflammation, was abnormally high as well.

She then had a lengthy conversation with the doctor about uric acid and its connections to many metabolic issues that in turn factor into conditions as diverse as heart disease, dementia, obesity, and cancer. She never knew about the close association between uric acid and metabolic syndrome and was eager to learn more. At the heart of the conversation was a surprising focus on fructose's secret relationship with uric acid. Joanna knew fructose didn't wear any health halo and wasn't winning any health awards, and, like many people, she assumed it could be consumed in moderation. But what this doctor shared with her turned a lot of what Joanna knew on its head. She soon realized that she didn't have a clue about fructose's true colors and the extent to which it was ruining her health. It was as if Joanna were listening to a whodunit about her own body's covert killer. Just as she didn't know about the unexpected relationship between uric acid and metabolic syndrome, she'd never before heard about uric acid's conspiratorial role in fructose's damaging effects. Joanna hung on to the doctor's every word, and after following his easy protocol for dropping her uric acid and bringing her blood sugar into balance, Joanna's health was transformed in a matter of months.

My hope is that your health will be, too, because the program I'll lay out in part 2 mimics what Joanna did to ameliorate her maladies and finally get her weight under control. Before we get to those details, though, we have a few more science lessons to cover, starting with public enemy number one: fructose. The story of fructose's connection to high uric acid is anything but sweet.

FAKE NEWS ABOUT FRUCTOSE

You might recall seeing alluring ads in the early 2010s, paid for by the Corn Refiners Association, that promoted high-fructose corn syrup's safety. The ad campaign was an attempt to stop the sharp decline in HFCS consumption and stem negative perceptions that had developed in the minds of many consumers. In one TV commercial that really stirred the pot, a father walks with his daughter across a cornfield and says that he's reassured by experts that high-fructose corn syrup is the same as cane sugar. "Your body can't tell the difference," he says. "Sugar is sugar."[1]

That didn't go over well with the Western Sugar Cooperative and other sugar processors, who sued the Corn Refiners Association, the Archer Daniels Midland company, and the Cargill corporation for false advertising, among other complaints. (Archer Daniels Midland and Cargill are global food corporations that process, among many other things, corn for HFCS.) They asked for $1.5 billion in damages, which prompted the corn refiners to countersue to the tune of $530 million.

The corn refiners' primary complaint was that the sugar processors were spreading misinformation about HFCS. A jury trial began on November 3, 2015.[2]

The war between Big Sugar and Big Corn is as fierce as they come, with billions of dollars at stake. The lawsuit unveiled how nasty the competitive rivalry is in the multibillion-dollar sweetener industry and the extent to which each side will go to claim market share in selling its sweet wares. It brought hundreds of pages of secret corporate emails and strategy documents into the public eye, putting on full display the lobbying, bullying, deceiving, mudslinging, and fearmongering that goes on behind the scenes. For years leading up to the trial, the corn refiners went to great lengths to change the growing narrative against them, going so far as to ask the FDA to let them call HFCS "corn sugar" so it sounded more natural. The FDA blocked that attempt in 2012.

In a bid to quell concerns that consuming HFCS leads to worse health consequences than consuming regular refined sugar does, the Corn Refiners Association spent around $10 million over the course of four years to help fund research led by Dr. James M. Rippe, a Massachusetts-based cardiologist who released a series of studies challenging the assertion that there are any particular health consequences associated with the corn-based sweetener.[3] Dr. Rippe was also paid a handsome $41,000-a-month retainer by the trade group to regularly send opinion pieces to local newspapers claiming that high-fructose corn syrup is no more dangerous than sugar. If that sounds a bit incestuous, I think it's even more sinister than that.

Although corporate support for product-based research is not unusual, when it comes to ingredients and products that significantly affect people's health, I believe the rules should be different. Why, for example, would you listen to a scientist who is paid by the tobacco industry to tell you that cigarette smoking in moderation is perfectly okay? You wouldn't. That's preposterous. But it happens frequently in the murky, self-promoting world of the food and beverage industry, within which each company is vying for your dollars. These companies are also elbowing one another for the attention of conglomerate food manufacturers that need sweeteners to make their own goods. It doesn't help that studies that claim the relationship between sweeteners (added sugars) and weight gain and diabetes is weak have generally been funded by the sugar and beverage industries.[4]

Ten days into the sugar–versus–high-fructose corn syrup jury trial, a truce was called, and the parties reached a confidential settlement. Interestingly, the joint statement on the settlement was neutral about whether sugar or HFCS is "healthier." Each side simply pledged to encourage the "safe and healthful use of their products."[5]

SUCROSE VERSUS FRUCTOSE: WHAT'S THE DIFFERENCE?

If you were quizzed about the science of sugar in the body, my guess is you might get a lot of questions wrong. Sugar in processed foods can be disguised by a long list of names (e.g., evaporated cane juice, cane juice solids, cane juice crystals, and so on), and I'll give you a cheat sheet for those names in part 2. For now, let's focus primarily on fructose, because it differs from other types of sugar and tangos with uric acid.

Pure glucose and fructose, monosaccharides, are the simplest forms of sugar, whereas sucrose — the white granulated stuff also known as table sugar — is a combination of glucose and fructose, thereby making it a disaccharide (two molecules linked together). After ingestion, sucrose is degraded in the small intestine by the enzyme sucrase, which releases fructose and glucose, which are then absorbed.

As I mentioned above, fructose is naturally found in fruit and honey as well as in agave and many vegetables, including broccoli, artichokes, asparagus, and okra. But rarely do we overdose on pure fructose from natural sources: whole, unprocessed foods contain fructose only in small amounts, and that fructose is absorbed slowly in the presence of fiber. So by and large, consuming these foods doesn't increase uric acid levels. What's more, many fruits contain nutrients and other molecules that off-set or counteract potential rises in uric acid, such as potassium, flavonols, fiber, and vitamin C (ascorbate), the latter of which actually has the power to lower uric acid while stimulating its excretion. Drinking liquid fructose in the form of fruit juice or other fructose-sweetened beverages is not the same as eating, say, an equivalent dose of that fructose from whole, fiber-rich fruits and vegetables. And when you gulp down a bever-age that has fructose in it, you're likely to drink a lot of it in a short period of time. This drives dramatic metabolic effects that you don't want. You won't necessarily feel them on the spot, but as they say, the body keeps score.

In the early 1900s, the average American ate around fifteen grams of fructose a day (the equivalent of one whole piece of fruit or a cup of blue-berries); we've almost quadrupled that intake today to north of fifty-five grams, mostly from unnatural sources—notably, high-fructose corn syrup.[6] Yes, let's be clear: despite the marketing, there is nothing natural about HFCS. Our fructose consumption, on average, amounts to more than thirteen teaspoons a day and constitutes nearly 10 percent of our total daily energy intake.[7] It's a major ingredient in soft drinks, pastries, desserts, and various processed foods. The sugar in the vast majority of soft drinks is at least 58 percent fructose, and the sugar in the three most popular soft drinks (Coca-Cola, Sprite, and Pepsi) can contain as much as 65 percent fructose.[8] As I'll soon explain, fructose, through the metab-olite uric acid, sends an urgent message to your body: "Make and store as much fat as possible!!!" No wonder bears getting ready to hibernate gorge on fructose-laden foods. They need to make as much fat as possible in order to survive the winter and live to see another spring.

Although estimates do vary and actual numbers can be hard to definitively calculate, the current consensus is that the average American consumes 94 grams of added sweeteners per day, quadruple the limit suggested by the guidelines put forth by the Office of Disease Prevention and Health Promotion (ODPHP), part of the US Department of Health and Human Services.[9] Yet there's no need for added sugar and no nutritional benefit that comes from it. What's more, the guidelines are sorely behind the times. Along with those from the ODPHP, the recommendations offered by organizations such as the American Heart Association and American Diabetes Association have lagged far behind the research. And I don't know any medical expert who says that we all have a healthy relationship with sugar.

It will take time for the gathering storm of scientific data that's proving the ills of sugar-sweetened drinks to change health guidelines in modern medicine. And the uric acid part of the story will probably elude most doctors' radar for a while. In one large meta-analysis of more than 154,000 people, which was reported in the *British Medical Journal* in 2019 but never made mainstream news, researchers demonstrated a powerful relationship between the consumption of sugar-sweetened beverages and both elevated uric acid and gout.[10] The people who drank the most sugar-sweetened beverages were more than twice as likely to experience gout than those who drank the least amount of sugar-sweetened beverages. And fruit juice consumption also increased the risk of gout. It's important to note that there was no association between whole-fruit intake and gout. This will factor into my dietary recommendations later on.

Although sweetened drinks and fruit juices are the main culprits in fructose overdose, people who don't drink anything but water may still get their fill of fructose through sauces, dressings, jams and jellies, snack foods, ice cream, crackers, cereals, candy, sweetened yogurt, soups, store-bought baked goods (e.g., muffins, cookies, pastries, and cakes), and various other processed foods. It finds its way, largely through those sauces and condiments, into fast-food fare such as burgers, chicken sandwiches, and pizza. It's even added to aspirin to make the bitter drug taste better. As I said, HFCS is everywhere.

> "Very simply, we subsidize high-fructose corn syrup in this country, but not carrots."
> —Michael Pollan, *The Omnivore's Dilemma*

Contrary to what Big Corn will tell you, fructose and glucose are not siblings with equal biological effects. Fructose is more like glucose's evil twin: when you eat glucose, your body uses it to produce energy; but when you eat fructose, it triggers changes in the body that favor the storage of energy in the form of fat. Put simply, glucose is the sugar involved in energy production; fructose is the sugar involved in energy storage. Once you understand how refined fructose is metabolized in the body, you'll come to see how it is indeed the worst sugar. And as you're about to find out, it's not the "safer alternative" to other sugars, despite what the food industry's most trustworthy people (doctors included) have said. Fructose is the twenty-first century's cloaked killer, much as tobacco and margarine were in the twentieth century. And uric acid, its ultimate metabolic product, does its evil bidding.

While it may not get digested and metabolized in the same way as other sugars, as my colleague the endocrinologist Dr. Robert Lustig describes it, fructose is like "alcohol without the buzz."[11] A longtime specialist in pediatric hormone disorders and a leading expert in childhood obesity, Dr. Lustig also calls fructose "a primary contributor to human disease," and he draws parallels between the damaging effects of fructose and alcohol's reverberations in the body.

When you compare excessive alcohol consumption to fructose, many similarities emerge: both promote the same dose-dependent toxic effects and trigger hypertension, insulin resistance, unhealthful blood fats, and fatty liver disease. Like alcohol, fructose induces changes in the energy-signaling capacity of the central nervous system through direct stimulation of our innate "hedonic pathway" as well as indirect stimulation of our "starvation pathway."

Let me slow this down a notch. First, our hedonic (pleasure) pathway is characterized by the drive to eat to obtain pleasure when we don't really need the energy, at least physiologically. We all know what it's like to have hedonic hunger—seeing a tasty treat and instantly wanting to devour it for its pure delight even though we're not physically hungry. Indeed, there are reward systems in the brain set up to induce feelings of gratification upon downing a bite of gooey chocolate cake. And my guess is that right now you're probably thinking how tempting that decadent cake would be. Maybe your mouth is watering. That's your hedonic brain trying to run the show. On the other hand, the starvation pathway is characterized by the processes I've described in which we're compelled to eat more because our bodies think we're starving when we're not!

Fructose is particularly treacherous in the starvation pathway because it disarms hunger cues and fails to help us feel full; as a result, we continue to gorge on food—no doubt a type of "mindless eating." In the presence of fructose, the body goes into hold-on-to-fat mode and does everything it can to self-preserve, under the false belief that it's starving. Meanwhile, insulin cannot work effectively, which further damages the whole enterprise while driving inflammation (more on this below). The combination of both hedonic and starvation pathway activation results in a vicious cycle of excessive eating, and you know what that means: weight gain, problems with blood pressure and blood sugar, and all the downstream effects that surely follow.

The major source of commercial fructose worldwide has not been fruit or honey—it's been table sugar derived from sugarcane and sugar beets. Table sugar was first processed in New Guinea and in the Indian subcontinent; it was a rare and expensive commodity that was introduced into Europe via Venice, Italy, and other trading ports during the Middle Ages. High-fructose corn syrup, which dominates today, was first produced by American biochemists Richard O. Marshall and Earl R. Kooi in 1957 at Oklahoma State University's Agricultural Experiment Station after they created an enzyme that chemically rearranged the composition of glucose in corn syrup and turned it into fructose.[12] Around a decade later it began to steadily creep into our diet because it's sweeter and cheaper to produce than table sugar, and thus it increasingly replaced the pricier sucrose. Starting around 1970, manufacturers began adding high-fructose corn syrup to their products, and in 1984, both Coca-Cola and Pepsi announced that they were switching from sucrose to HFCS in their soft drinks.

By the late 1970s, HFCS was everywhere and difficult to avoid: its consumption in the United States went from zero in 1970 to a whopping sixty pounds per person per year by 2000, accounting for half of every person's annual sugar consumption.[13] Long-term epidemiological studies now show that the concomitant rise in obesity and diabetes since the 1970s can be linked to the dramatic rise in HFSC consumption.[14]

During this meteoric escalation in fructose ingestion, there's been a parallel decline in the consumption of healthful fats after the US Department of Agriculture, the American Medical Association, and the American Heart Association erroneously advised against the consumption of all fat in favor of carbohydrates. The low-fat craze that took hold of the Western dietary world favored too many refined, sugary carbohydrates at the expense of healthful fats and proteins. Mind you, those healthful fats and proteins are what help make us feel full. And, as you'll see later on, certain fats, such as omega-3s, can counter, or offset, some of the negative effects of too much sugar—specifically, fructose.

The percentage of fat in people's diets has fallen from 40 to 30 percent over the past twenty-five years, while the percentage of carbs has gone up from 40 to 55 percent—all coinciding with an exploding obesity epidemic.[15] Notably, we've only just recently begun to understand that one of the fundamental ways fructose threatens our health is through—you guessed it—raising uric acid. Uric acid is the missing link between fructose consumption and illness. It's what separates fructose from all the other sugars.

Now, as I take you closer to understanding the behavior of fructose in the body and its clandestine relationship with uric acid, you may begin to view glucose as a hero. Don't fall for that, either. Glucose has a role in our lives as it relates to cellular energy, but this molecule, too, must be exquisitely managed. Like many molecules (and drugs) in the body, it can be an ally or a poison depending on its quantity, and we must establish a healthy relationship with it and control its levels for optimal health.

> The incidence of type 2 diabetes is 20 percent higher in countries with easy availability of HFCS than it is in countries where HFCS is not as available.[16] And by the year 2030, 7.7 percent of the world's population will be diabetic.[17]

FRUCTOSE METABOLISM AND URIC ACID OVERLOAD

The biochemistry of fructose's metabolism is complex and involves many molecules with long, tongue-twisting names. But here's what you need to know. First, fructose is absorbed from the gastrointestinal tract through a different mechanism from the one that processes glucose. As you know, glucose stimulates insulin release from the pancreas, but fructose does not. And this simple fact is precisely what has given clever marketing campaigns license to claim that because fructose doesn't elicit an insulin response, it can be considered a "safer" sugar. But despite what savvy marketing would have us believe, the effects of elevated fructose consumption are devastating as it relates to insulin, and uric acid plays a central role in this devastation.

Structurally, fructose and glucose look almost identical with the exception of a couple of chemical bonds. But these seemingly small variations make all the difference in the world. When glucose is metabolized by the enzyme glucokinase, the initial step in the process (phosphorylation of glucose) is carefully regulated, and levels of the body's most critical energy molecule—adenosine triphosphate (ATP)—are tightly maintained in the cell. This is not the case when it comes to fructose. When fructose is consumed, it is quickly absorbed into the bloodstream and siphoned off to the liver to metabolize. Within liver cells, the enzyme fructokinase begins its work, including the consumption of ATP.

Did you catch that last crucial fact? Because this process *uses* ATP, it means that fructose metabolism *depletes* energy resources. Rather than helping generate precious energy, it *steals* energy. And it consumes ATP in an unregulated way, as if no one is at the controls. If a cell sees a lot of fructose, its ATP levels can plummet by 40 or 50 percent.[18] Meanwhile, the downstream effect of fructose's highway robbery of ATP is not only mitochondrial dysfunction but also a rapid rise in the level of uric acid in the bloodstream. Fructose's drain on energy in cells provokes a Mayday signal that screams *We're running out of energy!* And this immediately compels the body to switch gears into energy-preservation mode: metabolism slows down to reduce the resting energy expenditure (i.e., you burn less fat), and any incoming calories are likely to go into storage (i.e., they're added to your fat).

Looking at this cascade more closely, I'll add that as fructose cycles through various steps in its metabolism, ATP gets converted to the molecule I mentioned in the previous chapter, AMP (adenosine monophosphate), and ultimately generates uric acid as an end product in this complicated chain of events. A self-perpetuating cycle ensues (what's technically called *feedback potentiation*) because the high level of uric acid further stimulates fructokinase.[19] Like a drug pusher, high uric acid keeps fructokinase in an activated state, sustaining the whole process that then goes on to exacerbate energy depletion and mitochondrial dysfunction, foment inflammation and oxidative stress, raise blood pressure, increase insulin resistance, and trigger the production of body fat—all things that would serve you well if you were a hunter-gatherer in a time of food scarcity.[20] But in the world in which we find ourselves, who needs this?!? In addition, as a survival signal, fructose triggers hunger and thirst, further pushing you to eat more; but as you do just that, you're shunting that potential energy into its most efficient storage form—fat.

Usually, there are physiological mechanisms in which the end products of biological reactions help turn off processes that threaten to go into overdrive or are no longer needed. This is called a negative feedback system: the end products reach a tipping point in volume and help stop their creation. Not so with fructose's metabolic products. Fructokinase has no negative feedback system; it keeps pushing the button to create uric acid. As a result, continued fructose metabolism further depletes energy and pumps out uric acid that is harmful at the cellular level. This out-of-control system may have worked well for our ancestors in times of food scarcity, and it continues to work for mammals about to migrate or hibernate. But it's the ultimate modern paradox: our innate survival mechanisms are killing us.

> Fructose consumption taps into our deepest DNA programming: our genes load the gun, and our environment pulls the trigger.

A lot goes on in the liver when fructose arrives for its metabolism. In addition to depleting energy, it also triggers *lipogenesis,* a process that produces liver fat. You read that right: fructose metabolism in the liver leads directly to fat production—chiefly, the formation of triglycerides, the most common type of fat in the body. When found at high levels in the blood, triglycerides are a major risk factor for cardiovascular events such as heart attacks as well as coronary artery disease. Elevated triglyceride levels have long been tagged as a hallmark of consuming too many carbs, but now we know which carb is the principal offender. In a 2017 review paper titled "Chronic Fructose Ingestion as a Major Health Concern," professor of nutrition Dr. Amy J. Bidwell of the State University of New York at Oswego stated it clearly: "The most detrimental aspect of fructose is its ability to be converted to fatty acids within the hepatocytes [liver cells]."[21]

Another fundamental takeaway: the accumulation of fat in the liver cells itself wreaks havoc because it directly compromises the ability of insulin to do its job and store glucose. Moreover, the generation of uric acid from fructose metabolism also causes oxidative stress to the pancreatic islets, which are small islands of cells in the pancreas that produce insulin. So while it is true that fructose does not directly elevate insulin, it ultimately increases insulin resistance through the back door of the liver with the aid of uric acid. This is precisely how fructose—and elevated uric acid—are linked to the development of diabetes and other metabolic disorders. Uric acid is not merely a by-product—it's an instigator of reactions that have harmful effects on metabolism and, in turn, the entire body.

I find it shameful that fructose was once marketed as a good, safe sugar for diabetics under the misguided thinking that it did not tap the flow of insulin and raise blood sugar. This notion is in direct conflict with science: fructose acts in stealthy ways through its behavior in the liver. Its unique metabolism, which culminates in the generation of elevated levels of uric acid, results in a constellation of bad outcomes—energy depletion, fat production, and impairments to the body's insulin system. All this ultimately triggers systemic inflammation and oxidative stress. Another biological blow.

In one of the most revealing studies to highlight the problem with fructose as opposed to glucose, a group of scientists from a diverse array of institutions, including the University of California at Davis, Tufts University, and the University of California at Berkeley, gave volunteers either glucose-sweetened or fructose-sweetened beverages that provided 25 percent of their calories for a ten-week period.[22] Both groups gained weight, but the fructose group had a much higher level of visceral adipose tissue (abdominal fat). We know that high levels of abdominal fat — the worst kind of body fat to carry around in excess — correlate with increased inflammation, increased insulin resistance, and conditions such as type 2 diabetes, Alzheimer's disease, and coronary artery disease. The study demonstrated that, crucially, it was the fructose group who experienced a striking rise in triglycerides and increased production of fat in their liver cells, which directly relates to insulin resistance. In addition, a variety of cardiovascular risk markers were also increased in the fructose group. In another similar study, conducted to chart the metabolic effects of ten-week consumption of fructose-sweetened beverages in women, the results were a carbon copy: dramatic increases in triglycerides, dramatic increases in fasting glucose levels, and compromised insulin resistance.[23]

Given uric acid's fat-promoting effects as a direct result of fructose metabolism, you can see now that it's not an innocent bystander.[24] It may as well be one of the prime suspects holding a smoking gun in these adverse biological events. Adding insult to injury, the breakdown of fructose in the liver generates more than elevated uric acid and the necessary building blocks for the synthesis of triglycerides; it also generates the structural materials for glucose production. In essence, it stimulates glucose production in the liver and, in doing so, turns on the spigot for insulin release from the pancreas as that glucose gets released into circulation. It's a vicious cycle, as you can likely see now. To put this all together, see the diagram below.

Effects of Fructose in the Liver

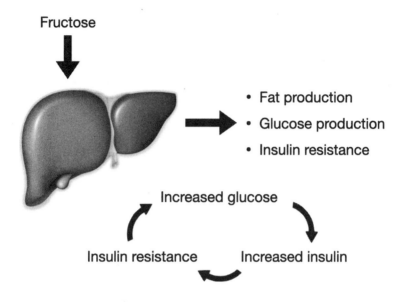

Fructose

- Fat production
- Glucose production
- Insulin resistance

Increased glucose

Insulin resistance   Increased insulin

Such findings have alarmed doctors in my field who study risk factors for Alzheimer's disease, prompting them to rethink the effects of fructose on the brain. They call fructose "a potential time bomb" for dementia risk, and I couldn't agree more.[25] And again, research has documented uric acid's hand in that risk. The alarm-sounding scientists, based at the UK's University of Cambridge and University College London, wrote: "The association between high fructose consumption and increased risk of cognitive impairment could also be mediated by the elevation of plasma levels of UA [uric acid] caused by high fructose intake." In their disruptive paper, the subhead "Fructose and Dementia: A Potential Time Bomb" caused a stir in the medical community.

The paper's authors go on to explain that an elevated level of uric acid is clear evidence that there's increased activity of an enzyme that has adverse downstream effects, including an increase in free radicals and a reduction in nitric oxide (NO) synthesis. You'll recall from the previous chapter that NO is essential to vascular health. It's also key to the health of the brain, where it's directly involved in the transmission of messages and memory formation. As I'll explain in detail in the next chapter, because insulin requires nitric oxide to stimulate glucose uptake in the body *and brain*, fructose-induced hyperuricemia has both direct and indirect roles in metabolic syndrome, a huge risk factor for brain dysfunction. Hence we have yet another link between uric acid levels and the risk of cognitive decline, a relationship demonstrated in plenty of studies.

FRUCTOSE HIJACKS HUNGER CUES, KEEPING URIC ACID PRODUCTION TURNED ON

One of the most misunderstood differences between glucose and fructose is the effect they have on appetite. And here's where fructose once again takes the lead in being more insidious. The two hormones that lord over our feelings of hunger and fullness are ghrelin and leptin. Put simply, ghrelin ("Go") triggers hunger, whereas leptin ("Stop") induces a sense of fullness. Ghrelin is secreted by the stomach when it's empty; it sends a message to your brain that you need to eat. Conversely, when your stomach is full, fat cells release leptin to tell your brain to stop eating. A now-seminal study published in 2004, which I've referenced numerous times in the past, showed that people with an 18 percent drop in leptin experienced a 28 percent increase in ghrelin, which translated to a 24 percent increase in appetite, driving them toward calorie-dense, high-carbohydrate foods, especially sweets, salty snacks, and starchy foods.[26] The study, led by researchers at the University of Chicago, was among the first to show the power of sleep in regulating our appetite hormones, because these striking changes in leptin and ghrelin were simply the result of sleep deprivation—the participants slept four hours a night for just two consecutive nights. As you'll see later on, this is one of the reasons why sufficient sleep is an important component of our program.

Clearly, you want these two hormones to be balanced and match your body's true energy needs so you don't undereat or overeat. Now, here's where fructose comes in: unlike glucose, which these hormones respond to, fructose reduces leptin and blunts the suppression of ghrelin.[27] In other words, fructose prevents you from reaching a feeling of fullness as you consume a meal. The result: greater appetite, more eating, and increased leptin resistance. You've deceived your body into thinking that it's on the starvation pathway. I've written a lot on this subject, but for readers unfamiliar with leptin resistance, here's the quick lowdown.

Leptin and insulin have a lot in common, though they tend to antagonize each other. Both are pro-inflammatory molecules. Leptin is an inflammatory cytokine in addition to playing a big part in the body's inflammatory processes. It controls the creation of other inflammatory molecules in the fat tissue throughout your body. And it helps explain why overweight and obese people are susceptible to inflammatory problems, including those that substantially increase the risk of chronic degenerative diseases in every part of the body from head to toe. Both leptin and insulin are the higher-ups in the body's chain of command, so imbalances tend to spiral downward and wreak havoc on virtually every system of the body beyond those directly controlled by these hormones.

What's more, leptin and insulin are negatively influenced by similar things, from sleep deprivation to refined-sugar overload. The more processed the sugar—fructose being at the top of the hit list—the more out of whack the healthful levels of leptin and insulin become. Just as continual abuse of the body's insulin-pumping and blood-sugar-balancing systems will eventually lead to insulin resistance, continual abuse of leptin signaling will do the same thing. When the body is overloaded and overwhelmed by substances that cause continual surges in leptin, the receptors for leptin stop hearing its message: they start to turn off, and you become leptin-resistant. Put simply, they surrender the controls, and you're left with a body vulnerable to illness and further dysfunction. So even though your leptin is elevated, it won't send a signal to your brain that you're full so you can stop eating. And if you cannot control your appetite, then you're at a much greater risk of contracting metabolic syndrome, which puts you at risk for other disorders.

Studies have also shown that elevated triglyceride levels—which, as you just learned, are a sign of too much fructose in the diet—cause leptin resistance. In fact, the strong relationship between fructose and leptin resistance has been well documented. As one group of researchers notes: "Because insulin and leptin, and possibly ghrelin, function as key signals to the central nervous system in the long-term regulation of energy balance, decreases of circulating insulin and leptin and increased ghrelin concentrations…could lead to increased caloric intake and ultimately contribute to weight gain and obesity during chronic consumption of diets high in fructose."[28]

In a 2018 study that explored these connections in lab animals, researchers documented stunning effects when they forced rats to generate fructose in their bodies.[29] They could do this by activating a well-known pathway from glucose to fructose using salt in the animals' diet. The outcome: leptin resistance and obesity in the rats. Let's think about that for a moment. If these researchers could spark internal production of fructose using a high-salt diet, that means that too much dietary salt could ultimately contribute to a bevy of conditions in people, from hypertension to fatty liver. We'll see in chapter 5 how salt can potentially trigger uric acid production—by sparking the conversion of glucose into its evil twin, fructose, in the body; call it the sugar swap. This is partially why high-salt diets are associated with obesity and the development of diabetes, among other metabolic maladies. It's pretty clear, and it's pretty terrifying: higher salt → higher fructose → worse leptin resistance → excessive appetite and overeating → obesity → insulin resistance → fatty liver.

Not a desirable chain of reactions.

One of the first studies proving the role of uric acid in fructose-induced metabolic syndrome dates back to pioneering work done on rats in 2005.[30] That's when a consortium of researchers fed a set of rats a high-fructose diet, recorded the physiological outcomes, and then experimented with uric-acid-lowering drugs on another set of rats. In the fructose-fed rats with no drugs to control uric acid, the results clearly showed the effects uric acid had on their development of metabolic syndrome's prime features (elevated insulin, elevated triglycerides, and elevated blood pressure). But in the set of rats treated with a drug to rein in their uric acid, guess what: there were no measurable changes to these metabolic markers.

Similar studies done on humans in order to observe the effects of high fructose consumption on blood pressure also point to uric acid's starring role in propelling staggering adverse changes.[31] How do we know that uric acid plays a prominent part? Because when uric acid is blocked artificially with drugs, the effects of the fructose on blood pressure is much lower by comparison.

Effect of Blocking Uric Acid in Men Fed a High-Fructose Diet

High-fructose drink

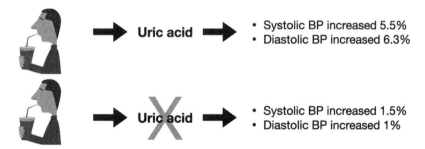

- Systolic BP increased 5.5%
- Diastolic BP increased 6.3%

- Systolic BP increased 1.5%
- Diastolic BP increased 1%

The plot thickens with another study, conducted in 2017, showing that HFCS affects dopamine signaling in the brain.[32] Although we already know from both human and animal studies that any damper on dopamine signaling can lead to compulsive overeating and obesity, this study documented HFCS's triggering of metabolic dysregulation and altered dopamine signaling *in the absence of obesity*. The authors warned that reduced dopamine signaling from HFCS could promote compulsive overeating, an addiction to food, and, in the long run, obesity. In other words, by consuming HFCS even at a healthful weight, you're entering the gates that lead to metabolic and weight chaos.

Findings like these make me think about other dopamine-related disorders, such as attention deficit hyperactivity disorder (ADHD), which now affects at least 10 percent of children in the United States between the ages of four and seventeen.[33] That's about 5.4 million children, more than half of whom are actively taking medication.[34] What if they cut back on their sugar intake, especially their intake of HFCS? Is it any wonder that parallel increases in obesity and ADHD are both associated with chronic sugar intake? Yet another study, conducted by the schools of medicine at Yale, Princeton, the University of Florida, and the University of Colorado, further connected the dots: reduction in dopamine activity points to increases in uric acid.[35] The team of scientists suggested that uric acid may reduce the number of dopamine receptors, thereby rendering dopamine less effective. They found that children with ADHD have higher blood levels of uric acid than children without ADHD. Although the connection between sugar consumption and behavioral issues such as ADHD have long been described in the literature and talked about anecdotally, we didn't know until recently about the relationship between dopamine signaling and uric acid levels. And even though researchers documented a link between elevated uric acid and symptoms of hyperactivity in otherwise normal children all the way back in 1989, clearly it took time for the whispers to be heard and the research further explored.[36]

My hope is that this knowledge will prompt us to treat these disorders, which increasingly affect our youth, through lifestyle medicine — not pharmaceuticals. Not so incidentally, although ADHD is often talked about in reference to kids, nearly ten million adults in the United States also grapple with this condition. For them, the solution could very well be the same: less sugar. Recent studies led by the National Institutes of Health have also tracked elevated uric acid among people with high impulsivity, including mild forms of ADHD and extreme conditions such as bipolar disorder.[37] Interestingly, in an experimental study of compulsive gamblers, uric acid concentrations increased while the gamblers played for money but not when they played checkers without betting![38]

A staggering 43 percent of the most popular videos posted by influencers between the ages of three and fourteen promote foods and drinks, and more than 90 percent of these products are unhealthful junk food, including fast food, candy, and soda.[39] Healthful or unbranded foods are only featured in a scant 3 percent of videos.

Speaking of children, I want to say a few words about fructose consumption and what we're beginning to see in adolescents. This demographic consumes more fructose than any other age group, but only in the past few years has it been studied for disease risk factors. The results have been troubling: just as in adults, it's been documented that high fructose consumption in children is associated with several markers known to increase the risk of cardiovascular disease and type 2 diabetes, and it appears that these relationships hinge on visceral obesity, or excess belly fat.[40] I don't think this comes as a surprise to anyone who studies these correlations within the context of the soaring rates of metabolic syndrome among the young. Although we like to think that adolescents are somehow saved or protected from the ravages of a poor, sugary diet and that they will go on to "outgrow" their penchant for sugar (and lose the resulting weight gain), I think that's a gravely ignorant way of thinking. We are setting them up for a host of health challenges in adulthood and programming them to live with chronic conditions. Moreover, these insults early in life set the stage for cancer, dementias, and premature death.

CHANGING THE STORY, AND ACKNOWLEDGING URIC ACID'S BIOLOGICAL PERSONA

I have had personal experience with the sugar industry's efforts to portray sugar as being less of a health threat than it really is. In 2018, I appeared on several national network television programs to promote the updated edition of *Grain Brain* five years after its original publication. On one popular morning program, which shall remain unnamed, my factually supported words about the health threats of sugar consumption were challenged practically the moment the conversation began. The producers had gone as far as to obtain a statement from the Sugar Association: "Sugar is best enjoyed in moderation and decades of research support this fact." I held my ground, compelled to challenge this blatant misinformation. I reflexively referenced the absurdity of believing the sugar industry, just as we shouldn't have believed the tobacco industry decades ago when it told us that smoking was healthful. Unfortunately, the folks conducting the interview seemed to miss the point.

In 2021, along with Stanford-trained physician and researcher Dr. Casey Means, I cowrote an open letter to newly inaugurated President Joe Biden for *MedPage Today*, a trusted online destination for people in the medical industry and readers who like to follow clinical news from scientific publications. It was titled "The Bitter Truth of USDA's Sugar Guidelines."[41] We called out the glaring disconnect: "The recommendations for added sugar in the 2020–2025 USDA dietary guidelines — released under the Trump administration — follow the sugar industry, the processed food industry, and the money. These recommendations fly in the face of science, and will continue to cause significant harm to American children and adults, with unfortunate health and financial ramifications for years to come." We urged the administration to reduce the USDA guidelines on the added-sugar quota to less than 6 percent of total calories from its current level of 10 percent and give Americans a fighting chance at health.

Reducing sugar consumption is essential to improving the health and productivity of all Americans. We especially pointed the finger at fructose in the form of high-fructose corn syrup, which is subsidized by Congress to the tune of nearly $500 billion. We wrote: "Diets high in sugar or blood sugar dysregulation are associated with mental illness, reduced cognition and learning, heart disease, Alzheimer's disease, ADHD, and suicide," not to mention cancer, stroke, infertility, chronic kidney and liver disease, erectile dysfunction, and preventable blindness. These outcomes contribute to an astronomically high degree of human and economic suffering. And the economic suffering is multifaceted, from high health-care costs to the fallout from a loss of productivity. People with type 2 diabetes, for example, are not only on the road to brain failure but may also have 44 percent less productivity at work.

When I posted another article on my website about the dangers of fructose, distinguishing between the fructose found in wholesome fruits and the refined, unnatural kind — while also calling attention to uric acid — the response from readers was swift. People have been confused about fructose for a long time, and barely anyone had heard about the uric acid part of the story. No sooner did I start this conversation about uric acid than I opened the floodgates to inquiries from people the world over seeking clarity, advice, and truth.

My mission in writing this book is to give you the unvarnished, albeit inconvenient, truth backed by the best unbiased science. For me, it boils down to this: forget the marketing and embrace what our most respected scientists are telling us. They're saying the same thing, over and over and over again: sugar is slowly killing us. And now the facts about fructose coupled with the uric acid plotline are rewriting the whole sugar narrative. That narrative contains a chapter about what the new scientific discoveries mean for the brain. Let's go there next.

CHAPTER 4

The U-Bomb in Your Brain

The Emerging Role of Uric Acid in Brain Decline

> *Overall, the human brain is the most complex object known in the universe—known, that is, to itself.*
>
> — E. O. WILSON

ON JUNE 7, 2021, the Food and Drug Administration approved a new drug called Aduhelm (aducanumab) for treating Alzheimer's disease, and the media lit up with headlines. It was the first new treatment approved for Alzheimer's in nearly twenty years, designed to slow the progression of memory loss and other cognitive issues in people with mild cognitive symptoms by reducing levels of beta-amyloid protein in the brain. The millions of people and their families who struggle with managing the illness cheered with renewed hope. The announcement sent shares of a select group of publicly traded biotech companies working on the neurodegenerative disorder on a wild ride. Pharmaceuticals giants that had long abandoned similar therapies under study suddenly revived their Alzheimer's drug programs. Billions seemed to be at stake as Big Pharma and investors eyed the next blockbuster class of drugs. But the news was not all positive. The initial fanfare you'd expect when a promising novel drug emerges to treat such a devastating disease with no known cure was quickly subdued by doubts and attacks on the drug's portrayal as a potential lifesaver. It is anything but.

Aduhelm, made by Biogen, was quickly and heavily criticized by many scientists, neurologists, and even the FDA's own independent advisory committee for being rushed through approval with little convincing evidence to show that it actually works (three of the FDA's experts resigned within days). Critics also pointed to the high cost of the drug ($56,000 a year for each patient), which needs to be delivered intravenously on a monthly basis, plus the fact that it requires patients to have regular MRI (magnetic resonance imaging) scans because it can cause swelling or hemorrhaging in the brain. The controversy also involved confusion over who should get the drug—everyone with signs of Alzheimer's or just those in the early stages? By July, under immense pressure, the FDA clarified that the drug should only be prescribed for people with mild memory or thinking problems because there was no data on its use in later stages of Alzheimer's. A week after that announcement, two of the nation's largest health systems, the Cleveland Clinic and Mount Sinai Hospital's Center for Wellness and Cognitive Health, announced that they would not administer the drug to patients. Others soon followed, including the Department of Veterans Affairs, excluding it from its formulary and going so far as to recommend against offering it.

The drama around Aduhelm reflects how desperate we are to end Alzheimer's and have at least *something* in our arsenal to combat the progression of this malady. We've made great strides in treating diseases such as heart disease, stroke, HIV/AIDS, and many types of cancer, but when it comes to dementias, particularly Alzheimer's, we remain stuck at a dead end. And the numbers are bleak: more than six million Americans are living with Alzheimer's today, and this number is projected to jump fourfold over the next forty years; it currently afflicts one out of every ten people in America age sixty-five or older and is on the rise. The latest estimates now rank Alzheimer's third behind heart disease and cancer as the leading cause of death for people in that age group. In 2021,

Alzheimer's and other dementias are projected to cost the nation $355 billion; by 2050, these costs could rise as high as $1.1 trillion. Anyone who has a loved one with this disease knows that it has devastating and costly consequences, not only for the afflicted but also for their families.[1]

So we are compelled to look at this issue from a different perspective. If we are dealing with a disease for which we have absolutely no meaningful treatment, doesn't it make sense to do everything possible to prevent it from manifesting itself in the first place? And what our best scientists are making clear is the simple fact that we have the tools, today, to bring this about. To be clear, there are steps we can take *right now* to dramatically reduce our risk for this disease.

What if you could prevent Alzheimer's from ever happening? That would be priceless, right? Well, all the data say we can do that using lifestyle medicine to keep our brain functioning on all cylinders long before pathology sets in and symptoms begin to show. According to some polls, people fear cognitive decline more than cancer or even death itself.[2] The thought of slowly withering away mentally to the point where you're unable to perform everyday tasks, yet you're expected to continue living for many more years, is just too overwhelming to imagine. Aduhelm will not save the day, but I have plenty of scientifically validated techniques to share that can help you build as resilient a brain as possible. And controlling uric acid is among the tools we must use.

Certain conditions—namely, increased blood glucose, insulin resistance, obesity, diabetes, hypertension, and inflammation—have all been strongly correlated with an increased risk for cognitive decline as well as brain shrinkage. As I wrote in *Grain Brain*, even a mild elevation of blood sugar imparts a significant risk of cognitive decline. And as I've also written, we've long known that a powerful predictor of cognitive decline is simply the size of one's belly (waist-to-hip ratio) and one's body mass index—the higher the BMI, the greater the risk. And now we can add elevated uric acid to the main list of risk factors.

Obesity is both a big predictor of elevated uric acid and a major risk factor for dementia; the two go together. In a twenty-seven-year longitudinal study looking back at more than ten thousand men and women, those who were obese when they were between forty and forty-five years old had a 74 percent increased risk of dementia later in life compared to those who maintained a normal weight or even those who were merely overweight.[3] If we could go back in time and test these individuals for their uric acid levels when they were in their forties, years away from showing cognitive deficits, my bet is we'd measure startlingly high levels. This has already been shown to be the case in other studies.

Consider, for one example, a 2016 Japanese study of a group of elderly people whose uric acid levels were tested within the context of risk for dementia: a high level of uric acid among the participants was associated with a *fourfold increased risk* of a dementia diagnosis. The researchers stated it succinctly in their conclusions: "Elevated serum UA levels are independently associated with cognitive deterioration."[4] There's that idea again: an *independent risk factor*. If obesity, type 2 diabetes, and hyperuricemia are each independent risk factors for dementia, imagine the exponential increase in risk when these conditions are *all* present in an individual.

While these researchers focused on the damaging effects of elevated uric acid on the brain's blood vessels, there are a number of downstream effects that demonstrate why high uric acid proves to be so threatening to the brain.[5]

It's important to emphasize that in many of the studies that document associations between elevated uric acid and negative outcomes for the brain, the definition of "high" uric acid is floating slightly above what your doctor would consider normal and could easily be dismissed as still within the normal range. As far back as 2007, researchers at Johns Hopkins University raised an alert flag when they found that "high-normal uric acid levels may cause barely detectable mini-strokes that potentially contribute to mental decline in aging adults."[6] (High normal is considered above 5.75 mg/dL in men and around 4.8 mg/dL in women.) Such findings are why I recommend lower limits for uric acid levels than the current guidelines (and most doctors) propose. Several studies conducted since 2007 have confirmed that "high normal" uric acid correlates with having 2.6 times the volume of white matter changes in the brain compared to people who have an average or lower uric acid level.[7] Structural changes, or lesions, in the white matter of the brain are not something you want—that's for sure. In adults age sixty and older, high but still "normal" levels of uric acid have been shown to render individuals 2.7 to 5.9 times more likely to score in the lowest twenty-fifth percentile in measurements of thinking speed and memory.

Although we tend to couch worries about cognitive decline in terms of aging adults, obesity is associated with poor cognitive performance in people of all ages.[8] And while we often wrongly assume that the young have the fastest, most agile, and most disease-free brains, plenty of studies reveal that poor memory, poor vocabulary, poor processing speed, and poor reasoning skills can be attributed to the effects of extra body weight on the brain. This phenomenon has been seen in children as young as five years old, and in fact obese children perform more poorly on academic tests compared to their normal-weight peers.[9] Children with metabolic syndrome suffer impaired abilities in spelling and arithmetic as well as impaired attention and overall mental flexibility. And we know that metabolic syndrome is associated with uric acid; elevated uric acid is commonly found in people with metabolic syndrome, whether they are five or seventy-five, significantly raising their risk for dementia later in life.

In research circles looking into the relationship between elevated uric acid and the risk of dementia, the treasure trove of data is a wake-up call. If you were to google "uric acid" and "cognitive decline," you would find a library of scientific papers, many of which have only been published since 2010 (and you'll find lots of extra citations listed in the endnotes). This is clearly emerging, leading-edge science. And if you were to read these papers, you'd come across talk of a connection between cognitive deficits and diabetes, which is precisely where uric acid enters the story as a villainous character.

TYPE 3 DIABETES

Nowadays, any talk about Alzheimer's disease brings diabetes into the conversation. In 2005, one year after chronic inflammation landed on the cover of *Time* magazine, studies describing Alzheimer's as a third type of diabetes began to make a quiet appearance in the scientific literature.[10] But the link between a sugary, fructose-heavy diet and Alzheimer's has only recently been brought into sharp focus: the newest research shows that fructose consumption increases the risk of dementia from a biochemical standpoint—and that uric acid may well be the lead actor. These studies are both worrying and empowering. To think we might be able to reduce the risk of Alzheimer's just by bringing uric acid levels under control is eye-opening. It has many implications for preventing not just Alzheimer's disease but other brain disorders as well.

What we're beginning to understand is that at the root of "type 3 diabetes" is a phenomenon in which neurons in the brain become unable to respond to insulin, which is essential for basic tasks, including memory and learning. We also think that insulin resistance may spark the formation of those infamous plaques present in Alzheimer's disease. These plaques are made up of an odd protein that essentially commandeers the brain and takes the place of normal brain cells. Some researchers believe that insulin resistance is central to the cognitive decline in Alzheimer's disease. It's all the more telling to note that people with prediabetes or metabolic syndrome have an increased risk of predementia and mild cognitive impairment, which often progresses to full-blown Alzheimer's disease. I should reiterate that once signs of disease set in, it's generally considered impossible to reverse course; the train has left the station and will most likely pick up speed.

The connection between diabetes and the risk of Alzheimer's does not mean that diabetes directly and always causes Alzheimer's disease, only that they may share the same origin. They can both develop from long-term dietary habits that lead to metabolic dysfunction and, further down the road, illness. Where do fructose and uric acid come into this picture? Research is sparkling with new insights that debunk misconceptions about the sugar that doesn't directly raise blood sugar but raises hell in the brain. And it does so in a multitude of ways.

First, as I said in the previous chapter, fructose-induced insulin resistance keeps the body locked in a mode in which blood sugar remains dangerously high. In the brain, insulin resistance prevents brain cells from receiving the energy they need. Insulin is a powerful *trophic* hormone, meaning that it nurtures neurons and is fundamental for brain energetics. Also called neuroenergetics, brain energetics refers to the system by which energy flows in the brain in order to take care of brain cells and meet their high demands for oxygen, fuel, and support. Rob brain cells of a vital caregiver, and they suffer — or, worse, die.

Second, the way the body metabolizes fructose leads to more uric acid production and depletes energy (ATP), which further sparks inflammation that can reach the brain (neuroinflammation). This metabolism can also occur directly in the brain: the biochemical machinery for metabolizing fructose has just recently been found to be present in brain cells like neurons and glial cells, which were not presumed to metabolize fructose.[11] This surprising new data has reversed old, prevailing dogmas about fructose metabolism in the brain.

Third, recall that in addition to depleting energy, fructose metabolism leads to reduced production of nitric oxide (NO), which you'll remember is a vital molecule for blood vessels, enabling them to function properly as well as transport insulin. By crippling NO activity, elevated uric acid consequently increases the risk of atherosclerotic disorders and vascular dementia while elevating blood glucose and increasing insulin resistance. Even subtle perturbations in the brain's insulin-signaling system will ignite neuroinflammation. And we know that fructose can act on specific areas of the brain involved in both the regulation of food intake and reward mechanisms (remember that hedonic pathway?) as well as on critical regions for learning and memory.[12] We'll circle back to uric acid shortly, but let's review some other biological facts first.

Studies conducted on mice are showing just what fructose does in the brain: it reduces synaptic plasticity in the hippocampus.[13] Translation: the cells in the brain's memory center are less able to make connections, an important part of the processes of learning and memory formation. At the same time, there's also reduced growth of new brain cells.[14] These two effects are the hallmarks of dementia. If you cannot process information well, learn and form new memories, or grow new brain cells to replace old or dying ones, you're on the road to serious cognitive decline and dementia. It's a simple as that.

The good news is that in these studies, in which mice were fed a fructose-based diet for weeks, developed metabolic syndrome, and showed signs of cognitive decline, the researchers were able to partially reverse the animals' condition by changing their diet and removing the fructose. Such an observation hints that there may be a window of opportunity during which we can reverse the course of the brain's decline — moving it away from the path toward dementia and back on the path toward health and superb cognition. But the reversal must start early: as I've mentioned, once serious disease takes root, it's very hard to erase the damage done or turn things around.

We also know that fructose compromises brain energetics in general, especially so where we want it most — in the mitochondria of the hippocampus. At UCLA's David Geffen School of Medicine, scientists declared: "[F]ructose consumption reduces neural resilience and may predispose the brain toward cognitive dysfunction and lifelong susceptibility to neurological disorders."[15] This is an important finding for two reasons. First, neural resilience is necessary for the brain's longevity and what's called *cognitive reserve* — its ability to stave off decline. It's like having an extra pair of shoes ready when your old ones wear out. People with high levels of cognitive reserve are known to avoid dementias even though their brains may show physical signs of decay (e.g., plaques and tangles).

We acquired this knowledge from autopsies performed on the brains of old people, some of whom made it past the age of one hundred and whose brains looked terribly sick and riddled with disease, yet they kept their mental sharpness intact to the very end. Their secret? During their lives they built neural roadways and byways, as it were, to make up for avenues that no longer functioned well. This is what makes the brain so remarkable—it's the most malleable, or plastic, organ in the body. Unlike other organs in the body that naturally show wear and tear with age, the brain can be improved upon as the years tick by, but only if we support it with the right inputs—especially those that involve metabolism.

Second, keep in mind that the brain is the most energy-demanding organ in the body. It may only constitute 2 to 5 percent of body weight, but it consumes up to 25 percent of the body's total energy *at rest*. So what are we doing to our beloved brains when we deprive them of energy? We're setting them up for dysfunction and failure. Leading-edge research indicates that compromised brain energetics is perhaps the most important mechanism underlying Alzheimer's disease. And chief among the wiliest offenders is plain old dirty fructose.

When researchers involved in the Framingham Heart Study, which I discussed in chapter 1, turned their attention to signs of what's called "preclinical Alzheimer's disease" in 2017, they showed just how harmful daily fruit-juice intake can be on the brain. To be sure, preclinical Alzheimer's disease refers to the period when individuals don't yet exhibit signs of cognitive decline, but if you were to look at their brains, you'd see something amiss. They are in a very early stage of the disease, which has yet to appear or present itself in their behavior and lack of cognition. This can be years or even decades before the disease pathology in the brain turns into outward symptoms (which is why capitalizing on preclinical time to prevent the start and progression of disease is so important). In this particular study, led by Boston University, the researchers studied thousands of people who underwent neuropsychological testing and magnetic resonance imaging to determine what effects, if any, sugar-sweetened beverages—from soda to fruit juice—had on their brains.

The test group was compared to a group that consumed less than one sugary beverage per day. The results speak for themselves.[16]

• Greater consumption of sugary beverages was associated with lower total brain volume, lower hippocampal volume, and lower scores on tests to evaluate memory recall.

• One or more servings per day of fruit juice were associated with lower total brain volume, hippocampal volume, and poorer test scores on memory recall.

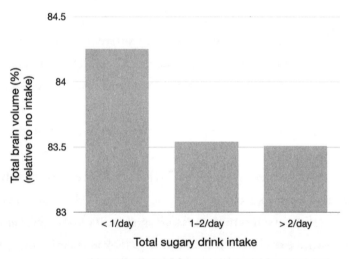

Sugary Beverages and Brain Shrinkage

Adapted from Matthew P. Pase et al., *Alzheimer's & Dementia* 13, 2017

Their conclusions pointed squarely to the effects of sugar, dominated here by fructose, on the brain: "These findings were striking given that they were evident in a middle-aged sample and were observed even after statistical adjustment for numerous confounding factors such as prevalent diabetes, total caloric intake, and physical activity. The magnitudes of the associations observed were the equivalent of *1.5–2.6 years of brain aging* for total brain volume and *3.5–13 years of brain aging* for episodic memory" (emphasis mine). (Episodic memory refers to the memory of specific everyday events.) In writing up their results, the authors cited other experiments that showed similar findings—the development of Alzheimer's disease pathology in conjunction with fructose consumption. So where does uric acid come into the scene?

Although this particular study didn't look at uric acid levels in the participants, other studies have done just that, showing time and time again that the important mechanisms by which fructose exerts its detrimental effects on the brain are assisted by uric acid.[17] This is an elusive missing link connecting the dots between fructose and brain degeneration. As fructose raises uric acid and compromises insulin signaling, brain cells lose their ability to properly use glucose.

This dysfunction in the brain's energetics helps explain why, for example, the ketogenic diet has proved effective as an intervention for Alzheimer's patients: it provides an alternative fuel—ketones.[18] When I interviewed fellow neurologist Dr. Matthew Phillips of New Zealand, who studies brain energetics in the context of Alzheimer's disease, he explained the power of using a ketogenic diet in the treatment of Parkinson's disease, which is also a disease of defects in the brain's energetics. My point being: this bioenergetics issue is a consequence of insulin resistance, and now we know the pivotal role of uric acid in this sad state of affairs.

Let's also not forget the UK study I briefly mentioned in the previous chapter. It highlighted fructose's and uric acid's joint, coconspiring forces in brain decline. The title said it all: "Increased Fructose Intake as a Risk Factor for Dementia." These scientists clearly showed that excess fructose consumption promotes the development of dementia: rats receiving the sugar swiftly developed insulin resistance and cognitive impairment. They further articulated that fructose impairs the brain's processing, learning, and memory capabilities, and, not surprisingly, they called out the role that uric acid is playing. Elevated uric acid is associated with increased free radical formation as well as decreased nitric oxide synthesis, which compromises blood flow, including precious blood flow to the brain. Further, decreased vascular nitric oxide directly compromises the ability of insulin to process blood glucose. And finally, these researchers found that decreased nitric oxide synthase, the enzyme that makes nitric oxide in the brain, reduces synaptic neural transmission and memory formation.

Synaptic transmission is the method through which a neuron connects with and speaks to its neighbor. This means that uric acid has more damaging effects related to nitric oxide than simply reduced blood supply and impaired insulin activity. It has direct compromising effects on the way one nerve communicates with another. In other words, uric acid helps send the brain into a metaphorical fuzzy state of static, like an old TV on channel 3 that cannot provide a clear picture. The brain's ability to hold fast, clear transmissions of messages across the synapses is fundamental to its health and functioning. Any interruption in that process is a major offense that will no doubt have serious downstream effects, including the risk of mental and cognitive decline.

To really grasp the contribution that uric acid makes to the development of cognitive decline, look no further than the effect that drugs to lower uric acid have on lowering the risk of developing dementia. In 2018, a retrospective study using Medicare claims data shone a light on the power of lowering uric acid to prevent dementia.[19] When comparing two popular drugs for elevated uric acid and gout—allopurinol and febuxostat—scientists at the University of Alabama discovered that, compared with a low allopurinol dose (< 200 mg/day), higher allopurinol doses and febuxostat at 40 mg/day were associated with a lower risk of a new diagnosis of dementia—by more than 20 percent. That's huge, especially in a world where we have no meaningful treatment for Alzheimer's disease whatsoever. Studies like that have stimulated a push to study the connection between uric acid and risk for dementia, and there is now serious interest in using drugs to lower uric acid as a means to prevent dementia. Although this was not an interventional trial against a placebo to determine who did or didn't get dementia, it was nonetheless a review of individuals who either were or were not taking a uric acid–lowering drug for other reasons, such as gout and kidney stones, and who seemed to benefit in terms of concomitantly reducing their risk of dementia. Future studies will provide further clues to the links and underlying mechanisms. Moreover, when I read studies like "Lowering Uric Acid with Allopurinol Improves Insulin Resistance and Systemic Inflammation in Asymptomatic Hyperuricemia," I know we're on track to understand a whole new approach to preventing and even treating brain disease, given the heavy risk factors that insulin resistance and systemic inflammation bring to the table.[20]

In a 2021 editorial for the *American Journal of Geriatric Psychiatry*, Duke University physician Dr. Jane P. Gagliardi writes: "Targeting modifiable risk factors is an important strategy in dementia management."[21] And elevated uric acid is indeed a huge risk factor we've only recently identified. As it's said in medical circles, when you change the soil, the seed doesn't grow. If we can control uric acid, among other important elements of the perfect "soil," we can support the optimal health and function of the brain.

While this research demonstrates a remarkable brain benefit for people taking uric acid–lowering drugs, this approach is not the intent of the LUV Diet. From this point forward, I'll cover the entire spectrum of drug-free things you can do today to take your uric acid level to a place where it doesn't threaten your brain health. We just need to keep certain things under control that are easily achievable through lifestyle—the strategies I'll be sharing in part 2. To bring this home, in the graph on page 110 I adapted data from the study done by the Johns Hopkins University scientists who raised the flag in 2007 about even mild elevations of uric acid being problematic and increasing the risk of cognitive decline among elderly adults.[22] As you can see, even mildly elevated (low-moderate) and high but still considered normal uric acid levels come with cognitive consequences.

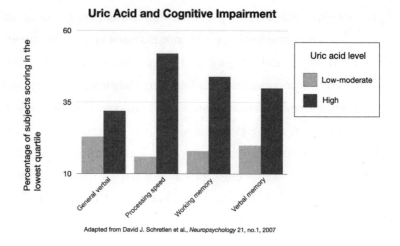

Uric Acid and Cognitive Impairment

Adapted from David J. Schretlen et al., *Neuropsychology* 21, no.1, 2007

To me, graphs like this one tell a lot of the story.

I began this chapter by presenting the sobering statistics related to Alzheimer's disease, along with where we are and where we are going. Remember that this is a disease for which there is no meaningful pharmaceutical treatment whatsoever. We have no choice but to focus on preventive strategies. And these strategies are being validated by the best research teams around the globe.

As a neurologist, I have a special interest in looking at the emerging research that makes clear that our day-to-day choices chart the health destiny of our minds. But my motivation in bringing out this information has another element. As I write these words, I'm taken back to the moments when I held my father's hands as I watched Alzheimer's disease take his life. This experience, far more than my mission as a neurologist, is what motivates me to share the other side of the Alzheimer's story, the part that consumers are not being told. The messaging that we should just live our lives and hope for a pharmaceutical fix is unfair and cruel. Imagine how I felt when I pleaded my case on national television about the importance of reducing sugar consumption as a brain-healthy lifestyle choice and was confronted by a statement from the sugar industry that basically reinforced the notion that we should go on our merry way, keep eating sugar, and hope for the best. We deserve better. You deserve better.

Now that we've beaten up sugar, particularly fructose, in the context of uric acid and health, the logical next question is: What else raises your uric acid level?

CHAPTER 5

Acid Rain

How Sleep, Salt, Psoriasis, Seafood, and Sitting Connect with Uric Acid

The value of experience is not in seeing much, but in seeing wisely.

— SIR WILLIAM OSLER, MD (1849–1919)

MORE THAN A CENTURY AGO, Sir William Osler was among the most forward-thinking physicians of his era. Now celebrated as the father of modern medicine, he was a keen observer who understood and taught the value of learning from patients as much as from textbooks. In his seminal book *The Principles and Practice of Medicine*, published in 1892 (the same year as Haig's book), he addressed gout, calling it a "nutritional disorder" and suggesting that the treatment of the chronic condition should be a low-carb diet in which "starchy and saccharine articles of food are to be taken in very limited quantities."[1] He also recommended restricting fruit intake in patients with gout to prevent recurrent arthritic attacks. Even then he was on to something about sugars and fructose, but he could not have known that there's a difference between biting into a piece of fresh fruit and drinking liquid sugar. And high-fructose corn syrup had yet to enter the world's stage.

Now that we understand how fructose—public enemy number one—raises uric acid levels, it's time to learn how other ingredients and habits can also stir the pot. Many factors can prevent you from clearing uric acid properly from the body, and the scientific library of evidence has been growing since the mid-1960s.[2] Some of these factors, which come from modern everyday life, will surprise you, but I'll give you the guidelines you need to manage them in a practical manner. Let's take a tour.

SLEEP IS MEDICINE

We're supposed to be slumbering for a third of our lives. And for good reason: we understand the value of sleep from a scientific perspective as we never have before. Cutting-edge laboratory and clinical studies alike have shown that virtually every system in the body is affected by the quality and amount of sleep we get, and you've probably already read about this in online media and in books, including my own. But here's the new piece of information you probably haven't heard: sleep's impact on the body has everything to do with its biochemical effects, including those that relate to uric acid.

Before we get to the connection between sleep and uric acid, let me offer a quick summary of sleep's established benefits: it can help us control how hungry we feel, how much we eat, how fast our metabolism runs, how fat or thin we get, how well we fight off infections, how creative and insightful we may be, how effortlessly we make good decisions, how well we cope with stress, how quickly we process information and learn new things, and how well we organize, store, and recall memories.[3]

The expression *Good night, sleep tight* has its roots to the nineteenth century but gained universal popularity when it became a lyric in a song on the Beatles' "White Album," in 1968. That's around the time when we slowly began to wake up (pun intended) to sleep's magical work in the body, but it would be several more decades before we would conduct the kind of controlled experiments that show that poor (not "tight") sleep triggers inflammation, impairs hormonal signaling and glucose regulation, and essentially dismantles a healthy metabolism. And the dismantling can be quick: the first controlled study that assessed the consequences of recurrent partial sleep loss on hormonal and metabolic variables involved forcing healthy young nondiabetic men to reduce their sleep time to just four hours a night for six consecutive nights.[4] On the fifth day, their tolerance for glucose was reduced by a whopping 40 percent compared to what it was when they were allowed to sleep longer. This landmark study was performed by Eve Van Cauter and her colleagues at the University of Chicago in 1999.

The first study to report a general association between insufficient sleep and mortality was actually published in 1964. It covered more than a million adults and found that those who slept for a solid seven hours had the lowest mortality rate. But it fell short of pinpointing all the underlying biological and even molecular events that occur during sleep. Since then, numerous studies have added to our understanding of the relationship between sleep and mortality and filled in a lot of the blanks, including explaining how sleep affects the behavior of our DNA.[5]

We didn't know about sleep's hidden connections to uric acid until more recently, although the anecdotal evidence had already been accumulating. People with gout tend to experience acute attacks at night during sleep, and the fact that uric acid levels peak early in the morning, when heart attacks are more likely to strike, further tells us something: sleep and uric acid share an intricate relationship.

Adequate sleep, which for the vast majority of us means at least seven solid hours, also influences our genes. In early 2013, scientists in England found that a week of sleep deprivation altered the function of 711 genes, including some involved in stress, immunity, metabolism, and inflammation.[6] Anything that negatively affects these important functions in the body affects everything about us, from how we feel to how we think. We depend on those genes to produce a constant supply of proteins for replacing or repairing damaged tissue, and if they stop working after just a week of poor sleep, it can accelerate all kinds of deterioration in the body. I'll come back to this relationship shortly; let's first gain a better appreciation for sleep's power.

Sleep is composed of a series of cycles that average around ninety minutes in length (though they can vary widely among people) during which your brain moves from deep, non-REM sleep to REM sleep. (REM stands for "rapid eye movement," and REM sleep is the unique phase of sleep characterized by random fast movement of the eyes.) Although the cycles are fairly stable throughout the night, the ratio of non-REM to REM sleep changes, shifting from non-REM to the lighter REM sleep the closer you get to daybreak. Some research has suggested that non-REM sleep is more rejuvenating than dream-infused REM sleep, but we need adequate amounts of both because each provides important benefits. While non-REM sleep helps the body physically recover and renew itself, REM sleep is key to learning and memory.

Although we may not notice the side effects of poor sleep on a genetic level, we certainly experience other signs of chronic sleep deprivation: confusion, memory loss, brain fog, low immunity and chronic infections, cravings for carbs, weight gain and obesity, cardiovascular disease, diabetes, and chronic anxiety and depression. All these outcomes are uniquely tied to sleep, both in how much of it you bank on a regular basis and in its ability to refresh your cells and keep systems in check. Do you reach deep, restorative sleep frequently enough throughout the night? Do you sleep through the night without disruptions? Do you wake up feeling refreshed? Do you keep a consistent schedule?

Aside from its effects on the way our genes behave, poor sleep directly increases our levels of powerful inflammatory molecules (cytokines) such as interleukin-6 and interleukin-1β, C-reactive protein, and TNF-alpha, as shown by studies done on humans who are deprived of sleep.[7] White blood cells are activated, too, a sign that the body is under stress and potentially prone to injury. As you know, these inflammatory markers correlate with risk factors for many diseases. Even a twenty-four-hour deprivation of sleep is associated with a dramatic increase in these inflammatory agents. Reducing sleep by as little as two hours (i.e., a six-hour night's sleep as opposed to an eight-hour night's sleep) is also associated with increased production of inflammatory chemicals. And just when you thought a good night's sleep was all about the number of hours, think again: if you lose out on restorative sleep or experience disturbances such as sleep apnea that poke holes in complete and sound sleep cycles, you're turning up the volume further on those inflammatory molecules.

In one particularly large 2016 review of seventy-two studies encompassing fifty thousand people, sleep disturbance was clearly associated with an increase in inflammatory markers.[8] Too much sleep was also shown to be a problem, because people who slept more than eight hours a night (long sleep) triggered an increase in inflammatory chemicals. And in other studies, excessive sleep has been associated with a 23 to 30 percent increase in all-cause mortality.[9] I should point out that too much sleep is now considered a potential early marker for cognitive decline, too. In 2017, the journal *Neurology* reported that sleeping more than nine hours a night could increase the risk of progressing to clinical dementia within ten years.[10] That's quite a statement, and it's all the more concerning when you know that the same study measured decreased brain volume in the long sleepers.

So clearly there has to be a sweet spot for leveraging sleep's benefits, and it appears that for most of us, seven to eight hours is it. But most of us can't even get that. Around 25 percent of Americans complain of occasional insomnia, and nearly 10 percent suffer from chronic insomnia.[11] This is about our children, too: the latest figures reveal that sleep insufficiency—simply not getting enough sleep for the body's needs—is epidemic among young people. Fully 30 percent of children six to eleven years old don't achieve restful, adequate sleep, and this certainly has played into the rise of metabolic syndrome in this age group.[12] In children who are short sleepers, their increased risk for obesity is a breathtaking

89 percent.[13] Poor sleep's impact on the risk of metabolic syndrome, in fact, is the other area where sleep medicine gets a lot of attention. Sleep is among the most influential activities in supporting critical bodily processes, from glucose metabolism and insulin signaling to hunger (ghrelin) and fullness (leptin) hormones.

Any conversation about sleep deprivation leads to a discussion about metabolism and the risk for obesity and diabetes. Study after study has shown that sleep deprivation increases insulin resistance and severely ups the risk for the whole spectrum of metabolic problems. How so?

Our sleep-wake cycles set the tone for our circadian rhythms, which in turn affect the rise and fall of hormones, fluctuations in body temperature, and the ebb and flow of certain molecules that contribute to our health and wellness. When our sleep patterns do not meet our body's physiological needs, several effects occur together, from complex hormonal changes in the body that increase appetite to an intense craving for junk food. You'll recall the groundbreaking study I described in chapter 3 that illuminated sleep's commanding role in balancing our hormones related to appetite and feelings of fullness. Imbalanced hunger hormones follow poor sleep, and the result is an undeniable craving for the wrong kinds of foods—foods that will then go to war with a healthy physiology.

A 2017 study of eighteen thousand adults showed that in prediabetics, logging fewer than six hours of sleep a night was associated with a 44 percent increase in the risk of developing full-blown diabetes, while getting fewer than five hours a night increased the risk by 68 percent.[14] The study concluded that "sufficient sleep duration is important for delaying or preventing the progression of prediabetes to diabetes." Remember that coronary artery disease, prediabetes, and diabetes are all inflammatory conditions that can go on to trigger other conditions. No wonder habitual sleep deprivation has been demonstrated to increase your risk of dying—from any cause—by as much as 12 percent.

SLEEP DEPRIVATION'S DESTRUCTIVE FORCES

Sleep deprivation increases the risk of all the following through a complex combination of biological pathways.

- Excess weight and obesity
- Insulin resistance, metabolic syndrome, and diabetes
- Memory loss, confusion, and brain fog
- Dementia and Alzheimer's disease
- Lowered immune function
- Cardiovascular events, including heart attacks
- Cancer
- Low libido and sexual dysfunction
- Low mood and depression
- Susceptibility to infection
- Impulsivity
- Addiction
- Shortened life expectancy

Now, I've barely mentioned uric acid in the previous paragraphs, but you can likely see where this is going. Because elevated uric acid is associated with the very conditions affected by sleep habits (or lack thereof), we know uric acid is among the players behind the scenes. And lo and behold, a study conducted in 2019 reveals a strong inverse association between the duration of sleep and uric acid concentration in the blood: sufficient quality sleep equates with a low uric acid level.[15] Other studies have confirmed this correlation, including those that show the inverse association: low-quality, short-duration sleep correlates with a high uric acid level.[16]

In people prone to gout, among the reasons for nighttime attacks are the physiological changes that take place during sleep that can catalyze the formation of uric acid crystals in the joints. These changes include a drop in body temperature, shifts in breathing patterns, and a drop in cortisol levels. Cortisol is an anti-inflammatory molecule whose production in the body goes down during sleep, so there's less of it to help out with gouty inflammation. Dehydration can also be part of the problem: as the body loses water during sleep through breathing and sweating, uric acid can become increasingly concentrated in the blood and can pool in the joints, where it crystallizes. But you don't have to suffer from gout to realize that you've got issues with elevated uric acid. Many people never experience a gout attack, but if you were to peer into their bodies at night during restless sleep, you might see their uric acid levels soaring and inflicting silent damage.

> A good night's sleep helps keep uric acid levels in check. The better you sleep and the more careful you are about getting as many hours of sleep as your body needs, the better you can manage uric acid levels.

For many people, falling asleep is not the problem—it's staying asleep and avoiding interruptions. Obstructive sleep apnea (OSA) is an incredibly common sleep disorder in which nighttime pauses in breathing disrupt the sleep cycle. It happens when the muscles that support the soft tissues in your throat, such as your tongue and soft palate, temporarily relax. The airway narrows and begins to cut off breathing until you're semiawakened to the problem; then the process likely repeats after you fall back asleep. The most common cause of OSA? Obesity, because extra weight in the neck area can trigger the cascade of events that lead to disordered breathing. We know now that people with OSA are more than twice as likely to develop dementia. They miss out on the vital sleep that sustains metabolic health—the kind of metabolic health the brain needs to thrive and remain disease-free.

One study showed a substantial rise in uric acid levels as sleep became increasingly disrupted by OSA—I've adapted the results in the graph below (the apnea-hypopnea index reflects the severity of the disrupted sleep; *hypopnea* simply refers to abnormally shallow or slow breathing).[17] This study happened to be conducted on people with type 2 diabetes whose average BMI put them in the overweight category, but it's not surprising to see OSA in these individuals—all three conditions often go hand in hand and have a common theme binding them together: metabolic syndrome.

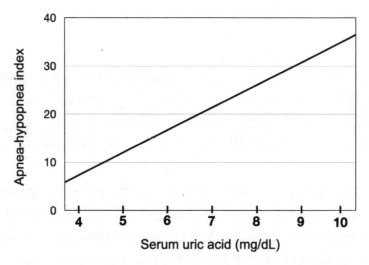

How Uric Acid Relates to Sleep Apnea

Adapted from Caiyu Zheng et al., *Disease Markers* 2019, April 3, 2019

Until recently, in order to gain a thorough understanding of the quality and quantity of their sleep, people needed to visit a sleep laboratory and undergo a polysomnogram. This is an incredibly valuable but complicated test to determine not just how long people are sleeping but also the quality of their sleep at its various stages. For example, it's important to determine how much time we spend in REM sleep, because this is the time when our memories are consolidated. Similarly, deep sleep is also critical, because this is the time when the brain activates its glymphatic system — the "shampoo-and-rinse cycle" that helps rid the brain of accumulated toxic metabolic waste products and various other elements, including the dangerous beta-amyloid protein that has been associated with Alzheimer's disease.[18] Interestingly, new research using sophisticated brain scans demonstrates that even one night of sleep deprivation is associated with higher levels of beta-amyloid in the brains of test subjects.

What is exciting is that nowadays we have the opportunity to easily obtain insightful metrics about the quantity and the quality of our sleep. With the proliferation of various wearable devices and their supporting apps, we can track all kinds of information, including what our heart rates and blood oxygenation levels are during exercise and even our blood sugar levels at any given moment. We can also track our sleep.

I'll offer more tips to help you end poor sleep in part 2. For now, let's move on to other instigators of elevated uric acid. Do not pass the salt...

SALT CAN SPRINKLE ON SYNDROMES

In many parts of the world, including in the United States, people's salt intake is north of ten grams per day when it should be a tiny fraction of that. Most people are aware that too much dietary salt increases the risk of high blood pressure as well as cardiovascular disease. It's also long been documented in the scientific literature that a high-salt diet is associated with increased frequency of obesity, insulin resistance, nonalcoholic fatty liver disease, and metabolic syndrome. Insulin resistance can be induced in humans in as little as five days by placing them on a high-salt diet.

However, the exact mechanisms of salt's actions on the body and its influence on metabolism have remained somewhat elusive until recently.

As I briefly mentioned earlier, we humans can make fructose endogenously—inside the body itself—by converting glucose to fructose. This occurs through the activation of a specific enzyme called *aldose reductase*. Research into this process using mice has explored the possibility that salt can activate this enzyme, which then increases the production of endogenous fructose.[19] And what this research has found is that a high-salt diet induces metabolic syndrome in mice. However, mice that are deficient in fructokinase, the enzyme essential to fructose metabolism, which keeps its finger on the button that generates uric acid, do not develop metabolic syndrome. Nor do they become obese. This suggests that blocking fructose metabolism—and uric acid production—saves the mice from developing metabolic problems.

Such a revelation shows not only that there is a relationship between salt consumption and fructose formation but also that the metabolism of fructose itself promotes the development of features of metabolic syndrome. In addition, these experiments have shown that in wild mice that are not deficient in fructokinase (meaning they will convert fructose to uric acid), a high-salt diet is associated with a cluster of problems: leptin resistance; uncontrolled, excessive eating that leads to obesity; insulin resistance; and fatty liver. And when researchers evaluated humans, the same cause and effects were recorded. One 2018 review evaluated thirteen thousand healthy adults and showed that a high-salt diet, defined as greater than eleven grams per day, *predicts* the development of diabetes and nonalcoholic fatty liver disease.[20] Let's remember that NAFDL is a harbinger of diabetes; these metabolic conditions are all interrelated. The take-home message is clear: it's bad enough that you're drinking fructose-sweetened beverages, but if you add sodium on top of it, you're rubbing salt in your wounds.

Note that we do not yet have enough solid research to suggest that salt stimulates fructose production in humans to a significant degree, but the evidence is mounting. Review papers covering several well-designed studies are now showing that dietary salt intake could be linked to the increasing incidence of metabolic syndrome—even after adjusting for total caloric intake. Salt has no calories, but it may stimulate appetite simply by triggering fructose production and its metabolism in the body. And the cascade starts as that endogenous fructose stimulates a bingeing response and leptin resistance, making us eat more. We do know that in rodents, fructose consumption stimulates the absorption of sodium, which then goes on to increase the metabolism of fructose by activating fructokinase. I see a vicious cycle here that future studies conducted on humans will likely validate scientifically. The journal *Nature*, which called special attention to the 2018 review I just mentioned, highlighted the scientists' conclusion: "Our findings challenge the dogma that salt restriction should be recommended only for the management of high blood pressure and lead us to propose that salt intake should be closely monitored in a variety of populations."[21]

I want to also mention that dietary salt, like uric acid, has been shown to compromise endothelial nitric oxide in laboratory animals, and this leads to cognitive dysfunction. We know that nitric oxide plays an important role in blood supply and vascular health, but it is also involved in preventing the formation of tau protein—the very protein that is a telltale sign of Alzheimer's disease. In 2019, *Nature* published a paper by a group at Weill Cornell Medicine's Feil Family Brain and Mind Research Institute whose title says it all: "Dietary Salt Promotes Cognitive Impairment." In their paper, the authors explained that the mechanism works via a busted nitric oxide pathway that permits the accumulation of those infamous tau clumps.[22]

My hope is that future research in humans can better define these multilayered interplays between salt and our physiology and redefine healthful levels of salt consumption. Both sugar and salt are dominant ingredients in everyday fare for the vast majority of Americans. Not only are these ingredients dehydrating on their own, they also disable the body's normal functioning and raise uric acid when consumed in excess.

DRUGS THAT UP YOUR ACID

Certain medications increase uric acid.[23] I won't go into all the details of how this happens for each drug; suffice it to say that it involves an increase in the reabsorption of uric acid, a decrease in the excretion of uric acid, and an increase in the production of purines, which then become degraded into more uric acid in the bloodstream. These are the most common mechanisms, but note that chemotherapy drugs, by virtue of their cytotoxicity (ability to kill cancer cells), also increase uric acid by liberating purines when these cells are destroyed (more on this shortly).

Below is my comprehensive list of drugs that can raise uric acid. Clearly, the decision to discontinue, reduce, or maintain any of these medications should be made in consultation with your health-care provider.

- Aspirin (in doses of 60–300 mg daily)
- Testosterone (in testosterone-replacement therapy for men)
- Topiramate (e.g., Topamax, an anticonvulsive)
- Ticagrelor (e.g., Brilinta, a blood thinner)
- Sildenafil (e.g., Viagra)
- Omeprazole (e.g., Prilosec, for acid reflux)
- Cyclosporine (an immunosuppressant)
- Niacin (vitamin B_3; e.g., Niacor)
- Acitretin (e.g., Soriatane, to treat psoriasis)
- Filgrastim (e.g., Neupogen, to treat low white blood cell count)

- L-dopa, or levodopa (e.g., Sinemet, to treat Parkinson's disease)
- Theophylline (e.g., Theo-24, to treat lung diseases such as asthma and chronic bronchitis)
- Diuretics (water pills)
- Beta-blockers (e.g., propranolol and atenolol)

Many people forget to revisit their medicine cabinets once or twice a year to take inventory of their true needs. They get used to popping pills when in fact they could do away with them entirely. I'll give you one prime example that I hear about routinely: drugs to combat acid reflux — the proton-pump inhibitors, or PPIs (e.g., Nexium, Prilosec, Protonix, and Prevacid). Although these drugs don't raise uric acid as directly as some of the others listed above do, an estimated fifteen million Americans use PPIs to treat gastroesophageal reflux disease (GERD) and could be putting themselves in harm's way collaterally.

These drugs block the production of stomach acid, something your body needs for normal digestion. Not only do they leave people vulnerable to nutritional and vitamin deficiencies and infections, some of which can be life-threatening, they also put people at an increased risk of heart disease and chronic kidney failure, which in turn will affect the body's ability to excrete uric acid. And they do a number on your beneficial gut bacteria, which also can adversely affect your body's clearance of uric acid. Study after study shows that in individuals who take PPIs for gastrointestinal symptoms such as heartburn, not only do 70 percent of them not realize any benefit, they also all experience adverse changes to their gut's microbiome.[24] And it happens quickly — within a week. These drugs can effectively ruin the integrity of your digestive system — and your metabolism. The good news is that if you're a long-term sufferer of GERD, the LUV Diet may well help remedy the condition. Your gut bugs will rejoice and further help you achieve target uric acid levels.

ALCOHOL AND XYLITOL

Although xylitol is not a drug per se, I want to call it out specifically because it's a common sugar substitute in many food products. Because it has a much lower glycemic index than sucrose and fewer calories per gram, it's marketed as a healthful alternative to regular and artificial sugars, and many diabetics are told to favor it over other sugars. It finds its way into many baked goods, chewing gum, and toothpaste. Xylitol is a natural sugar (technically a sugar alcohol, a type of carbohydrate that does not actually contain alcohol) and can be found in small, insignificant amounts in fibrous fruits and vegetables. But it's long been known to provoke an increase in uric acid by stimulating the breakdown of purines in the body, and I think we'd do well to avoid it when it's added to food products.

Alcohol is classified as a drug, but it can be enjoyed in moderation with careful attention to the type of alcohol you drink, because some types raise uric acid levels more than others do. Beer, for example, confers a larger increase in uric acid than liquor does, whereas moderate wine drinking does not increase uric acid levels. Biochemically, alcohol increases uric acid in three main ways: (1) it may be a source of purines, which produce uric acid when broken down by the body; (2) it causes the kidneys to excrete alcohol instead of excreting uric acid, thereby leaving more uric acid in circulation; and (3) it increases the metabolism of nucleotides, an additional source of purines that can be turned into uric acid.

Interestingly, the reason beer is the worst type of alcohol is that it is made with brewer's yeast and as such is high in purines (that said, I'll share tips on finding purine-free beers in part 2). Not only do people who drink a lot of beer get abdominal obesity (beer belly), they also develop fatty liver, high blood pressure, and unhealthful triglyceride levels. Unlike other forms of alcohol, such as spirits and wine, beer delivers a dual punch: it's high in purines *and* it contains alcohol, which promotes even more uric acid production. Alcohol is metabolized in a similar way to fructose in that it converts ATP to AMP and paves the way for the formation of uric acid.

So the type of alcohol you drink does indeed make a difference, as does your sex.[25] Turns out that in women, wine consumption is associated with a decline in uric acid, while there's no measurable effect in men. The current thinking is that some of the nonalcoholic components in wine, such as its polyphenols, with their antioxidant properties, could be working in women in ways that protect against elevated uric acid. That's not to say that women are given carte blanche in wine consumption. I'll offer specific advice in part 2.

PURINE-RICH FARE

As you've learned, many foods naturally contain purines, which get metabolized into uric acid. The most concentrated source of purines is animal products: red meat such as beef, lamb, and pork; organ meats such as liver and kidney; and oily fish such as anchovies, sardines, and herring. Lentils, peas, beans, and many fruits and vegetables also contain purines. But here's the thing: just because foods are high in purines does not mean that they are going to raise uric acid. There are many nuances to cover in part 2, where I outline my LUV Diet and present dietary adjustments you can make that will keep your uric acid level down.

Although eating a ton of red meat, anchovies, organ meats, sugar-sweetened drinks, and alcohol will definitely up your risk for elevated uric acid and its related conditions, you're not going to overdose on peas, asparagus, and spinach and blame your high uric acid on those nutritional gems. Several large studies prove that there's no relationship between vegetable consumption, even consumption of vegetables that are high in purines, and elevated uric acid. In fact, some purine-containing foods, including vitamin C–rich whole fruits, fibrous vegetables, and certain soy and dairy products, can *protect* you from elevations

127

in uric acid. Soy gets an asterisk, however, because you should be careful about GMO-sourced soy. (I'll provide guidance about that in part 2.)

To put this into perspective, let's consider a large review conducted in 2018 that evaluated nineteen cross-sectional studies in order to determine the risk of gout relative to the consumption of various foods.[26] Below is a list of foods that both increased and decreased the risk.

- Seafood: 31% increased risk
- Red meat: 29% increased risk
- Fructose: 114% increased risk
- Alcohol: 158% increased risk
- Dairy products: 44% *reduced* risk
- Soy products: 15% *reduced* risk
- Vegetables: 14% *reduced* risk
- Coffee: 24% *reduced* risk (in men only; see more below)

Even casting the risk of gout aside, when the researchers connected the dots between these categories of foods and the risk of hyperuricemia, or elevation in uric acid, the percentages tracked very similarly: seafood, red meat, alcohol, and fructose led the way in upping risk, and coffee, dairy products, and soy products led the way in reducing risk. Coffee came out the winner for men, reducing the risk of gout and hyperuricemia significantly, but in women it seemed to marginally increase the risk of hyperuricemia (though not gout). In part 2, I'll detail what this means for both men's and women's consumption levels.

One thing I'd like to point out is that we all experience five basic tastes: sweet, salty, sour, bitter, and savory (umami). *Umami* literally means "pleasant savory taste" or "deliciousness" in Japanese and owes its mouthwatering quality mostly to glutamate, an amino acid classically found in monosodium glutamate, or MSG. All high-purine foods are umami foods; when your mouth waters for the taste of savory umami, you're craving purine-rich fare.[27] These foods are tantalizingly good and keep us coming back for more, putting us on that hedonic pathway. Umami supports gorging and storing even when there's no real famine looming in the future.

Food manufacturers love to use umami in the form of MSG to enhance flavoring and stimulate food intake, but the vast majority of these foods provoke elevations in uric acid for two main reasons. One, as I mentioned, MSG is found in foods high in purines. And two, MSG is commonly manufactured with additives that are converted to uric acid, such as inosinates and guanylates. Research shows that giving MSG to mice induces obesity if it's given early in life.[28] In addition, serving adult mice MSG causes them to develop insulin resistance, elevated triglycerides, high blood pressure, and increased waist size—all features of metabolic syndrome and all explainable in the context of uric acid. In human trials, a study of healthy adults who were followed for a little over five years showed that a high intake of MSG was correlated with high body mass index as the participants' weight soared.[29] Several human studies have also linked a high intake of MSG with hypertension.[30]

The underlying mechanisms of these outcomes are still under study and likely involve several pathways, including those affecting the pancreas, glucose metabolism, and overall blood sugar control. In addition, MSG can disrupt the body's energy balance by increasing the palatability of food and disturbing leptin signaling. Research also demonstrates that MSG triggers the release of inflammatory chemicals such as interleukin-6 and TNF-alpha, which in turn stoke more insulin resistance.[31] And a 2020 Chilean study showed that MSG given to obese rats led to elevations in blood cholesterol, glucose, and uric acid levels.[32] High levels of uric acid in obese rats are to be expected, because the extra weight makes it harder for the kidneys get rid of the metabolite. But other biological events could be taking place in the presence of MSG that elevate the acid. Note that MSG-induced obesity and hypertension alone will keep uric acid levels higher than normal because these conditions prevent the kidneys from efficiently excreting the acid.

We've all gotten the message that MSG is not a beneficial ingredient and that we shouldn't be consuming a lot of it, especially when it's hidden in highly processed fare. In the past, it's been wrongly accused of triggering headaches and migraines. But it won't escape being blamed for elevations in uric acid. This is one ingredient we'd do well without.

HEALTH CONDITIONS LINKED TO ELEVATED URIC ACID

You already know that metabolic disorders are specifically tied to elevated uric acid. Following are a few more conditions to add to the list.

Psoriasis: The connection between psoriasis, psoriatic arthritis, and gout has been documented for decades. But only recently have scientists found that the common denominator there is elevated uric acid, a by-product of the rapid skin-cell turnover and systemic inflammation seen in people genetically prone to psoriasis. To be sure, psoriasis is an immune-related chronic inflammatory skin disorder, and 25 percent of patients who have the condition also suffer from joint disease (psoriatic arthritis).

In a large 2014 study that drew almost 99,000 participants from two large databases and encompassed nearly 28,000 men and 71,000 women, the researchers found that men with psoriasis are twice as likely to develop gout as men without the condition; that women with psoriasis are 1.5 times more likely to develop gout than women without the condition; and that men and women who have both psoriasis and psoriatic arthritis are five times more likely to develop gout than their healthy counterparts.[33]

Research is under way to fully understand the underlying intertwined mechanisms behind these connections. But no doubt they share complex interactions involving systemic inflammation and metabolic dysfunction, which also plays into immune function. In 2020, a group of French researchers gave a name to the condition of having both gout and psoriasis—*psout*—and called for more studies in the hope that people with psoriasis will be able to manage their condition simply by controlling their uric acid levels.[34]

Renal insufficiency and chronic kidney disease: Renal insufficiency (the inability of kidneys to filter waste) and chronic kidney disease (CKD) afflict a significant portion of the population. Kidney disease, which follows renal insufficiency, affects an estimated thirty-seven million people in the United States, or 15 percent of the adult population—more than one in seven adults—and approximately 90 percent of people with CKD don't even know they have it. One in three American adults (approximately eighty million people) is at risk for CKD. The connection should make sense: when your kidneys are not up to speed with filtering and excreting waste products such as uric acid, guess what—uric acid builds up.

Hypothyroidism: An estimated twenty million Americans have some form of thyroid disease, and according to the American Thyroid Association, more than 12 percent of the US population will develop a thyroid condition during their lifetimes. We've known about the relationship between hypothyroidism and elevated uric acid since 1955. But it wasn't until 1989 that the relationship between elevated uric acid and both hypothyroidism *and* hyperthyroidism was described.[35] As I mentioned previously, the lack of proper levels of thyroid hormones (in the case of hypothyroidism) will compromise uric acid excretion and jack up the level of uric acid in the blood.

In hyperthyroidism, elevated thyroid function leads to the breakdown of tissues and hence the release of purines, which then become uric acid during their processing. I should also add that the thyroid is a master regulator of metabolism and can be heavily influenced by leptin—one of the hormones that has recently been tagged as a regulator of uric acid. You will recall that both an imbalance or deficiency of leptin and elevated uric acid levels are predictors of metabolic syndrome and that the two are intimately connected.

Lead poisoning: When the English physician Alfred Baring Garrod discovered, in 1848, an abnormal increase of uric acid in the blood of patients with gout, it marked the first time the condition was described as being caused by excess uric acid. Nobody had made that connection before. This was a period when increased reports of gout in England were largely attributed to lead poisoning, and Garrod was well aware of the association between lead and gout and kidney disease. Lead essentially prevents uric acid from being excreted by the kidneys, thus leading to the buildup. Exposure to lead in Garrod's era was fairly common, because it made its way into many alcoholic beverages (so you can immediately see the double whammy there). Many popular alcoholic drinks of the day, including hard apple ciders and fortified wines such as port and sherry, were manufactured and stored in lead-containing equipment and barrels. People's daily swill was laced with lead: at the same time, sugar consumption was markedly increasing with its introduction into liquor, tea, coffee, and desserts (though the invention of high-fructose corn syrup would have to wait another century or so).

Today, we are much more aware of the dangers of lead poisoning and try to control sources of the heavy metal. But it still lurks, and it turns out that very low levels of exposure can result in elevated uric acid. In a study published in the *Annals of Internal Medicine* in 2012, researchers reported that the risk of gout is increased even among adults whose blood lead levels *are several times lower than what is considered acceptable by the CDC.*[36]

There is no such thing as a safe, acceptable level of lead in the body, and lead is difficult to eradicate. If you live in an old dwelling with peeling, lead-laden paint, you may want to test for lead. It also behooves all of us to make sure we avoid lead-tainted water, which plagued Flint,

Michigan, from 2014 to 2019. These kinds of contaminations are bound to happen again, and we often don't know about the leaks until the damage is done.

Tumor lysis syndrome: If you're being treated for cancer, you could develop what's called *tumor lysis syndrome*. Although very rare, the condition is characterized by the constellation of metabolic disturbances that occurs when a large number of tumor cells die quickly, usually as a result of chemotherapy. Among these metabolic derangements is the release of purines, which become metabolized into uric acid. Remember that anything that has to do with tissue (cellular) breakdown will raise uric acid. Which means that other events can cause this, too, such as physical trauma, excessive exercise, and even fasting. The reason for the uptick during fasting should sound familiar: fasting tells the body that food is scarce, and uric acid is the body's signal to go into preservation mode — conserve energy and break down tissues when necessary for energy (thereby releasing purines).[37] Because of this, it's important to time your uric acid testing appropriately after fasting.

There are many benefits to fasting, however, when timed right, as you'll see in the next chapter: it can help restore insulin sensitivity, assist with weight loss, and activate the process of autophagy, which clears out cellular debris. Uric acid levels usually go back to baseline twenty-four hours after the fast is over. I'll show you how to practice intermittent fasting in part 2, and I'll encourage people who want to lose weight by adopting a very low-calorie ketogenic diet with significant carbohydrate restriction to do so. Like fasting, ketogenic diets can cause a transient uptick in uric acid, but the overall goal of weight loss makes them worth a try, and the typical return to normal levels of uric acid after going off the keto diet makes the temporary rise okay for most people. You just need to monitor your levels closely, especially if you have a history of gout or kidney issues. For people who don't want to add a ketogenic element to this program, the LUV Diet will more than suffice for both weight loss and lowering uric acid.[38] Put simply, you do not need to go keto to reap the benefits of the LUV Diet. This diet checks all the boxes for managing uric acid smartly and improving your overall physiology to restore and reignite radiant health.

LACK OF REGULAR MOVEMENT (A.K.A. SITTING TOO MUCH)

Is it really any surprise that leading a sedentary life is bad for you? I have written extensively about the magic of movement, from the fact that it keeps our metabolism humming and turns on genes linked to longevity to its positive impact on brain health and the prevention of every ill that can strike us. We are designed to be athletes, which is to say that natural selection drove early humans to evolve into supremely agile beings — we developed long legs, stubby toes, big brains, and intricate inner ears to help us maintain balance and coordination while walking on just two feet as opposed to four. Our genome, over the course of millions of years, evolved amid constant physical challenges to our efforts to find food. In fact, our genome *expects* frequent exercise to sustain life. Unfortunately, too few of us respect that requirement today. And we have the chronic illness and high mortality rates to show for it. Experts calculate that nearly 10 percent of the world's death rate is attributable to increased sedentary lifestyles,[39] and the World Health Organization calls physical inactivity a leading cause of disease and disability.[40]

A lot of media have covered the "sitting is the new smoking" angle. The study that made the most headlines was a 2015 meta-analysis and systematic review published in the *Annals of Internal Medicine* showing that sedentary behavior was linked to premature death from all causes, as well as to an increased risk of cardiovascular disease, diabetes, and cancer.[41] While that may not sound surprising, this was found to be true regardless of how much physical activity was performed in a lifestyle otherwise dominated by sedentary behavior. In other words, a one-hour workout will not make up for sitting the rest of your day. Neither will being a weekend warrior and avoiding exercise the rest of the week. In addition, routine movement to break up sedentary behavior has been shown to prevent illness and death. And it doesn't have to be all that much movement: another 2015 study that evaluated people over a period of several years, for example, revealed that getting up from a chair every hour for a mere *two minutes* of light activity was associated with a 33 percent reduction in the risk of dying prematurely from any cause.[42]

Take the two-minute challenge: if you get up off your derriere every hour for a mere two minutes of light activity (jump up and down, do a few squats and lunges, take a fast walk around the block), experts say you'll reduce your risk of dying from anything by 33 percent! That's a minuscule sacrifice of time for a longer life.

Several effects coalesce when the body is engaged in physical activity. First, exercise is a potent anti-inflammatory. It also improves insulin sensitivity, helps manage blood sugar balance, and reduces the glycation of proteins — a biological process in which glucose and proteins become tangled together, causing tissues and cells to become stiff and inflexible. We know this to be true from studies of the effects of exercise on hemoglobin A1c, which is also a marker of glycation. Exercise also has proved to induce the growth of new neurons in the brain and help us increase mental sharpness, build cognitive reserve, and avoid decline.

In the past few years, researchers have finally begun to study the role exercise plays in uric acid levels, and not surprisingly, they have come across the same U-shaped curve I described in chapter 1: too much strenuous exercise can cause an increased turnover of tissue ATP (adenosine triphosphate), leading to an increase in the purine pool, the immediate precursor of uric acid; but too little exercise increases the risk of elevated uric acid as well. In one of the first studies of its kind to note the association between sedentary behavior and hyperuricemia, a group of researchers in South Korea found in 2019 that people who spent ten or more hours a day sitting were more likely to have hyperuricemia than those who spent fewer than five hours a day being inactive.[43] This was no small study — it looked at more than 160,000 healthy men and women. The researchers also calculated that the risk of elevated uric acid levels was reduced by 12 percent in low- and moderate-intensity physical activity and by 29 percent in high-intensity physical activity. And while we don't know all the underlying biology yet, we know that sedentary behavior and hyperuricemia are both connected to insulin resistance and obesity and that the combination of physical movement and weight loss can result in dramatic improvements in uric acid levels.[44]

I'm not going to worry too much about the exercise fanatics out there who engage in regular activity, sometimes rigorously enough to break down tissues and raise uric acid. I'm more concerned about the majority of the population — the people who don't break a sweat or challenge their bodies enough physically to reap the benefits of movement. The good news is that there are plenty of easy, accessible, and affordable ways to get adequate and enjoyable physical exercise. I'll be giving you some ideas in part 2.

CHAPTER 6

New Habits to LUV

The Acid-Dropping Power of Five Key
Supplements, CGM Technology, and
Time-Restricted Eating

Eat to live, not live to eat.

— SOCRATES

IF YOU READ A HEADLINE that said, SUGAR LEADS TO EARLY DEATH, BUT
NOT DUE TO OBESITY, what would you think was the culprit? It sounds like
a trick, because we all know that obesity follows too much sugar, and
obesity kills.

That was the headline of a news release put out by the American
Association for the Advancement of Science in March of 2020, when a
new study led by the MRC London Institute of Medical Sciences in the
UK countered the common belief that obesity resulting from too much
sugar was the prime reason why people with a sweet tooth die prematurely.[1] The researchers showed that an early death from excess sugar
consumption was related to the buildup of uric acid and not, contrary to
conventional wisdom, the result of the diabetes-like metabolic issues that
we typically associate with sugar-rich diets.

Of course, this finding surprised the researchers, who concluded that premature death from sugar overload was not necessarily a direct consequence of obesity itself. Although the study involved fruit flies, which are surrogates for humans in laboratory studies, collaborators from Kiel University, in Germany, replicated the results in humans, showing that dietary sugar intake is associated with decreased kidney function and increased purines in the blood, which in turn lead to an increase in uric acid levels.[2] And those high uric acid levels go on to inflict harm that cuts life short. Flies fed a high-sugar diet, like their human counterparts, show many hallmarks of metabolic disease—they become fat and insulin-resistant. But now we need to acknowledge that a stealthy culprit in these outcomes, including premature death, is elevated uric acid. Which again means that you don't have to be obese or have obesity-related metabolic issues to lose out on life if your uric acid levels are constantly in overdrive.

Now that you've gotten a panoramic view of uric acid's role in biology and the factors that trigger dangerous elevations, let's examine ways to bring this sneaky offender under control, starting with five key supplements well documented in scientific literature to directly lower uric acid.[3]

FIVE ACID-LOWERING SUPPLEMENTS

Quercetin: Quercetin is an important dietary polyphenol, a family of micronutrients that includes the flavonoids, which have potent antioxidant, anti-inflammatory, and antipathogenic properties. It is a pigment that gives color to many plants and acts as an immune regulator that may prevent or slow down the development of degenerative diseases. It is present in various foods, mainly fruits and vegetables such as apples, berries, onions (especially red onions), cherry tomatoes, and broccoli and other green leafy vegetables. Apart from its antioxidant and anti-inflammatory properties, quercetin has been shown to help control mitochondrial processes. And new research shows that quercetin supplementation may have beneficial effects on neurodegenerative diseases in particular: in laboratory mice models that are engineered to mimic signs of Alzheimer's disease, it reduces the adverse buildup of the plaque proteins associated with the disease. It also inhibits AGE formation in the body. (AGEs, short for "advanced glycation end products," are harmful compounds formed in the body as the result of a bad chemical reaction that takes place under certain circumstances, and their abbreviated name is apt because their accumulation *ages* you inside and out; more on this shortly.)

Now, here's what makes quercetin a jewel for lowering uric acid: it inhibits the actions of an enzyme called *xanthine oxidase*, which is required during the final step of the body's production of uric acid. Anything that can inhibit this enzyme will reduce production of uric acid (and yes, this is how uric acid–lowering drugs such as allopurinol work — they, too, interfere with the activity of the enzyme). In a prominent 2016 study of healthy adults whose uric acid levels were high but still within the "normal" range, a month of daily quercetin (at 500 mg per dose) resulted in significantly lowered levels.[4] Quercetin's acid-lowering effects were more dramatic in people with above-normal uric acid levels. The authors stated that "quercetin may be a promising approach to lower uric acid levels in individuals with above-optimal blood uric acid, for those at high risk and have not yet developed any disease or for patients recovering after therapy." Further, in studies of individuals at high risk for cardiovascular events, quercetin has also been shown to lower blood pressure and LDL levels in the blood.[5]

I recommend a dose of 500 mg per day.

Luteolin: Like quercetin, luteolin owes its acid-lowering powers to its ability to inhibit xanthine oxidase. Incredibly, luteolin has been shown to have uric acid–lowering properties on par with those of allopurinol. It has also been shown to prevent dysfunction of beta cells in the pancreas. Because elevated uric acid can cause direct damage to the pancreas, whose beta cells are key for insulin production, this is an important find-ing. In a 2017 Japanese double-blind, placebo-controlled study of people with mild hyperuricemia, those who received the luteolin supplement wound up with significantly lower uric acid values than the people in the control group.[6]

In addition to being found in chrysanthemum flower extract, this fla-vonoid is naturally concentrated in many fruits and vegetables, especially green peppers, celery, citrus fruits, and broccoli. Herbs such as thyme, peppermint, rosemary, and oregano contain luteolin. Like most flavo-noids, luteolin packs a powerful punch: it has anti-inflammatory and antioxidant properties and shows signs in animal studies of conferring cardioprotective and neuroprotective benefits. Studies are also under way to explore luteolin's anti-cancer power.[7]

I recommend a dose of 100 mg per day.

DHA: Perhaps no other molecule has received as much attention in my field as DHA, or docosahexaenoic acid, an omega-3 fatty acid. DHA is an important building block for the membranes surrounding brain cells, particularly the synapses, which lie at the heart of efficient brain function. It helps reduce inflammation in the brain and throughout the body and appears to increase brain-derived neurotrophic factor (BDNF), the brain's preferred "fertilizer" for new neurons. DHA also fights inflam-mation in the gut caused by a poor diet. And it can block the damaging effects of a diet high in sugar, especially fructose, and help prevent meta-bolic dysfunction.

The DHA-fructose relationship is particularly intriguing and rele-vant to the control of uric acid. In chapter 4, I mentioned a 2017 study conducted by UCLA scientists about fructose's damaging effects in the brain through the lens of uric acid participation. This team of researchers also found that DHA can help offset those negative effects, calling DHA the ultimate fructose-fighting fatty acid.[8] What they did in their nifty experiment was first to train rats to escape from a maze. Next, they divided the rats into three distinct groups: one was given water mixed with fructose; another received the same water-and-fructose mixture but also a diet rich in DHA; and the third drank plain water without fructose or DHA. Six weeks later, the researchers put the rodents to the test, watching them try to escape from the same maze. Which group struggled? The rats that had consumed water mixed with fructose got through the maze at about half the speed of the rats that drank only water, showing that the fructose had affected their memory. But the rats that were served a water-fructose mixture in combination with a diet rich in DHA finished the maze *at the same speed* as the group that received only water. This was clear evidence that the DHA protected against the negative effects of the fructose.

DHA also plays in important role in regulating the way vascular endothelial cells function. Recall that excess uric acid compromises nitric oxide production and function, leading to reduced vascular health and a reduction in the ability of blood vessels to properly dilate (and support optimal insulin signaling within the vessels). DHA's significant positive effects on vascular endothelial cells make it a potent counterbalance to the adverse effects of elevated uric acid.

In 2016, the *American Journal of Clinical Nutrition* reported that DHA beat out another popular omega-3 fatty acid, eicosapentaenoic acid (EPA), in terms of its anti-inflammatory properties.[9] (Though it's okay to buy DHA that is combined with EPA.) Our bodies can manufacture small amounts of DHA, and we are able to synthesize it from a common dietary omega-3 fat, alpha-linolenic acid. But it's hard to get all the DHA we need from the food we eat, and we can't rely on the body's natural production of it, either. We need at least 200 to 300 mg daily as a minimum, but most Americans consume less than 25 percent of this target and would do well to go beyond this bare minimum. Opt for a fish oil supplement or choose DHA derived from marine algae.

I recommend a dose of 1,000 mg per day.

Vitamin C: You know vitamin C for its long-documented benefits in supporting immunity. Vitamin C, also called ascorbic acid, must be obtained from food because we cannot manufacture this vital nutrient ourselves. It's necessary for the growth, development, and repair of all tissues—from blood vessels and cartilage to muscles, bones, teeth, and collagen. Vitamin C is also key to many bodily processes, including wound healing, the absorption of iron, and the proper functioning of the immune system.

In the treatment and management of gout, vitamin C is frequently hailed as a hero.[10] And for good reason: a number of studies show that vitamin C's uric acid–lowering powers are enough to help protect even people susceptible to gout flares. In a study of almost 47,000 men over a twenty-year period published in the *Archives of Internal Medicine,* researchers from the University of British Columbia found that those taking a vitamin C supplement had a 44 percent reduced gout risk.[11] And in a rigorous meta-analysis conducted by scientists at Johns Hopkins University that synthesized the findings from randomized controlled trials published in more than two thousand publications, the results were unanimous: "Vitamin C supplementation significantly lowered SUA [serum uric acid]."[12]

Why might vitamin C be effective? According to the Johns Hopkins study, vitamin C increases the urinary excretion of uric acid, may decrease uric acid reabsorption in the kidney, and, interestingly, because vitamin C is a powerful antioxidant, may reduce damage to tissues that would have led to more uric acid production. Part of the reason so many vitamin C–rich citrus fruits are beneficial for lowering uric acid surely involves this micronutrient's role.

I recommend a dose of 500 mg per day.

Chlorella: You may not have heard of chlorella before, but it is a single-celled freshwater medicinal alga. There are many species, but the one most studied for lowering uric acid is *C. vulgaris,* which is easy to find in supplement form. Chlorella is commonly used to help ameliorate features of metabolic syndrome because it's well known to help lower blood sugar and C-reactive protein. It's also known to lower triglycerides, boost insulin sensitivity, and improve liver enzymes. It's a great detoxifier, too, binding to pesticides and heavy metals in the bloodstream to help eliminate them from the body.

In a 2017 study that used chlorella to treat patients with nonalcoholic fatty liver disease, researchers found remarkable differences between people taking chlorella versus those on a placebo after eight weeks.[13] In addition to recording drops in fasting glucose, inflammatory markers, and uric acid, and in addition to signs of improved liver function in the patients who received the chlorella (as opposed to the patients on the placebo), the chlorella group experienced meaningful weight loss. Remember, NAFLD patients are at risk for weight gain because they have insulin resistance and actively produce fat as a result of their condition (90 percent of patients with NAFLD have at least one of the features of metabolic syndrome). If a supplement can do all that in people with NAFLD, imagine what it can do in someone without the condition. Chlorella is a biological supercharger.

Chlorella has other applications as well, thanks to its anti-inflammatory effects. Studies, for example, are currently making a case for its use in treating depression, which is increasingly being viewed as an inflammatory disorder. In a six-week pilot study of patients with major depressive disorder, researchers documented significant improvements in those taking chlorella in addition to standard antidepressant therapy.[14] Their physical and cognitive symptoms of depression as well as anxiety symptoms eased.

I recommend a dose of 1,200 mg of C. *vulgaris* per day.

I'll be reminding you of the recommended dosages of these five key supplements in part 2, where I lay out the program week by week. You'll start taking your supplements in the prelude to week 1. For now, let's move on to two other useful tactics to consider in your overall transformational plan: continuous glucose monitoring (CGM) and time-restricted eating (TRE). Both CGM and TRE will help you in your quest to drop acid and optimize your entire physiology from head to toe. These are important supplemental strategies in the grand master plan of action.

TEST BLOOD SUGAR REGULARLY WITH CGM TECHNOLOGY

I cannot emphasize enough the importance of keeping blood sugar under control. As a reminder, blood sugar (glucose) is a key substrate of human metabolism, serving as a raw material that our cells can use to produce the energy required to power all cellular processes. Our body works hard to keep blood sugar within a narrow range, equivalent to about a teaspoon's worth of sugar in the entire bloodstream, because too much or too little of it can cause problems for the body and make our metabolic processes less efficient. Up to this point in the book, I've primarily focused on uric acid, but I would be remiss not to spend a little more time on blood glucose and its damaging effects when it's out of balance. Bear with me, because this is all relevant to managing your uric acid. It's like a giant spider's cobweb: when you pull on one thread, the entire net moves. We cannot pull on the metaphorical thread of uric acid without considering the interwoven threads of blood sugar. Both metrics help complete the complex pattern.

Given how many deleterious effects excess glucose can have, it's not surprising that the vast majority of the chronic diseases associated with elevated uric acid are also rooted in poor glucose control. It would be biologically hard to have one of these parameters—uric acid or blood glucose—well under control while the other is not. The two biomarkers that reflect both blood sugar and purine metabolism collaborate in the totality and intricacies of the body's biology. One can make the argument that fully nine of the ten leading causes of death in the United States are connected to or exacerbated by dysregulated blood sugar—all of them except accidents![15] And, by extension, given uric acid's central participation in metabolic processes, dysregulated uric acid or chronic hyperuricemia is a coconspirator in this situation. We used to die primarily of infectious diseases and starvation, but now we die primarily of metabolic-related diseases.

As you know by now, glucose is a product of the breakdown of the carbohydrates we eat in our diets. When glucose enters the bloodstream, it signals the pancreas to release insulin, a hormone that tells cells to absorb the glucose, thus allowing the cells to process it and thus restoring blood sugar concentration to its ideal narrow range. Some of the glucose brought into cells is processed by the mitochondria to form energy (called ATP) that our cells can use. Excess glucose is stored in the muscle and liver as chains of glucose called glycogen. Glucose can also be converted into fats (typically triglycerides) and stored in fat cells. Conversely, the body, if necessary, can also manufacture glucose from fat or protein through a process called *gluconeogenesis.*

You're probably also familiar with the fact that glucose causes insulin resistance when it's constantly flooding the body (typically, through an overconsumption of hyperprocessed foods filled with refined sugars), provoking direct, perpetual spikes in insulin levels. Eventually our cells adapt by reducing the number of receptors on their surfaces that respond to insulin. In other words, our cells desensitize themselves to insulin as if they are revolting against its deluge. This causes classic insulin resistance, and the pancreas responds by pumping out more insulin. So high levels of insulin become needed for sugar to be taken up by the cells. This creates a cyclical problem that eventually culminates in type 2 diabetes.

But glucose isn't the only villain in town. As I've said, the leading research of the day now tells us that uric acid plays a prominent role not only in promoting insulin resistance and diabetes but also in stoking more glucose-insulin activity, which further intensifies and compounds the metabolic problems.

By definition, people with diabetes have high blood sugar because their bodies cannot transport sugar into cells, where it can be safely stored for energy. And this sugar in the blood presents many problems. Following is a brief rundown.

Inflammation: Chronic high blood sugar triggers inflammation through many pathways, from the release of inflammatory molecules to the expression of inflammatory genes and the effects of weight gain, which typically follows in sync with high blood sugar as excess glucose becomes fat. And we know that excess fat, particularly around the waist, promotes immune cell activation and secretes large amounts of pro-inflammatory chemicals. Diabetes, which is fundamentally a disease of glucose dysregulation, is itself a severe pro-inflammatory state.

Glycation: When "sticky" glucose molecules attach to proteins, fats, and amino acids (e.g., DNA) in the body, a chemical reaction occurs called glycation, which produces advanced glycation end products (AGEs). These bind to receptors called RAGEs (receptors for advanced glycation end products), and this leads to inflammation, which promotes chronic illness. The A1c test for average blood sugar over a ninety-day period measures glycated protein (hemoglobin), so in a real sense A1c is also a marker of inflammation. To get a glimpse of AGEs in action, simply look at the skin of someone who is prematurely aging—someone with a lot of wrinkles, sagginess, discoloration, and a loss of radiance. What you're seeing is the physical effect of proteins hooking up with renegade sugars. High blood sugar also causes blood vessels to produce damaging AGEs, stirring up cardiovascular problems. We also can consume AGEs in foods that have been exposed to high temperatures, such as during grilling, frying, and toasting. People who follow a typical Western diet consume lots of AGEs, but you won't be eating any of these bombs on the LUV protocol.

Oxidative stress: High blood sugar has long been implicated in the generation of excess free radicals—those rogue reactive molecules that can damage cells. It is thought that many of the complications seen in diabetes are directly caused by overproduction of *reactive oxygen species,* a specific type of free radical resulting from high glucose levels. Even brief episodes of high blood sugar cause tissue damage by both generating free radicals and decreasing the amounts of antioxidants produced in the body. And too much free radical activity generates an unbalanced state I call oxidative stress. Such a state may impair nitric oxide signaling, which, as you've learned, helps blood vessels dilate and utilize glucose. What's more, high blood sugar can also cause oxidation of free fatty acids stored in your fat cells, which contributes to more inflammation. Finally, excess glucose causes the oxidation of low-density lipoprotein (LDL, the bad cholesterol), increasing the risk of plaque buildup in your blood vessels.

Mitochondrial dysfunction: Any insult to mitochondrial function can set countless health conditions in motion, because cells that can't generate energy effectively will not function well. I covered this above, when I explained how fructose metabolism drains energy (ATP) in the cells and hampers mitochondria, the cells' precious energy generators. Remember that those reactive oxygen species inflict damage on the mitochondria, and as a result the cells' ability to process fuel into energy is reduced. And this can lead to accumulation of toxic fat metabolites in the cell. These fat metabolites then gum up the inside of the cell and impair the insulin-signaling pathway, further insulting the cell's energy balance.

Changes in gene expression: Experiments in which fasting blood sugar levels have been acutely elevated have been shown to modify the expression of hundreds of genes involved in a wide variety of cellular process, from energy metabolism to the immune response. Some of the changes in genetic expression include those that lead to additional inflammation.

* * *

The message is clear: we need to keep our blood sugar in balance. You won't be able to control uric acid without controlling blood sugar. In recent years, doctors and researchers alike have called for continuous monitoring of blood sugar even among people without insulin resistance or diabetes. Why? Because studies dating back nearly twenty years show that high blood sugar, even if it's only slightly elevated, is associated with an increased risk of cardiovascular events, cancer, and even death, long before a diagnosis of type 2 diabetes is made. And now we're seeing this with uric acid as well: chronic high levels *precede* and *predict* these same deleterious outcomes.

Currently, in the United States, blood glucose levels are used in order to detect the presence of prediabetes and diabetes. The US Preventive Services Task Force recommends blood glucose screening for adults between the ages of forty and seventy who are overweight or obese, whether or not they have symptoms of diabetes. But there's a growing trend to screen everyone regardless of weight or risk for diabetes. At least 50 percent of people whose blood glucose number qualifies them as prediabetic will eventually develop diabetes, and the vast majority of them aren't aware of their condition![16] The same goes for elevated uric acid: a great percentage of the population is walking around with elevated levels that may be in the normal range today, but they may not know they've crossed the threshold until it's too late and they've developed a metabolic condition.

In one landmark paper published in the *New England Journal of Medicine*, a group of Israeli researchers showed that as fasting glucose increases from less than 81 mg/dL up to 99 mg/dL, there is an increase in the risk of developing diabetes, sometimes by as much as 300 *percent*, despite the fact that this range qualifies as normal fasting glucose.[17] What's more, the researchers revealed a sharp increase in the risk of cardiovascular disease, heart attacks, and thrombotic stroke as fasting glucose increases. This rise in risk begins at less than 90 mg/dL — well below the traditional normal fasting-glucose-level cutoff of 100 mg/dL. The takeaway: the idea that a fasting glucose less than 100 mg/dL is safe and risk-free is flawed, if the intention is to help people stay as healthy as possible.

One of the challenges with current diagnostic testing of blood glucose is that it does not pick up metabolic issues early enough. Studies show that in individuals who ultimately develop diabetes, the levels of insulin secretion are higher, and insulin sensitivity is lower, *three to six years before diagnosis* in comparison to people who did not develop diabetes.[18]

Another fact I should point out is that sustained high glucose levels may not be nearly as bad as large swings in glucose levels, or what's known as *glycemic variability* or *glycemic excursions*. It's thought that excessive peaks and dips in glucose can lead to tissue-damaging metabolic by-products such as free radicals, damage to blood vessels, damage to the nervous system, inflammation, and activation of the stress-hormone cascade (called sympathetic nervous system activation). Glycemic variability increases as people move along the continuum from normal glucose regulation toward diabetes. As people become more insulin-resistant, they will tend to show more variability in glucose levels. This is another reason why it's important to track your blood glucose. You can spot those spikes and dips and take them into account. Clearly, for best health, you want to eat in a way that produces minimal glycemic fluctuations, and the LUV Diet will help you achieve that.

Traditionally, a fasting blood sugar measurement is taken after fasting for eight hours, which is easy to do overnight. But for the reasons I just mentioned, you can do a heck of a lot more with a continuous glucose monitor (CGM), an incredible technology that I encourage you to try even if you don't have diabetes or don't think you have problems with blood sugar balance. Daily finger sticks to spot-check glucose levels do provide some information, but they only give you a snapshot of a single point in time rather than a dynamic picture of how things change over the course of a day. They can't tell you much about your personal glycemic variability.

This is where CGM technology comes in. Dr. Casey Means says CGM is like "a full-length movie of glucose, giving more information and context."[19] Dr. Means is cofounder and chief medical officer of the pioneering metabolic health company Levels, which offers CGM equipment that syncs with a nifty app (LevelsHealth.com). Full disclosure: I sit on the board of the company and am thrilled to watch these advanced technologies finally reach the hands of people outside the medical community. To drive home the difference between measuring blood glucose at a single point in time versus using CGM, Dr. Means likes to point to a 2018 Stanford University study (that she was not part of) in which researchers found that even individuals considered normal by standard glucose metrics exhibit high glucose variability on CGM, and in fact they reach prediabetic ranges 15 percent of the time.[20] So if you're not checking blood glucose during those spikes, you won't detect levels that qualify for prediabetes.

In another rather alarming study out of New Zealand and Belgium, conducted in 2016, researchers homed in on a group of athletes over the course of six days. Using CGM, they found that four out of ten study participants spent more than 70 percent of the total monitoring time above healthful glucose levels, and three of ten participants had fasting glucose levels in the prediabetic range.[21] Granted, this was a small study, but similar results have been found in larger investigations: one reported that 73 percent of the healthy nondiabetic participants had glucose levels that were above normal—in the range of 140 to 200 mg/dL at some point during the day.[22] I should add that glucose can start killing beta cells (the cells that produce insulin) at levels below 140: one study found that people with fasting blood glucose between 110 and 125 mg/dL (within the official prediabetic range) had already lost as much as 40 percent of their beta cell mass.[23]

Although CGM is not yet used as a diagnostic tool, I predict that we'll see this happen in the near future. But you can get ahead of the imminent trend and empower yourself today with this technology, because you can use the device to optimize your diet so that you can stabilize glucose and minimize glycemic variability. A diet like the one featured in this book controls glucose levels and helps limit extreme glucose elevations after meals, or what's called postprandial hyperglycemia. If you can keep tabs on your blood glucose and watch how high it goes after a meal, you can make precise, personalized adjustments to your diet. This in turn will ultimately help you control uric acid.

Don't forget, however, that many things affect glucose levels and insulin sensitivity beyond diet, from health conditions you might have to the medications you take, the pace of your circadian rhythm, how much you exercise and sleep, and even your stress level. Not only does chronically high blood glucose impair your stress response system, chronically high stress can also affect your body's ability to use its available glucose. In mice, for example, acute psychological stress (in the form of getting repeatedly shocked on the foot and then needing to escape from a cage) leads to substantially reduced clearance of glucose after a glucose load as well as to acute insulin resistance.[24]

Many diabetics are well versed in using these compact medical systems that continuously monitor their glucose levels in more or less real time. They involve inserting a small sensor onto your abdomen (or arm), with a tiny plastic tube the size of a human hair that gently penetrates the top layer of skin. An adhesive patch holds the sensor in place, allowing it to take glucose readings in interstitial fluid (the fluid that surrounds cells in the body) throughout the day and night. The sensors typically have to be replaced every ten to fourteen days. They transmit real-time readings wirelessly to a smartphone that displays your blood glucose data. I highly recommend checking them out and considering adding CGM technology to your health and fitness regimen. For more specifics on these devices and brand recommendations—in addition to Levels—go to DrPerlmutter.com.

CGM BRINGS PRECISION AND ACCOUNTABILITY INTO THE PICTURE

In a perfect world, controlling sugar intake in order to manage blood sugar would be easy. But we don't live in a perfect world. According to the International Food Information Council Foundation, 59 percent of Americans say that conflicting information about nutrition makes them doubt their food choices.[25] "As a society," Dr. Means explains, "we find it challenging to make healthy choices consistently, and wearable technology may be able to give us the feedback to keep us on track and help us cut through food marketing claims and confusing nutrition recommendations, and create a personalized, empowered plan for ourselves. In addition, keeping your glucose levels constant is more complicated than just following a list of 'eat this, avoid that' foods."[26] I couldn't agree more.

We might try to obtain feedback on our diets by monitoring our weight, but small changes on the scale are difficult to tie to specific foods. Similarly, blood tests for cholesterol and glucose levels can give us some feedback on our diets, but the results often reflect a multimonth (or multiyear) continuum. If your numbers are out of range, a doctor might tell you to "eat better," advice that lacks the specificity necessary to change behavior. But with wearable technology such as a continuous glucose monitoring device, it's possible to directly match an action with its consequence. If you eat a bag of potato or tortilla chips and see a huge glucose spike, for example, you know what caused it.

Furthermore, tracking glucose continuously can give you a partner in accountability that is helpful in sticking with goals. And it won't be just glucose that you'll be tracking in the future. Companies like Levels are developing systems that merge many data points, from other useful biomarkers such as uric acid and inflammatory molecules to activities such as sleep and exercise.

TIME-RESTRICTED EATING

When you eat is just as important as *what* you eat. At least that's what the data say. Here's how to think about it: every hormone, brain chemical, and genetic expression in your code of life — your DNA — behaves differently throughout a twenty-four-hour day, and your body's rhythms, including your eating and sleeping patterns, have an impact on this behavior. Even your gut's microbiome follows the circadian rhythm of the body: when you go without food for several hours, for example, your gut environment changes, and that influences the composition of gut bacteria and how the microbiome collectively behaves.

Think about it: our ancestors did not have the luxury of eating several meals and snacks a day, and they certainly didn't break their fast every morning with a bounty of food (they had to hunt and forage for it during the day, likely eating a larger meal in the late afternoon or evening). Our modern meal practices are more a product of culture and habit in the land of plenty than anything else. Although we've been told in the past to eat frequently to prevent our bodies from going into starvation mode and to keep our metabolisms humming, the theory behind this advice could not be further from the truth. The human body is designed for recurrent fasting. I would go so far as to say that the human body prefers and *expects* recurrent fasting. It's how it automatically resets, refreshes, and deglitches itself, just as a cold hard reboot of your computer does. As Benjamin Franklin said, "The best of all medicines are resting and fasting." Put simply, temporarily denying your body nutrients through the safe practice of time-restricted eating is one of the best ways to boost the integrity of your cells.

Dr. Satchidananda (Satchin) Panda of the Salk Institute for Biological Studies, author of *The Circadian Code,* knows a thing or two about honoring one's physiological clock through the practice of time-restricted eating (TRE), or what some people refer to as intermittent fasting.[27] He has dedicated his life to research about TRE. In fact, he is credited with figuring out that the section of the hypothalamus called the suprachias-matic nucleus (SCN) lies at the center of the body's master clock and receives input directly from light sensors in the eyes. Dr. Panda figured out how these eye-based sensors work as well as how cellular timekeepers in other parts of the body function to keep the entire body on schedule. He also discovered a novel blue-light sensor in the retina that measures the ambient light level and sets the body's innate time clock so it knows when to go to sleep and wake up every day.

In the process of exploring how the liver's daily cycles work, Dr. Panda found that mice who ate within a restricted amount of time—a period between eight and twelve hours in duration—became slimmer and healthier than those who ate an equivalent number of calories within a larger window of time.[28] This showed that timing does indeed matter: confining caloric consumption to an eight-to-twelve-hour period, as people did just a century ago, can help stave off high cholesterol, dia-betes, and obesity. Panda also discovered that the circadian clock even moderates the immune system. Mice that lacked an essential circadian molecule had higher levels of inflammation than other mice.

Additional research about time-restricted eating and metabolism conducted by Dr. Panda and other scientists around the world indicates that limiting your meals to an eight-to-twelve-hour window can improve insulin sensitivity, blood pressure, fat metabolism (ahem: fat burning), and the function of the kidneys, liver, brain, pancreas, gut (digestion and microbiome), and immune system. Most relevant to our message, it low-ers inflammation and helps drop uric acid over the long term because of its beneficial effects on weight management and metabolism. The tempo-rary rise in uric acid during the short-term fasting period—which is just that, short-term—is worth it for the end result: less weight, more meta-bolic health, and easier management of uric acid.

In the fall of 2021, Dr. Panda published a study that narrowed the timing further, to an eight-to-ten-hour window, showing again that eat-ing your daily calories in that time frame is a powerful strategy for preventing and managing chronic diseases such as diabetes and heart disease.[29] It also improves sleep and overall quality of life. He brought up a good point when interviewed for his latest findings: TRE requires less mental math than counting calories; it's easy to follow and supports the synchrony of the body's internal programming.[30]

During the fasting period, cells are under mild stress, which is a "good" kind of stress, and they respond to that stress by enhancing their ability to cope with it and, in turn, resist disease. As I noted above, although fasting may cause a temporary rise in uric acid, the result is worth it because the benefits of fasting eclipse the transient elevation in uric acid. Even if you practice TRE on a regular basis, the recommendations I outline in part 2 will not lead to chronic hyperuricemia. You won't be taking this to extreme routinely.

The average overweight person who grazes all day and consumes a lot of carbohydrates is used to continually burning glucose rather than fat at the cellular level. Such a person probably has insulin resistance, too, which you know now is both caused by and leads to chronically high insulin levels, which in turn leads to fat storage and suppression of fat mobilization — meaning that the fat stays locked in fat cells. The average American eats over at least a twelve-hour period. In fact, in a study conducted by Dr. Panda using the myCircadianClock app, which he developed, he found that more than half the adults using the app ate over the course of fifteen hours or more every day![31] This type of around-the-clock eating is a setup for metabolic disaster, not to mention a guaranteed risk factor for hyperuricemia, weight gain, obesity, insulin resistance, diabetes, inflammation, and chronic disease.

There are many different forms of time-restricted eating. But a simple way to implement this practice is to find an eating window during which you consolidate your caloric intake for the day. I recommend starting with a twelve-hour window and then aim to narrow it down to ten, then perhaps to eight hours, lengthening the interval of your fast (I'll present sample schedules in part 2). It typically takes twelve hours after your most recent meal to fully enter a fasted state and begin to reap the biological benefits. This is why skipping breakfast on occasion is an easy and practically effortless way to reach a fasted state as you take advantage of your natural overnight abstinence and delay the first meal of the day for a number of hours. Healthy people who have no underlying medical conditions and are not taking diabetes medications can fast for long periods of time without suffering from hypoglycemia, because nondiabetic hypoglycemia is exceptionally rare and usually tied to certain drugs.[32]

And don't even think that fasting makes you vulnerable to losing muscle mass. Turns out that growth hormone *rises* during periods of fasting, which can help preserve muscle. The release of growth hormone while fasting makes evolutionary sense: when our ancestors went without food for long stretches, they had to remain physically and mentally strong or they wouldn't be able to find food, thus risking extinction. And contrary to popular wisdom, your metabolism does not slow down during a fast. It may even speed up, especially the longer the fast. In studies of people who fast for up to seventy-two hours, research shows that they activate their fight-or-flight sympathetic nervous systems and release metabolism-revving biochemicals such as adrenaline (epinephrine), norepinephrine, and dopamine.[33] Again, this makes evolutionary sense: we want the sympathetic nervous system activated during the day so that we can find food and water, and then we rely on the rest-and-digest parasympathetic nervous system in the evening, during a meal.

One final point I want to make about TRE: when the body enters a prolonged fasted state, autophagy, which I defined in chapter 1, is triggered. This is an important cellular process that helps the body clean and detoxify itself. And guess what triggers autophagy: AMPK, the antiaging molecule that turns our bodies into fat-burning machines. When AMPK is activated, it also tells cells to remove internal pollutants via autophagy. And through autophagy, we give a boost to our immune systems and greatly reduce our risk of developing cancer, heart disease, chronic inflammation, and neurological disorders from depression to dementia.

We also help support our mitochondria, because autophagy happens to regulate the functions of our cells' energy generators.

Much of what we know about autophagy has come from studying yeast, mice, and rats. But pilot studies of humans are beginning to show us the potential power of TRE in promoting autophagy: one interesting 2019 study from the University of Alabama at Birmingham and the Pennington Biomedical Research Center documented TRE's positive effects on improving glucose levels, markers of the circadian clock, aging, and autophagy in humans.[34] A group of overweight adults participated in a randomized crossover study in which they ate between 8:00 a.m. and 2:00 p.m. (what's called early TRE) and between 8:00 a.m. and 8:00 p.m. (the control schedule). This took place for four consecutive days. All participants underwent continuous glucose monitoring, and blood was drawn to assess their cardiometabolic risk factors, hormones, and gene expression in whole blood cells.

While it was easy for the researchers to track the positive metabolic effects of TRE by testing blood chemistry for things such as glucose, insulin, and fats, they also managed to document the effects it had on the expression of genes known to be related to circadian rhythm and autophagy. Compared to the control schedule, on which participants could eat between 8:00 a.m. and 8:00 p.m., the TRE schedule gave partipants metabolic rewards in the form of better blood glucose control, fat metabolism, and expression of genes related to the circadian clock and longevity. In their conclusions, the researchers stated that TRE may also increase autophagy and have antiaging effects in humans.

Granted, this was a very small study looking at only a handful of people, and most studies of autophagy to date demonstrate that it may take a full two days of fasting in humans to spark autophagy in any meaningful way. But I think it's worth mentioning this important process, which future studies will explore and tell us how, exactly, we can turn autophagy up in the body without having to go days without eating. In addition to fasting, other habits such as exercise and adequate sleep, which are part of the LUV protocol, will help spur autophagy. It's important to know that this process is not like a hard on-and-off switch. It's more like a dimmer switch — it's always on to some degree in the body, but we want it turned up more often than it is in most of us. And the combination of TRE, proper movement, and sufficient sleep will help in this regard.

Food. Sleep. Supplements. Movement. Mother Nature. Meal timing. These will be among your core focal points in the LUV plan of action, along with a few optional but highly recommended additions such as testing (notably for uric acid and blood glucose) and fasting for a day before you begin the program. Although this program spans just three weeks, it's your launchpad for a whole new way of life. Get ready...

U-TURN: THE LUV PLAN OF ACTION

Now that you've gotten this far in the book, congratulations. That was a lot of science, I know. But you've discovered one of the most cutting-edge tools for priming your body to live a healthy, lean, long life: dropping acid. As in uric acid. If you haven't already begun to change a few things based on what you've read (put down that soda pop!), now is your chance. In this section of the book, you'll follow a structured three-week program, during which you'll rehabilitate your metabolism on the LUV Diet (remember, LUV stands for "lower uric values"); bring in some companion habits that support the makeover in the form of restful sleep, regular movement, immersion in Mother Nature, and optimum meal timing; and learn to turn this new blueprint into a lifelong habit.

Shockingly, only 12 percent of Americans—one in eight people—are considered metabolically healthy.[1] The other 88 percent display one or more features that indicate metabolic dysfunction. By definition, a metabolically healthy person is someone who has healthful levels of blood glucose, triglycerides, and high-density lipoprotein (HDL) cholesterol, along with healthful blood pressure readings and waist measurements—*without the need for any medications.* That's a high standard that most people don't meet. Let's be part of that minority club and help improve those numbers. Because every cell type needs energy to function, metabolic dysfunction doesn't discriminate. When metabolic fitness is poor, the effects can be both vast and diverse, both subtle and overt. By measuring uric acid, your new tool for managing your overall health, you'll stay within your target range for healthy metabolism and ultimately avoid any imminent misfires in your biology that can spell trouble and trigger the development of a number of conditions.

The goal, of course, is to arrive at a place where your metabolism is humming and you feel vibrant and energetic. Beyond uric acid control, this will result in significant improvement in the way your body functions across the board. You're bound to gain much better control of your blood sugar and insulin levels, inflammatory markers, blood pressure, and even blood fats. In turn, you'll reduce your fat mass and waistline, not to mention your risk factors for all manner of disorders and diseases. And you'll earn plenty of mental rewards, too: more confidence, more motivation to push through the stress of life with ease, and more inspiration to be productive. All told, your life will just be better and more fulfilling.

Achieving lifestyle changes, even small ones, can feel overwhelming at first. You might worry about how you can avoid your usual habits. Will you feel deprived and hungry? Miss your beloved sugary drinks and desserts? Will you find it impossible to keep this new behavior up forever? Is this program doable, given the time you have and the commitments you've already made? And can you reach a point where following these guidelines is second nature?

This program has the answers. It's simple and straightforward and offers the right balance between structure and adaptability to your personal preferences. You will finish my three-week program with the knowledge and motivation to stay on a healthful path for the rest of your life, with your uric acid under control. The closer you stick to my guidelines, the faster you will drop your acid and experience positive results.

You have the power to break the metabolic mayhem that's probably been going on in your body for years and turn your metabolism around to your advantage. Remember, you want to activate AMPK—the fat-burning, cell-cleaning switch. It all hinges on controlling your uric acid levels.

It's a good idea to check with your doctor before beginning this program, especially if you have any health issues. This is particularly important if you're going to opt for the one-day fast, outlined on page 169. Over the course of the next twenty-one days, you will achieve three important goals. You will

* learn how to monitor your uric acid and blood glucose regularly;

* shift your body away from uric acid triggers, including those in your diet as well as those resulting from habits such as poor sleep and lack of adequate exercise; and

* establish a new rhythm and maintain these healthful habits for life.

You'll start by making simple dietary edits and add specific supplements known to help lower uric acid. Then you'll focus on sleep, exercise, exposure to nature, and time-restricted eating. I've broken the program down into three weeks, in which each week is devoted to paying attention to specific goals. In the days leading up to the first week ("Start Your Engines"), I encourage you to see your doctor and have certain tests performed that will give you a baseline picture of your metabolic health. You'll also use this time to learn about and start your acid-dropping supplements, think about continuous glucose monitoring (for reasons you'll soon come to know), and consider a one-day fast to kick-start the program.

During week 1, "How to Make Over Your Metabolism on the LUV Diet," you'll start my menu plan and execute my dietary recommendations as well as begin to test your uric acid and blood glucose. This is where you'll come to appreciate the power of food as medicine. Many foods contain natural compounds that act as pharmaceuticals in the way they lower uric acid. An important fact: the level of uric acid in your bloodstream depends on how much of it is made and how much of it is excreted. Remember, the final step in your body's production of uric acid depends on the action of the enzyme xanthine oxidase. Anything that can inhibit this enzyme will reduce production of uric acid. This is how uric acid–lowering drugs such as allopurinol work. But there are natural inhibitors of xanthine oxidase in foods, as I've noted, typically those that contain certain types of flavonoids found in many fruits and vegetables. Flavonoids are natural substances (phytonutrients) found in plants that have powerful antioxidant and anti-inflammatory properties. They are made by plants to help protect them but have lots of applications in human medicine, too.

During week 2, "Sleep, Movement, Nature, and an Eating Window," I'll encourage you to start a regular workout program and give you ideas for increasing your movement throughout the day. I'll also offer tips for improving your sleep habits, leveraging the power of Mother Nature, and meal timing.

During week 3, "Learn to LUV and Live High," you'll turn your attention to putting all the elements of this program together as I equip you with strategies for permanently establishing these new behaviors in your life. This is not just a three-week program — it's also a model for life, and these first three weeks constitute the breaking-in period as you follow this new template.

Don't second-guess your ability to succeed at this: if you need to take more time to establish this new way of eating, feel free to lengthen the program. Take two weeks to focus solely on the dietary component, then bring in your support staff — exercise and attention to sleep habits. Go at your own pace. Use these three weeks as your launchpad. The payoffs will be well worth the time and effort you put into this process. And you'll never go back to the old habits that keep you stuck in metabolic pandemonium. Say hello to a LUV-ly life.

CHAPTER 7

Prelude to LUV

Start Your Engines

To keep the body in good health is a duty . . . otherwise we shall not be able to keep the mind strong and clear.

— GAUTAMA BUDDHA

MELISSA, A BUSY BUSINESS OWNER and mother of two, was just forty years old when she noticed blips in her thinking and memory that were worrisome enough to prompt her to seek help. As a health-conscious woman who thought she ate pretty well and enjoyed lifting weights and doing cardio several days a week, she could not make sense of her chronically low energy and "brain fog," as she called it, which left her incredibly forgetful. Recent conversations seemed to vanish from her mind, and she'd have to set alarms every day just to remember when to pick up her kids from school. By six o'clock in the evening, Melissa felt ready for bed — mentally drained and physically exhausted. At the same time, her evening routines were riddled with anxiety as she cared for a son who had frequent temper tantrums. And despite conscientious attention and tweaks to her diet, she increasingly found herself unable to suppress sugar cravings and took to binge eating, especially in the evening. She revved up her workout routines, tried to improve her sleep, and even paid a visit to a naturopath.

Alas, nothing worked until she discovered my books and learned how to boost brain health through diet. No sooner did she cut out wheat, gluten, and sugar, particularly the fructose that snuck into her diet without her realizing it, than she began to positively shift her biology and experience tremendous improvements in her body—and brain. She also cut back on her meat consumption and moved toward a plant-based diet.

"I feel amazing," she wrote, bravely sharing her story on my website, where I love to collect and feature real-life success stories from people who take my lessons to heart. "I have a clear mind. In fact, I feel it getting clearer every day. I think I forgot what it was like to have a clear head! I am starting to remember where I put things, or a conversation I just had. The brain fog is completely gone. My uncontrollable food cravings are gone. I'm eating less. I'm not binge eating or getting stressed out at dinnertime. I simply eat like a normal person." Melissa felt triumphant in being able to wake up every morning feeling mentally sharp and good about herself. She finally felt balanced, something she had always struggled with. Best of all, as Melissa reshaped her dietary habits, which mimicked the LUV Diet, and as she brought her new way of eating home to her family, she noticed changes in her children's behavior as well—far fewer temper tantrums and behavioral issues. It was a win-win for the whole family.

Testimonials like this are the reason why I continue to write and teach as well as design effective, practical programs to help people just like Melissa and their families. After all, it's never just about an individual. When one person in a household makes lifestyle changes, the shift often carries over to others. Think about that as you move forward and execute my strategies. I trust that no matter what conditions currently ail you and your loved ones, you'll find collective relief and a new formula for living. And if you think you and yours are already healthy, get ready to turbocharge. There's always room for improvement.

LAB TESTS

Prior to beginning the dietary program, it helps to have the following
laboratory studies performed, if possible. I've included target healthful
levels where appropriate. Most of these tests can now be performed in
pharmacies that have on-site clinics with licensed nurses who can get
you results quickly. Or if you've had a visit with your doctor recently, you
can call and ask for a copy of your routine laboratory tests: all the measurements below are typically part of the usual regimen during checkups
or visits for a particular problem.

Test	Ideal Level
Fasting blood glucose:	<95 mg/dL
Fasting insulin:	<8 µIU/mL(ideally, <3 µIU/mL)*
Hemoglobin A1c:	4.8 to 5.4%
C-reactive protein:	0.00 to 3.0 mg/L (ideally, less than 1.0 mg/L)
Uric acid:	5.5 mg/dL or below

Understand that it may take several months to see dramatic improvement in some of these metrics, especially the hemoglobin A1c, which
indicates your average blood glucose level for approximately the preced-
ing three months (also called HbA1c). But if you follow this program
from day 1, you should see positive changes in your uric acid, blood glucose, and insulin levels within three weeks, which will motivate you to
keep going. Remember that men generally have higher levels of uric acid
than women do for two main reasons: they tend to eat more meat, and
estrogen helps keep uric acid levels down in premenopausal women (after
menopause, uric acid levels go up). Most labs will not flag a level of uric
acid until it hits 7.5 mg/dL, and such a flag is only meant to sound the

---

* The abbreviation "µIU/mL" means "micro international units per milliliter."

alarm for the risk of gout and kidney issues. But we can do better than that. This is about way more than gout and kidney conditions.

As you might expect, the two tests I encourage you to perform on yourself are uric acid and blood glucose, though you can still follow this program and exclude the testing altogether if that's just not your thing or if you want to wait until you've found your rhythm with the main program by itself. If you've never had the above tests done (or don't know if you have), that's okay, too. I realize that I'm speaking to a broad audience, including "biohackers"—people who pay close attention to their health and track their data religiously with all the latest technology—as well as those who don't rely on blood tests and track other, less granular metrics, such as how they feel and look, how well they sleep at night, and their levels of energy. And that's fine. Do what suits your personal needs. Perhaps this lifestyle program is enough to start, and you'll introduce testing later on.

For people who want to start testing with this program, plan to test your uric acid level at least once a week and then at least every two weeks thereafter. A brand I recommend for uric acid testing is called UASure and is available online (UASure.com); it's an easy and quick way to measure the level of uric acid in your blood at any given time with a painless prick of your finger. The kit costs around $70, and it's well worth the investment. As I previously noted, aim to test first thing in the morning, before any meals or exercise. Pick a day and mark it on a calendar.

For blood glucose, test yourself once a week at a minimum, also first thing in the morning before eating or exercise (mark this on a calendar, too, and note that it's fine to do both uric acid and blood glucose testing at the same time). Your local pharmacy likely sells several different brands of tests. And for people who want to take this practice to a more precise, high-tech level with continuous glucose monitoring (CGM), which I explained in chapter 6, please don't hesitate! CGM technology is a far more helpful tool that automatically checks your blood glucose levels throughout the day. This helps you find patterns in your levels as they change. You can always start with traditional glucose spot-testing and add CGM technology to your routine further down the road. Again, follow your personal preferences.

Remember that uric acid can go up after you eat foods high in fructose, alcohol, or purines; it can also be affected by fasting and by following the keto diet. Acute and intense exercise, such as training for a triathlon, running a marathon, or engaging in high-intensity interval training (HIIT), can raise uric acid *temporarily* if there's muscle injury. But don't forget that regular exercise is associated with lower uric acid in the long run. The benefits of exercise far outweigh any risk of a transient rise in uric acid. Uric acid may also fleetingly increase with heat stress, so if you're someone who uses, for example, a sauna or steam room, you might see a bump in the short term. When you document your levels, just note what's going on in your environment so you can track your body's response and make insightful connections.

START YOUR SUPPLEMENTS TO DROP ACID

You will be starting a daily regimen of nutritional supplements specially designed to drop acid. The supplements I list below are not the only ones to consider, but here I'm focused on the superstars—those that are well documented in the scientific literature for their ability to drop acid. (Refer to chapter 6 for all the scientific details.)

These supplements can be found at health food stores, most drugstores and supermarkets, and online. You can learn more about supplements on my website, at DrPerlmutter.com. It's usually best to take the supplements at the same time every day so you don't forget; for many people, the best time is the morning.

Quercetin:	500 mg per day
Luteolin:	100 mg per day
DHA:	1,000 mg per day

Vitamin C:	500 mg per day
Chlorella:	1,200 mg *C. vulgaris*

OPTIONAL BONUS SUPPLEMENTS: PROBIOTICS

As I explained in part 1, the health of your gut's microbiome affects everything about your metabolism, and people who suffer from chronic elevated uric acid tend to harbor unhealthy biomes. There's a lot you can do to nourish the health of your intestinal microbiome, including eating probiotic-rich fermented foods such as kimchi and cultured yogurt and adding prebiotic-rich foods to your plate. Prebiotics are like fertilizer for your microbes, helping them grow and reproduce. They can be found in common foods such as garlic, onions, leeks, and asparagus (and many prebiotic foods inhibit the enzyme needed for making uric acid, so you're getting a double benefit). You can also support your gut bugs by avoiding genetically modified organisms (GMO) and eating organic food whenever possible. In animal studies, the herbicides used on GMO crops have been shown to negatively alter the microbiome.

I've written extensively about the microbiome and offered recommendations for supplementation in the book *Brain Maker*. Because probiotics decrease inflammation in the body and improve sugar and uric acid metabolism, they can be a welcome addition to your supplement regimen. I highly recommend them but have made them optional because I find that many people do not like taking more than five supplements a day. Studies are under way to understand the specific connection between probiotic supplementation and lowering uric acid, particularly to identify the strains that are best at dropping acid. The link may be less direct than it is with the other supplements on the list. Nonetheless, probiotics will help support healthy digestion, metabolism, inflammation levels, and in turn uric acid levels, so I do encourage adding them to your regimen if possible.

To find the highest-quality probiotics, go to a store known for its natural supplement section and speak with the salesperson most familiar with the store's array of brands—someone who can offer an unbiased opinion. Probiotics are not regulated by the FDA, so you don't want to end up with a brand whose claims don't match the actual ingredients. Prices can vary wildly, too. The store rep can help you navigate all the nomenclature, because some strains are sold under more than one name. Most products contain several strains, and I encourage my patients to seek supplements that contain at least twelve different strains in a high-potency, broad-spectrum probiotic formula. Specifically, you'll want to seek strains from the *Lactobacillus*, *Bifidobacterium*, and *Bacillus* genera. These are the ones with the best research and data behind them. Make sure you're also buying probiotics that are labeled hypoallergenic and non-GMO. Probiotics should be taken on an empty stomach right before a meal.

OPTIONAL FAST

Ideally, you'll start week 1 after fasting for one full day. Fasting is an excellent way to speed up your body's metabolic transformation and provide a foundation of sorts. For many people, fasting on a Sunday (after eating a last meal on Saturday evening) and beginning the diet program on a Monday morning works best. Or you could have your last meal on a Friday night and start the program on a Sunday morning.

The fasting protocol is simple: no food but lots of water for a twenty-four-hour period. Avoid caffeine, too. If you take any medications, by all means continue to take them (but if you take diabetes medications, please consult your physician first). If the idea of fasting is too daunting for you, simply wean yourself off the items on the No list (page 176) for a few days as you prepare your kitchen. The more addicted your body is to uric acid–raising sugar and carbs, the more challenging this will be. When you've established the LUV Diet for life and want to fast for further benefits, you can try a seventy-two-hour fast, but be sure to check with your doctor ahead of time, especially if you have any medical conditions to consider. I recommend fasting at least four times a year, for at least twenty-four hours each time, during the seasonal changes (e.g., the last week of September, December, March, and June). While fasting, you can skip testing your uric acid levels until twenty-four hours after the end of the fast. Or, if you feel like experimenting to see how the fast affects your uric acid levels, test before, during, and after.

OPTIONAL KETO

If you'd like to modify the LUV Diet to meet a ketogenic formula, I explain how to do that at DrPerlmutter.com. I refrained from doing this in the book because most people will not opt to go keto, and following the core LUV Diet is enough to start the transformation. However, let me offer a brief introduction to this diet for readers who are unfamiliar with it.

The ketogenic diet is one of the most talked-about diet trends today, and as a clinician, I have recommended the diet both as a prescribed intervention for patients suffering from a wide variety of ailments and as a general suggestion for people looking to optimize their metabolism, weight, cognitive health, and uric acid levels.

You've probably heard celebrities, athletes, and neighbors raving about the benefits of this dietary approach. Studies back up its rapid growth in popularity: a ketogenic diet has been shown to reduce the risk of heart disease, improve insulin sensitivity and glycemic control in both type 1 and type 2 diabetes, help individuals struggling with obesity to lower their BMI, and even improve or control symptoms of debilitating neurodegenerative conditions such as Parkinson's disease and epilepsy. There is even some evidence to suggest that a ketogenic diet can play a role in the treatment of cancer. If it is implemented properly, a ketogenic diet can be a very powerful tool in the fight against a variety of chronic diseases. In the treatment and management of gout, there is promising evidence that the diet may help reduce the joint inflammation character-istic of the disease. But the most powerful benefit of the keto diet for anything related to uric acid is its effect on weight loss. Put simply—and I've been reiterating this throughout the book, so it shouldn't come as a surprise—weight loss is the most effective way to lower uric acid levels and prevent gout flare-ups. And for many people, ketogenic diets are the ticket to dropping weight...and, in turn, dropping acid.

While the ketogenic diet may sound new, it parallels the way many of our ancestors ate before the advent of agriculture allowed for the domes-tication of staple crops such as wheat and corn, which are high in carbo-hydrates and sugar, particularly in their processed forms. Our ancestors ate a wide variety of wild plants and animals as well as fewer carbohy-drates and less sugar than we eat today. This diet forced our ancestors' bodies into a state of ketosis, in which we burn fat, or ketone bodies, for fuel as opposed to carbohydrates—the main goal of the ketogenic diet.

In order to achieve ketosis, one must consume a diet high in health-ful fats and dramatically low in sugar and carbohydrates. The optimal macronutrient ratio will vary from person to person. Some will thrive on a diet in which they get roughly 80 percent of their calories from health-ful fats and 20 percent from carbohydrates and protein. Others may do better in the range of 60 to 75 percent of calories from fat and slightly more protein. I encourage you to experiment to find what works best for you. Note that because ketogenic diets tend to emphasize meat-based proteins, they can add to your incoming purine pool and aggravate uric acid production. But you *can* have it both ways—reap the benefits of going keto without adding more uric acid triggers—if you choose wisely. And you'll be doing just that on this program, with a focus primarily on above-ground leafy and fibrous vegetables and low-purine meat as a side dish. What's more, you can go keto even as a strict vegetarian.

If you want to learn more about the ketogenic diet with step-by-step instructions, go to my website to access a library of information plus my e-guide to this incredibly powerful dietary and lifestyle choice. In order to cycle in and out of keto while following the LUV Diet, you'll have to make wise substitutions, including LUV-friendly carbohydrates such as fruits and wild rice.

Although high amounts of ketones correspond to high levels of uric acid, research demonstrates that the temporary elevation of uric acid rapidly improves once carbohydrates and proteins are added back to the diet following the defined period of ketosis. The short-term elevation of ketones while you're on the diet may compete with uric acid for excretion, so that there is less excretion of uric acid during ketosis. But the good news is that ultimately, once the weight is lost, uric acid levels drop below where they were at the beginning of the diet. In other words, the weight loss achieved by the ketogenic diet results in a drop in baseline uric acid levels.

In a 2020 study in which a group of women were placed on a very low-carbohydrate ketogenic diet for three months, there was an average weight loss of nearly 20 percent, with notable reductions in fat mass.[1] That effect alone would help with dropping uric acid, and indeed at the conclusion of the study, uric acid levels were measurably lower than they were at the start.

The point I am making here is that in the short term, a ketogenic diet may be helpful in achieving your goal of lowering uric acid, but please be aware that uric acid may be elevated during the period of weight loss while in ketosis—especially if you take the ketogenic diet to the extreme, as some people like to do. Generally, for people cycling in and out of mild ketosis, there shouldn't be any significant or meaningful elevation of uric acid. Further, in my opinion, following a very low-calorie ketogenic diet with significant carbohydrate restriction to achieve weight loss is a good choice. The endgame is worth enduring slight temporary elevations in uric acid. My only cautionary notes are for people with a history of gout or kidney stones: if you fall into this category, carefully monitor your uric acid while fasting or following any diet that is ketogenic.

Week 1: Dietary Edits to Lower Uric Values

How to Make Over Your Metabolism on the LUV Diet

The doctor of the future will give no medicine, but will instruct his patients in care of the human frame, in diet, and in the cause and prevention of disease.

— THOMAS A. EDISON

ONE IN FIVE DEATHS GLOBALLY is now attributed to poor diet.[1] And poor diet, as you now know, is linked to the dangerous buildup of uric acid, which wreaks havoc on the body. This means that eleven million people are unnecessarily wiped off the planet each year because they do not eat or have access to foods that support health and prevent disease. That's more deaths from diet than from tobacco use, high blood pressure, or any other health risk. What's more, the nutrition guidance that has been doled out over the last several decades is simply not useful.

If nine of the top ten causes of death today are attributable to the downstream effects of poor diet, then we can say that diet is *the* leading cause of chronic disease in the world. It plays into every disease imaginable, from depression to dementia and even cancer. We don't think about the relationship between what we eat and our risk for certain illnesses. We know that smoking causes lung cancer, but how does eating too many doughnuts or cheeseburgers with soda pop increase our chances of developing Alzheimer's disease, heart disease, and cancer? The links are not so obvious.

Food is essential well beyond its role in nutrition. We've long known that food is information. The foods we consume send signals to our life code, our DNA. Everything we put in our mouths has the potential to change the expression — behavior — of our genes. Think about that fact alone: you have the ability to alter, for better or worse, the activity of your DNA! We call this alteration, brought about by the effects of extrinsic influences, *epigenetics*. And as it turns out, more than 90 percent of the genetic switches in our DNA that are associated with longevity are significantly influenced by our lifestyle choices, including the foods we eat and the drinks we consume. One illustrative example I routinely give: a diet rich in refined carbohydrates decreases the activity of the gene that makes brain-protective BDNF, the essential protein in the brain for supporting neuronal survival and growth, but when we eat healthful fats and proteins, that activity increases, producing more BDNF.[2] More BDNF means more healthy brain cells. Who doesn't want that?

It makes sense that our DNA works best with an ancient diet. For more than 99 percent of the time we have existed on this planet, we have eaten a diet much lower in refined carbohydrates, higher in healthful fat and fiber, and much more nutrient-dense in general than the diets we eat today. And we didn't eat processed or fast foods then, either; we ate what we could find in nature. In fact, our modern-day Western diet works against our DNA's ability to protect health and longevity. And we experience the consequences of this mismatch every day.

But even though you can quit smoking, you can't quit eating. And unfortunately, it's unlikely that our food environment is going to drastically improve anytime soon. What's more, most doctors think that serious metabolic and weight issues are impossible to treat, so they often dodge the subject with patients.

Nutrition is barely taught in medical school. Even in my day, I kept waiting for the nutritional part of my medical education. It never came. Upon seeing the critical connections between health and nutrition, I became a fellow of the American College of Nutrition and now serve on its scientific advisory board. We have to take matters into our own hands. This is a public health crisis that only we citizens and consumers can solve. And now we have a new entryway to achieving optimal health: dropping acid. If elevated uric acid precedes and predicts biological mayhem and future risk for most chronic diseases, then we must start paying attention to this important metabolite. Think of it as giving you a preview of a traffic signal that screams "Stop" long before you find yourself racing through a dangerous intersection. It's the new bellwether of health. Welcome to the LUV program, which must prioritize diet first and foremost.[3]

THE LUV DIETARY PROTOCOL

Below are the top ten rules to follow on the LUV Diet.

1. Go gluten- and GMO-free.

2. Eat mostly plant-based meals featuring whole acid-dropping fruits and vegetables.

3. Consume no refined carbs, added sugars, or artificial sweeteners.

4. Do not eat organ meats.

5. Limit serving sizes of purine-heavy meat and fish, especially sardines and anchovies.

6. Eat nuts and seeds.

7. Eat organic eggs.

8. Confine yourself to small amounts of dairy products, if you choose to consume them at all.

9. Be generous with extra virgin olive oil.

10. Incorporate acid-lowering "offsets" (e.g., cherries, broccoli sprouts, coffee).

Why go gluten-free? Well, you can read all about gluten in *Grain Brain*, but the main reason to avoiding gluten-containing foods is that gluten exacerbates inflammation in the body. It also is contained in a lot of sugary, carbohydrate-heavy, uric acid–raising foods that we'd do well to avoid. When you nix gluten, knowing what to eat to feed a healthy metabolism becomes much easier.

At the end of this chapter, you'll find a one-week sample meal plan to help you see how to put the above guidelines into practice. Now here come the LUV Diet rules categorized by No, Yes, and In Moderation.

No

Start by removing the items on the following list.

• All sources of gluten, including whole-grain and whole-wheat forms of bread, noodles, pastas, pastries, baked goods, crackers, and cereals (see my website or *Grain Brain* for the full list and all the scientific details about why to remove gluten).

• All forms of processed carbs, sugar, and starch, including chips, crackers, cookies, pastries, muffins, pizza dough, cakes, doughnuts, sugary snacks, candy, energy and snack bars, ice cream, frozen yogurt, sherbet, jam, jelly, preserves, ketchup, commercial marinades and sauces, commercial salad dressings and pasta sauces, processed cheese spreads, juices, dried fruit, sports drinks, soft drinks and soda pop, fried foods, agave, sugar (white and brown), corn syrup, and maple syrup. See the note below about honey.

- All artificial sweeteners and products made with artificial sweeteners, including sugar substitutes that are marketed as "natural": acesulfame potassium (Sunett, Sweet One), aspartame (NutraSweet, Equal), saccharin (Sweet'N Low, Sweet Twin, Sugar Twin), sucralose (Splenda), and neotame (Newtame). Also avoid any sugar alcohols that are marketed as healthful alternatives to regular and artificial sugars. In addition to xylitol, which I called out on page 126 within the context of raising uric acid, beware of others such as sorbitol, mannitol, maltitol, erythritol, and isomalt. Also see the note below about artificial sweeteners. But don't panic: I have positive things to say about a new sweetener on the market that you've probably never heard of—allulose; it is a wise choice in addition to a few other options when a little sweetness is called for.

- Margarine, vegetable shortening, and any commercial brand of cooking oil, including soybean, corn, cottonseed, canola, peanut, safflower, grapeseed, sunflower, rice bran, and wheat germ oils—even if they are organic. People often think vegetable oils are derived from vegetables. They are not. The term is incredibly misleading, a relic from the days when food manufacturers needed to distinguish these fats from animal fats. The oils typically come from grains, seeds, and other plants, such as soybeans. And they have been highly refined and chemically altered. The majority of Americans today get their fats from these oils, which are pro-inflammatory. Do not consume them.

- Processed meats, including bacon, sausage, ham, salami, prosciutto, smoked meat, canned meat, dried meat, hot dogs, corned beef, and cold cuts. Most processed meats contain high levels of purines and additives that can ultimately cause inflammation.

- Organ meats (the consumable organs of animals, also called offal), including liver, heart, brains, kidney, tongue, tripe, and intestines. Most organ meats come from cows, pigs, lambs, goats, chickens, and ducks. Tripe is the lining of an animal's stomach and most often comes from cattle. Sweetbreads are also considered organ meats and are neither sweet nor a type of bread; they are made from the thymus gland and pancreas. Although organ meats are nutrient-dense, they are also among the most purine-dense, uric acid–raising foods you can eat.

- Nonfermented soy products (e.g., tofu and soy milk) and processed foods made with soy. Look for "soy protein isolate" in the list of ingredients and avoid soy cheese, soy burgers, soy hot dogs, soy nuggets, soy ice cream, and soy yogurt. Note that soy products that are fermented — including natto, miso, and tempeh — are acceptable if they are organic and non-GMO; they provide a source of protein for vegetarians and are suitable for plant-based meals.

SNEAKY NAMES FOR SUGAR

Following are commonly used names for sugar on food labels (tip: any ingredient ending in "ose" is a type of sugar). Find sugar's hiding spots by looking for its unfamiliar names.

Agave syrup	Brown sugar
Anhydrous dextrose	Buttered sugar/buttercream
Barley malt	Cane juice (crystals)
Beet sugar	Cane sugar
Birch syrup	Caramel
Blackstrap molasses	Carob syrup
Brown rice syrup	Coconut palm sugar

Coconut sugar	Golden sugar/syrup
Confectioners'/powdered sugar	Grape juice concentrate
	Grape sugar
Corn sweetener	High-fructose corn syrup (HFCS)
Corn syrup	
Corn syrup solids	Icing sugar
Crystal dextrose	Invert sugar
Crystalline fructose	Lactose
Date sugar	Liquid fructose
Demerara sugar	Malt syrup
Dextrin	Maltodextrin
Dextrose	Maltose
Diastatic malt	Maple syrup
Ethyl maltol	Molasses
Evaporated cane juice	Muscovado sugar
Evaporated corn sweetener	Nectar*
Florida crystals	Palm sugar
Fructose	Panela sugar
Fruit juice	Raw sugar
Fruit juice concentrate	Refiners syrup
Galactose	Ribose
Glucomalt	Rice syrup
Glucose	Saccharose
Glucose syrup solids	Simple syrup

---

* Nectars include all fruit nectars, such as peach and pear nectar, agave nectar, and coconut nectar.

Sorghum syrup	Treacle
Sucanat	Turbinado sugar
Sucrose	White granulated sugar
Sugar beet syrup	Xylose
Sugar cane juice	Yacon syrup
Tapioca syrup	Yellow sugar

The five most commonly used sweeteners are corn syrup, sorghum, cane sugar, high-fructose corn syrup, and fruit juice concentrate.

Yes

The following items can be consumed liberally. Go organic, non-GMO, and local with your whole-food choices wherever possible; flash-frozen is fine, too.

- Healthful fats, including extra virgin olive oil, sesame oil, coconut or MCT (medium-chain triglyceride) oil, avocado oil, grass-fed tallow and organic or pasture-fed butter, ghee, coconuts, olives, cheese, cottage cheese, nuts and nut butters, whole eggs (see note below), and seeds (flaxseed, sunflower seeds, pumpkin seeds, sesame seeds, chia seeds).

- Herbs, seasonings, and condiments. You can go wild here as long as you watch labels. Kiss ketchup and chutney goodbye, but enjoy mustard, horseradish, tapenade, and salsa if they are free of gluten, wheat, soy, and sugar. There are virtually no restrictions on herbs and seasonings: be mindful, however, of packaged products that are made at plants that process wheat and soy. Cultured condiments, such as lacto-fermented mayonnaise, kombucha mustard, sour cream, fermented hot sauce, relish,

180

and fermented salsa, are rich in probiotics. Kimchi, a fermented vegetable (usually cabbage), is also an excellent choice.

- Whole fruits, including avocados, bell peppers, berries, cherries, pomegranates, cucumbers, tomatoes, zucchini, squashes, pumpkins, eggplants, lemons, and limes. Note that fruits high in sugar, such as apples, bananas, peaches, plums, apricots, melons, mangoes, papayas, pineapples, grapes, kiwifruits, and oranges, are okay, but the low-sugar fruits listed first should be prioritized. Virtually all fruits, when consumed in their whole, unadulterated state, are associated with a decreased risk of both metabolic syndrome and elevated uric acid—see the note below. The only fruit to avoid is the dried kind, which contains concentrated fructose that may raise uric acid.

- Vegetables, including leafy greens and lettuces, collards, spinach, broccoli (and broccoli sprouts—more on this below), kale, chard, cabbage, onions, mushrooms, cauliflower, brussels sprouts, sauerkraut, artichokes, alfalfa sprouts, green beans, celery, bok choy, radishes, watercress, turnips, asparagus, garlic, leeks, fennel, shallots, scallions, ginger, jicama, parsley, water chestnuts, celery root, kohlrabi, and daikon.

- Plant sources of protein, including cooked legumes such as black beans, kidney beans, pinto beans, fava beans, navy beans, lentils, peas, and chickpeas, and fermented, non-GMO soy products such as tempeh and miso.

In Moderation

Animal sources of protein must be consumed in moderation or avoided.

- Limit seafoods high in purines—sardines and anchovies—to a maximum of once weekly. Although most people don't consume large amounts of anchovies at once, be careful about anchovy-based fish sauces and Caesar salad dressings.

- Most starchy (sugary) vegetables and those that grow below the ground, including peas, carrots, parsnips, sweet potatoes, and yams can be consumed in moderation—a couple of times weekly.

- Limit the following to no more than four to six ounces two to three times per week: wild fish, including salmon, cod, sole, mahi-mahi, grouper, and trout; shellfish and mollusks, including shrimp, crab, lobster, mussels, clams, and oysters; grass-fed meat and poultry, including beef, lamb, pork, bison, chicken, turkey, duck, ostrich, and veal; and wild game.

- For a touch of sweetness: dark chocolate (at least 70 percent cacao), allulose, natural stevia, honey, and monk fruit (see note below).

LUV NOTES

A Note About Sugar Substitutes, Allulose, Honey, and Other Natural Sweeteners

Although we used to think that sugar substitutes such as saccharin, sucralose, and aspartame didn't have a metabolic impact because they don't raise insulin, it turns out that they can indeed wreak havoc and cause the same metabolic disorders as real sugar does. How? By changing the microbiome in ways that favor bacterial imbalances (dysbiosis), blood sugar imbalances, and an overall unhealthy metabolism.

Ever since the journal *Nature* published a landmark study in 2014 establishing the link between sugar substitutes and dysbiosis, other studies have replicated the findings.[4] Consuming artificially sweetened "diet" drinks can heighten the risk of diabetes via dysbiosis: some studies show a doubling of the risk for people who drink two diet beverages a day. And you know what that means in terms of the risk of metabolic chaos, not to mention the risk of degenerative disorders such as Alzheimer's disease. In 2017, the journal *Stroke* released a bombshell paper that revealed the risk for stroke, Alzheimer's, and dementia in general among people who drank artificially sweetened drinks.[5] What they found was quite remarkable: participants who drank one or more artificially sweetened drinks per day had almost three times the risk of stroke and three times the risk of Alzheimer's disease.

Within the context of uric acid specifically, here's what to keep in mind: it's important to avoid anything that interferes with your body's ability to break down and filter compounds and toxins, and that includes sugar substitutes. Remember, too, that some substitutes, particularly xylitol, can directly raise uric acid levels by stimulating the breakdown of purines in the body, so be on the lookout for this one. It's an ingredient in many foods and personal care products, even in things labeled "naturally sweetened," so read the full list of ingredients to spot it. Although you're not likely to consume too much xylitol from sugar-free gum, toothpaste, and mouthwash, it sneaks into baked goods, peanut butter, drink powders, candy, pudding, condiments such as ketchup and barbecue sauce, and commercial pancake syrup. Medications and vitamins that are designed to melt in your mouth also may contain this sugar, though the amount is minuscule and you don't have to worry too much about drugs that you may need. More problematic is the xylitol found in common food products.

You'll see that many of my recipes call for allulose, a sugar you can sweeten up to. Allulose is a sugar that resembles fructose (some call it pseudofructose), but it has little to no effect on blood glucose or insulin levels; the body absorbs allulose but does not metabolize it into glucose, so it is virtually calorie-free. New research shows that in humans, allulose has a favorable impact on blood glucose and may *improve* insulin sensitivity.[6] In addition, studies reveal that allulose may exert an anti-inflammatory effect on adipocytes—fat cells—the source of inflammatory cytokines that drive metabolic syndrome and, in turn, the risk of elevated uric acid. Allulose is found naturally in some foods, such as figs and raisins, but you can buy it in both granulated and liquid forms online. The brand I enjoy is RxSugar, which is certified organic and has zero net carbs.

In the past, I have written about honey and recommended that people avoid it at all costs. This position was based on the fact that honey has a very high sugar content. In fact, the actual fructose content in most batches of honey is around 40 percent, but this percentage can range between 21 and 43 percent depending on how and where the honey is harvested and processed. When digging deeper into the literature about this sweet nectar from nature, I discovered that research supports the idea that it may not be so bad after all. We may be able to make a small space for honey in our lives. So have I changed my position on honey? Yes, and that's a reflection of the way scientific research continues to inform us.[7]

Approximately 85 percent of the solids in honey are a combination of dextrose (another name for glucose) and fructose. A variety of other sugars also make up honey, alongside trace elements and minerals, including zinc, copper, iron, manganese, chromium, selenium, magnesium, calcium, and potassium. Honey contains vitamins, including vitamins B_1, B_2, B_3, B_5, and B_6 as well as vitamins A, E, and C. It also has flavonoids as well as quercetin and luteolin, both of which, as you know now, can significantly help lower uric acid levels. So it is fair to say that honey is far more than a sweetener made from sugar. Its unique composition varies greatly depending on soil and climate conditions and other aspects of the environment, including, as you might expect, the flowers from which the honey is made. Unfortunately, there are no standardized methods for producing honey or verifying its quality.

As I mentioned, one of the most important goals of this book is to help you keep your blood sugar under control. And it turns out that there are good data indicating that honey may also help you toward that goal. Honey does not appear to be significantly dangerous in terms of glucose metabolism. In fact, several human trials have indicated that honey consumption is associated with improved insulin response and decreased blood glucose levels. Some researchers have gone so far as to characterize honey as a "novel anti-diabetic agent" in terms of its effects on both the liver and pancreas, where it has been shown to improve blood sugar control, and the gastrointestinal tract, where it positively modifies the gut microbiota.[8] These are effects we wouldn't expect from a fructose-heavy sugar product. But like whole fruits, which don't raise uric acid, thanks to their complex components, honey falls into a special category because of its intrinsic chemical makeup.

Although more studies are needed to understand honey's benefits and potential risks, I'm convinced by the current evidence that we can enjoy a touch of honey in moderation. Put simply, you're not going to enter the danger zone with a teaspoon of honey added to a dish or drink for a touch of sweetness. And honey is a well-known anti-inflammatory, antioxidant, and antibacterial agent that has been used in medicine for centuries. Just be judicious and use it sparingly. Opt for raw honey whenever possible, which may offer more benefits than the processed, pasteurized variety. You can add a dollop to yogurt or tea, for example.

Another popular sweetener that burst onto the scene in the 2010s is agave syrup, or agave nectar. This one deserves a warning label. Agave syrup is produced from many species of agave—notably, blue agave—a type of succulent. This is the same plant from which tequila is made. But don't let the word *nectar* when it's attached to *agave* fool you into thinking it's honey's more healthful twin. Unlike honey, agave is highly processed and contains quite a bit more fructose. In fact, it may contain anywhere from 75 to 90 percent fructose, and it lacks many of the nutrients found in honey. This sweetener should remain on the No list.

The only sweeteners that make my Yes list are allulose, natural stevia, the occasional dollop of honey, and monk fruit. Never heard of monk fruit? Monk fruit is another sweetener used as a substitute for table sugar because it contains zero calories and does not affect blood sugar. It is derived from a small round fruit native to Southeast Asia that looks like a melon. It has been used for centuries in Eastern medicine as a cold remedy and digestive aid, and now, coming in at between 150 and two hundred times sweeter than table sugar, it's being used to sweeten foods and beverages. It's sold in granulated, liquid, and powdered forms. It takes its name from the thirteenth-century Buddhist monks who first used it. All my recipes use allulose when a sweetener is needed, because it's less expensive than monk fruit, but you can easily substitute monk fruit for the allulose—or mix them together—and experiment with the different tastes and textures. My hope is that you begin to play with these sugars and learn to incorporate them safely into your daily menus.

A Note About Gluten-Free Grains

When gluten-free grains are processed for human consumption (e.g., when whole oats are milled and when rice is prepared for packaging), their physical structure changes, and this may result in increased inflammation in the body. For this reason, amaranth, buckwheat, rice (brown and wild, but not white), millet, sorghum, and teff should be consumed in moderation. Watch your portions, too. I prefer wild rice, which is technically a reed, when I need a small side dish.

A Note About Fruits and Vegetables: Focus on Fiber and Bust Uric Acid with Broccoli Sprouts and Cherries

Despite their (low) fructose content, fruits and vegetables do not elevate uric acid, and certain of them can help prevent elevations, thanks to their inherent chemical compounds and fiber content. Fiber, especially inulin, which is found in many vegetables, including onions, leeks, artichokes, and asparagus, slows the release of sugars in the body while nourishing the microbiome and promoting its actions. Inulin is a type of fiber that's not digested or absorbed in the stomach and acts as a prebiotic — it stays in the bowel and helps certain beneficial bacteria grow. This special fiber has long been found to enhance the composition of the gut bacteria, and it's abundant in the LUV Diet. Now that we have evidence that uric acid is disruptive to the gut bacteria and the integrity of the gut lining, leading to inflammation, we must do what we can to support the health and function of our gut bugs. Inulin has even been shown to help offset the adverse metabolic effects of a fructose-laden diet.[9]

The more fiber you consume, the better. And even though many vegetables, such as spinach, peas, asparagus, cauliflower, mushrooms, and broccoli, do contain high levels of purines, they do not raise uric acid and can be safely eaten. According to the World Health Organization, 1.7 million deaths worldwide (2.8 percent) are attributable to low fruit and vegetable consumption.[10] Moreover, insufficient intake of fruit and vegetables is estimated to cause around 14 percent of gastrointestinal cancer deaths, around 11 percent of heart disease deaths, and around 9 percent of stroke deaths globally. Now, about those broccoli sprouts and cherries in particular . . .

The cruciferous vegetable family — broccoli, broccoli sprouts, brussels sprouts, and others — contains an important precursor molecule that creates a superhero compound in the body called *sulforaphane*, which is currently taking research circles by storm.[11] Sulforaphane is one of the most important offsets of elevated uric acid and confers a multitude of benefits for general health. How so? Well, it has to do with its relationship to a certain pathway in the body that, when activated, triggers the expression of more than two hundred genes that play a role in reducing inflammation, increasing the body's production of antioxidants, and even enhancing our ability to detoxify when challenged by toxins.[12] It's called the Nrf2 pathway. Technically, Nrf2 is a class of proteins that induce the expression of certain genes — in this case, genes responsible for anti-inflammatory and antioxidant processes. The pathway is basically a sensing system that tells the body that it needs to take action to protect itself. Normally, Nrf2 exists inside the cell but outside the nucleus. When the cell senses oxidative stress, however, the Nrf2 pathway lights up, and critical genes within the nucleus jump into action to cause an increase in antioxidants.

Because uric acid does some of its damage by increasing the production of damaging free radicals as well as increasing inflammation, anything to combat these consequences helps the whole enterprise. The unchecked activity of free radicals leads to damage to our DNA, our proteins, and fat. Several well-studied activators of the Nrf2 pathway include coffee, exercise, turmeric, and, notably, sulforaphane. Sulforaphane may be one of the most potent activators of this incredibly important pathway. Sulforaphane itself is neither an antioxidant nor an anti-inflammatory agent, but it's an activator of the Nrf2 pathway, which then triggers antioxidant and anti-inflammatory activities. Where can we get a good dose of sulforaphane? From broccoli sprouts.

To be clear, there is no sulforaphane to speak of in broccoli sprouts. What broccoli sprouts have is a chemical called *glucoraphanin*, which is the precursor molecule from which sulforaphane is made. This turns out to be very important. The conversion of glucoraphanin to sulforaphane requires a specific enzyme called *myrosinase*. This enzyme is released when, for example, broccoli sprouts are chewed. Then the enzyme is allowed to come into contact with glucoraphanin, and — voilà — sulforaphane is formed.

This process is actually a defense mechanism for broccoli sprouts and other plants. As the leaves are eaten by insects, for example, sulforaphane is produced to ward off the invading bugs (apparently, sulforaphane is quite distasteful to them). The sprouts are nutritionally superior to the "adult" vegetable because they contain fifty to one hundred times more sulforaphane than mature broccoli and other cruciferous vegetables. If they are hard to find at your local grocery store, you can easily sprout them yourself; they look just like alfalfa sprouts but are very different when it comes to flavor and nutritional content. (For a step-by-step lesson in growing broccoli sprouts, go to DrPerlmutter.com.) Although you can buy sulforaphane supplements, the ideal way to bring active sulforaphane into the body is to chew broccoli sprouts. Simply add a handful of them to a salad, spread, or smoothie, or use them as a soup garnish. I'll show you how to work with these versatile gems in my recipes, featured in chapter 11.

For decades, people prone to gout have sworn by tart cherries and tart cherry juice to prevent gout attacks. The evidence was anecdotal, but now we know from new research findings that in people who live with gout, a mere half cup of cherries per day can reduce the risk of flares by 35 percent.[13] Clearly, something is going on here, and we finally have a clue as to how cherries, despite being relatively high in fructose compared to other fruit, exert their acid-dropping effects. The secret is that they contain high levels of two types of flavonoids that famously act like uric acid–lowering drugs: anthocyanins and quercetin.[14] These compounds are also highly anti-inflammatory and fight oxidative stress. Although varieties of tart cherries such as Montmorency and Balaton contain more anthocyanins than sweet cherries such as Bing, new studies show that Bing cherries can increase the excretion of uric acid quite significantly. They also have been shown to result in a significant reduction in uric acid in the bloodstream after consumption. Added bonus: they appear to lower C-reactive protein.

Although many people choose to drink tart cherry juice, I recommend avoiding the juice altogether because it so often contains added sugar and absolutely no fiber. You can certainly seek out 100 percent unsweetened tart cherry juice, but I'd prefer you stick with either whole fresh tart or Bing cherries or try a cherry extract in supplement (tablet) form. This is ideal for people who don't like the taste of cherries. Other fruits and vegetables that have acid-dropping properties, because they contain compounds to inhibit xanthine oxidase, include pomegranates, blueberries, green peppers, celery, red onions, and walnuts. As an aside, many herbs and spices also contain acid-dropping compounds—notably, cardamom, cloves, thyme, peppermint, rosemary, and oregano.

MARKET MEDICINE TO LUV

Pomegranates

Blueberries

Cherries (tart and Bing)

Broccoli and broccoli sprouts

Red onions

Walnuts

Green peppers

Celery

In the herbs and spices department: Cardamom, clove extract, thyme, peppermint, rosemary, and oregano

In the beverage department: Coffee and green tea

A Note About Dairy and Eggs

Whole cow's milk and cream can be used in recipes or in coffee and tea (avoid skim milk because of the lack of fat to offset the sugar content). If you opt for milk alternatives such as oat or almond milk, watch out for products with added sugar and choose unsweetened varieties. Eggs and unsweetened full-fat yogurt are fine. Choose probiotic-rich yogurt that contains plenty of live, active cultures. Whole eggs, including the yolks, are an excellent source of high-quality protein and fat, are low in purines, and come with many extra nutrients to make them a nutritional gold mine. In fact, they contain all the essential amino acids we need to survive, and they're loaded with vitamins, minerals, and antioxidants. Egg salads, hard-boiled eggs, frittatas with vegetables…eggs are among the most versatile, satisfying, near-perfect foods around. Ideally, choose organic pasture-raised eggs.

A Note About Snacks to LUV

It helps to avoid snacking in between meals, and because of the high satiety factor of the meals I recommend, you're not likely to find yourself hunting ravenously for food in between meals. But if you must snack, I've included a few delicious recipes starting on page 265 that won't break your metabolism, including smoothies that contain acid-lowering ingredients. Below are some other ideas.

* A handful of raw nuts (with the exception of peanuts, which are legumes and not nuts). Or go for a mix of nuts and olives, including acid-dropping walnuts.

* Chopped raw vegetables (e.g., bell peppers, broccoli, cucumber, green beans, or radishes) dipped in hummus, guacamole, goat cheese, tapenade, or nut butter. Or try my Brussels Sprouts Kimchi (page 268) or Crudités with Cashew Sriracha Mayo (page 267).

* Half an avocado drizzled with olive oil.

* Two hard-boiled pasture-raised eggs, regular or fermented (try my Turmeric-Fermented Hard-Boiled Eggs, on page 265).

* One piece or serving of whole fruit (e.g., cherries, grapefruit, orange, apple, berries, melon, pear, grapes, kiwifruit, plum, peach, or nectarine).

* One serving of full-fat Greek-style yogurt topped with fresh berries and chopped walnuts (or try my Cinnamon Turmeric Yogurt, on page 266).

Drinks to LUV

I can't praise coffee enough, and yes, this is self-serving, because coffee brings me a lot of pleasure. Decades of research now confirm that a cup or two of coffee a day might keep the doctor away. When the *Annals of Internal Medicine* reported news about two massive longitudinal studies completed in 2017, one of which involved ten European countries and more than half a million people followed for more than sixteen years, the results were convincing. Participants who drank the most coffee had the lowest risk of dying—of anything. The men's risk was reduced by 12 percent, and the women's risk was reduced by 7 percent.[15] And "higher consumption of coffee was associated with lower risks of death, and in particular, mortality due to digestive and circulatory diseases." Significantly, in women, high levels of coffee consumption correlated with reduced A1c levels as well as reduced C-reactive protein levels.

In the second study, led by the University of Southern California, which sought to examine coffee's powers among an ethnically diverse group of people between the ages of forty-five and seventy-five over a nearly twenty-year period, the results echoed the findings above: higher consumption of coffee was associated with lower risk of death—notably, from various types of cancer.[16] Both studies show that coffee might be protective, but here's the interesting part: it's not the caffeine that gets the credit. Polyphenols and other bioactive compounds in coffee have antioxidant properties, and coffee's well-documented association with reduced insulin resistance, inflammation, and biomarkers of liver function is attributable to these compounds, unrelated to the caffeine. Moreover, coffee contains xanthines, chemicals that can inhibit xanthine oxidase, which, as you'll recall, is the enzyme required for the production of uric acid.

And in a third large study, using data amassed from 14,758 participants in the United States enrolled in the third National Health and Nutrition Examination Survey, researchers from the University of British Columbia and Harvard found an inverse relationship between coffee consumption—both caffeinated and not—and uric acid levels: uric acid decreased with increasing coffee intake.[17] Their findings ruled out other factors that could have skewed the results, including the participants' weight, alcohol consumption, and diuretic use. They did not see this relationship between tea consumption and uric acid. So if you don't like to drink coffee because of its caffeine content, decaf can be just as beneficial for dropping acid.

In chapter 5, I mentioned a meta-analysis spanning nineteen studies that revealed increased uric acid levels among coffee-drinking women, but that did not translate to any negative effects, nor did it increase the risk of gout. The authors were quick to point out the need for future randomized controlled trials to understand potential differences between men and women in terms of their risk for hyperuricemia and gout within the context of coffee consumption. The slightly increased risk of hyperuricemia observed among the coffee-drinking women could have very well been an "artifact"—an inconsequential finding resulting from the way the authors made their calculations (using several studies, each conducted differently). What we do know is that a robust body of evidence beyond this study has repeatedly validated a strong association between coffee consumption and a reduced risk of hyperuricemia (and gout) among both men and women.

I'm a huge proponent of coffee for all adults and believe the benefits far outweigh any risks, unless of course you have any adverse reactions or allergies to the drink—these are rare but do affect some people. You can drink decaf and still reap acid-dropping benefits. Most Americans down a couple of cups of coffee a day, and I'm all for it. The one thing to be careful about, however, is ensuring that your caffeine consumption does not affect your sleep quality. It's helpful to switch to decaf coffee or caffeine-free teas in the afternoon. A good cutoff time is 2:00 p.m.

Although tea does not drop acid to any measurable degree in clinical studies, we know it contains other compounds that can contribute to healthy physiology and metabolism. Green tea earns an extra halo. The reason why green tea's star polyphenol—epigallocatechin-3-gallate (EGCG)—is so effective at giving tea its antioxidant and anti-inflammatory properties is because it triggers the all-important Nrf2 biological pathway.[18] Another tea to keep on your list is kombucha tea. This is a form of fermented black or green tea that contains naturally occurring probiotics. Fizzy and often served chilled, it's been used for centuries to help increase energy, and it may even help you lose weight in addition to contributing to the health of your gut microbiome, which in turn aids in keeping uric acid in check.

For every caffeinated beverage you consume, drink an extra twelve to sixteen ounces of water to balance its dehydrating effects. I find it helpful to keep a large container of water near me throughout the day. It may seem like a lot, but aim to drink half your body weight in ounces of purified water daily. For example, if you weigh 150 pounds, that means drinking around 75 ounces—the eight-glasses-a-day maxim. But bear in mind that you do get a lot of water from the foods you'll be eating on this plan, so don't follow this rule too strictly. If your urine is clear and light as opposed to dark yellow, you're drinking enough.

For added fun, I've included recipes for a few beverages you can mix up at home, starting on page 269. I've got a great Raw Cacao Almond Cold Brew Coffee you can stir up on a weekend morning, and a Tart Cherry Lime Mocktail you can blend up later in the day. If you're someone who has had a long love affair with soda pop and sugary beverages, see if you can nix those entirely and replace them with my Raspberry Mint Lemonade.

WATER DOES A BODY GOOD

The old wives' tale that drinking eight glasses of water a day will help you stay skinny is partly true. It turns out that water helps counterbalance some of the negative effects of sugar, especially fructose. While I should hope that you're not going to be eating any processed fructose from this point on, it's nice to know that water can help offset its adverse effects. It also offsets the effects of excess sodium. My menu is low in sodium by design, but when you return to preparing your own recipes and eating out rather than using my recipes, you'll likely encounter more sodium. Remember that high-salt diets are not just about blood pressure — they are also associated with obesity, insulin resistance, the development of diabetes, and, yes, elevated uric acid. Even if you avoid fructose, a high salt intake may trigger your body to produce fructose and spur production of uric acid. This is when having the right balance of water to counter these effects is critical.

As for alcohol, my rules are pretty straightforward: limit wine consumption to a glass a day if you so choose — preferably red, because it contains more polyphenols than white wine — and avoid or severely limit purine-filled beers. Some studies show that one beer a day is associated with a 50 percent increased risk of gout and a rise of uric acid to the tune of nearly half a milligram per deciliter (0.4 mg/dL).[19] If beer is your favorite alcoholic beverage, seek purine-free varieties. These began to make a splash in the market in 2014, and now there are many beers available with little to no purine content. Sapporo and Kirin, for example, have lines of purine-free beer. These join the burgeoning low- and no-alcohol alternative beer market. When it comes to spirits such as vodka and whiskey, these have substantially less purine content but can raise uric acid, so be careful with these drinks. Use uric acid testing to see how your body responds.

You might find it helpful to keep a food journal throughout the program in addition to logging your uric acid and blood glucose values (if you choose to test). Write down what you like and what you don't like so you can personalize your choices as you go along while sticking to the main guidelines. I also recommend that you avoid eating out during these three weeks so you can focus on getting the dietary protocol down. This will prepare you for the day when you do eat out and have to make good decisions about what to order (for more information, see page 222). These first three weeks will also reduce your cravings so there will be less temptation when you're looking at a menu filled with ingredients that can sabotage your metabolism. It's virtually impossible to go to a restaurant or even a salad bar in a market or buffet table at a party without running into added sugar and hidden refined fructose.

A SAMPLE SEVEN-DAY LUV MEAL PLAN

During week 1, focus on mastering your new eating habits. You can use my recipes and follow my sample seven-day meal plan below or venture out on your own in your kitchen, as long as you follow the guidelines. I've included easy, no-recipe meals in the plan for breakfast, lunch, dinner, dessert, snacks, and drinks, so you can pick and choose. Each meal should contain a source of healthful fat and low-purine protein as well as at least one offset that will drop acid (e.g., quercetin-rich vegetables or a handful of tart cherries). Remember that you can use butter, organic extra virgin olive oil, or coconut oil when you pan-fry foods. Avoid processed oils and cooking sprays unless the spray is made from organic olive oil.

If you want more servings, double or triple any recipe. Some of these recipes are more time-consuming to make than others, so plan ahead and feel free to swap one for another if you're short on time.

For even more ideas, go to DrPerlmutter.com for a gallery of additional recipes and plenty of additional resources. Finally, try skipping breakfast a couple of days a week, which will enhance your metabolic makeover. I've made that suggestion on two of the days below.

Monday

- Breakfast: Coconut Pudding (page 232) with one or two soft- or hard-boiled eggs

- Lunch: Chicken Salad with Broccoli-Sprout Pesto (page 242)

- Dinner: Three ounces of roasted organic chicken or wild-caught fish with a side of greens and vegetables sautéed in butter and garlic

- Dessert: Half a cup of berries topped with a drizzle of unsweetened cream or honey

Tuesday

- Breakfast: Skip!

- Lunch: Mixed green salad with dandelion greens, raw cut vegetables, and two hard-boiled eggs, dressed with Tart-Cherry Vinaigrette (page 252)

- Dinner: Harissa-Roasted Halibut with Roasted Zucchini, Tomatoes, Peppers, and Blistered Red Onions (page 256) and a side of salad greens dressed with extra virgin olive oil or other LUV Diet dressing

- Dessert: Two to three squares of dark chocolate

Wednesday

- Breakfast: Greek Farm Egg Cups (page 239) and one slice Cherry Almond Loaf (page 238)

- Lunch: Za'atar Chickpea Salad (page 248) with three to five ounces of roasted turkey, chicken, or wild-caught fish

- Dinner: Thyme-Roasted Pork Tenderloin (page 251) with half a cup of wild rice and unlimited steamed vegetables

- Dessert: One apple, sliced and topped with a sprinkle of cinnamon or cardamom

Thursday

- Breakfast: Yogurt with Ginger Carrot Marmalade (page 233)

- Lunch: Jackfruit Lettuce Tacos (page 249) with three to five ounces of roasted turkey, chicken, or wild-caught fish

- Dinner: Rainbow Vegetable-Noodle Salad (page 260) with a side of greens and vegetables sautéed in butter and garlic

- Dessert: Two to three squares of dark chocolate

Friday

- Breakfast: Skip!

- Lunch: Roasted Spaghetti Squash with Broccoli-Sprout Pesto (page 261) and a side of three to five ounces of grilled grass-fed steak

- Dinner: Grilled Halibut with Tomatoes and Hearts of Palm (page 255) with half a cup of wild or brown rice and unlimited steamed or roasted broccoli

- Dessert: Half a cup of berries topped with a drizzle of unsweetened cream or honey

Saturday

- Breakfast: LUV Pancakes (page 236)

- Lunch: Turkey Patties with Leek and Mint (page 243) and a side salad of mixed greens and raw cut vegetables, dressed with Tart-Cherry Vinaigrette (page 252)

- Dinner: Instant Pot Steak Shawarma Stew (page 253)

- Dessert: Three-quarters of a cup of sliced peaches or nectarines dipped in three squares of melted dark chocolate

Sunday

- Breakfast: Broccoli Sprout, Green Pepper, and Red Onion Frittata (page 238)

- Lunch: Whole Roasted Cauliflower with Green Tahini Dressing (page 247) with a side salad of mixed roasted vegetables

- Dinner: Roasted Cod with Broccolini (page 259) and half a cup of wild or brown rice

- Dessert: Two squares of dark chocolate dipped in one tablespoon of almond butter

Abiding by the LUV dietary principles is easier than you think. And once you learn how to make substitutions in some of your favorite dishes, you'll be able to cook your own recipes and return to your classic cookbooks. The LUV recipes will give you a general sense of how to apply the guidelines to virtually any meal and help you master the art of acid-dropping cuisine.

Although I encourage you to follow my seven-day meal plan so you don't have to think about what to eat during the first week on the program, you can design your own protocol by choosing the recipes that appeal to you. Most of the ingredients are widely available. Remember to go grass-fed, organic, and wild whenever possible. When choosing olive or coconut oil, reach for the extra-virgin varieties. Although all the ingredients listed in the recipes were chosen to be gluten- and sugar-free, always check labels to be sure, particularly if you're buying a food processed by a manufacturer (e.g., mayonnaise and mustard). You can never control what goes into a product, but you can control what goes into your meals.

Be patient with yourself as you get used to this dietary code, which will speak directly and kindly to your genome—and your metabolism. This first week is your starting point, but it may take a few weeks to break old dietary habits and learn how to make smart substitutions. If, for example, you're someone who has been addicted to sugary beverages, then just switch to beverages that meet the LUV protocol and make that your main goal in the first week. Do whatever you need to make this transition. If you take this one step, one meal at a time, you'll eventually get to your destination: a healthier body with optimum control of uric acid.

CHAPTER 9

Week 2: Companions to LUV

Sleep, Movement, Nature, and an Eating Window

Every one should be his own physician. We ought to assist, and not to force nature. Eat with moderation . . . Nothing is good for the body but what we can digest. What medicine can procure digestion? Exercise. What will recruit strength? Sleep.

— Voltaire

When Marcus was diagnosed with mild cognitive impairment at just fifty-eight years old, he took the diagnosis seriously and vowed to fight back before it progressed to anything more serious. It was his wife and teenage children who started noticing his unusual forgetfulness, lapses in judgment, anxiety, and changes in mood and overall behavior. They encouraged him to seek help. Although he had no family history of premature cognitive decline or Alzheimer's disease, his neurologist urged him to work hard at improving his lifestyle habits in a bid to stave off further decline, not to mention a graver diagnosis such as dementia. The neurologist warned him that many of her patients didn't have any history of neurological problems, yet they went on to develop cognitive issues for reasons that likely stemmed from environmental factors rather than genetic ones. This doctor happened to be well versed in the relationship between uric acid and the risk of neurodegeneration. Laboratory tests showed that indeed, his uric acid was on the high side, and although Marcus was not obese, he did qualify as overweight with metabolic syndrome.

Marcus saw himself as an active person who loved casual bike riding on weekends, but he knew his beer-drinking days were over and that it was time to focus on improving his nutrition, being more active throughout the week, and solving his chronic insomnia problem, which had started when he turned fifty. Eight years of poor sleep were catching up with him. When he asked the neurologist to recommend a book he could read to educate himself, she mentioned *Grain Brain,* and it helped set him on the right path. Marcus changed his eating style and habits—and his life.

I have never met Marcus and was never part of his treatment, but his transformation was so profound that he shared his experience with me on my website. Within weeks of upping his exercise habits and cutting carbs, sugar, and wheat (and his beloved uric acid–raising beer), everything about him improved—including his mental faculties. Even his chronic insomnia abated, particularly once he dropped the weight and cured his sleep apnea, which had previously caused disruptions in his sleep.

It's extraordinary to think we can halt—or, dare I suggest, *reverse*—the progression of cognitive decline just through simple lifestyle hacks. The key, however, is to fix uric acid bedlam as soon as possible, preferably long before any symptoms present themselves. And now research reveals a clear and direct association between elevated uric acid—one parameter of metabolism—and the risk of cognitive deficits. As you read in chapter 4, chronically high uric acid may induce oxidative stress and inflammation in the brain, damaging cerebral tissue. And high uric acid directly insults the brain's memory center, the hippocampus, and several of the studies I've cited demonstrate uric acid's role in brain shrinkage.

This was likely a root cause of Marcus's mental blips at such a young age. Luckily, he took action fast and managed to turn things around before serious illness permanently established itself beyond repair.

Colleagues of mine who routinely diagnose cognitive problems in patients, from mild impairment all the way to full-blown Alzheimer's disease, are now testing for uric acid as part of their cutting-edge screening protocol. My friend and fellow neurologist Dr. Dale Bredesen has achieved remarkable results in his own patients when they rebalance their metabolisms by adjusting lifestyle factors, including micronutrient levels, hormone levels, and sleep quality. As he said to my podcast audience, a disease like Alzheimer's, as it is currently treated, is not one condition but several. These conditions are driven by various mechanisms and typically manifest themselves in various ways and at various ages. But all are dramatically influenced by imbalances in metabolic factors that can trigger "downsizing" in the brain, as he calls it. And among these factors is—you guessed it—the level of uric acid coursing through the body.

Now that you're in your second week, my hope is that you have the nutritional playbook down and the medicinal power of food already working inside you. If you are using a continuous glucose monitor, don't forget to take as many notes as possible so you can chart patterns in your levels throughout the day and in response to your environment. In this second week, you'll bring your focus to three other habits that will drop acid: sleep, exercise, and time-restricted eating. These are your lifestyle companions to LUV. You can repeat the first week's seven-day menu plan to make it really easy or start to incorporate other recipes from chapter 11.

SLEEP HYGIENE

It's no longer a mystery that quality sleep is vital to health. As Dr. Casey Means shared with me in conversation, "Sleep might be our greatest metabolic hack, and loss of sleep is one of the easiest ways to thwart our metabolic health." Sleep affects every organ system and every disease state. And while we've all known anecdotally that not getting enough sleep is a threat to health, not until recently have we gained a new understanding as to *why*—and it relates to uric acid.

Within just the past few years, sleep research has finally moved into the territory of tracking uric acid levels among patients who sleep poorly, and you know from chapter 5 that the results are in: elevated uric acid is consistently documented in poor sleepers. To be sure, the definition of poor sleep ranges from not getting enough sleep and lacking proper time in deep, restorative sleep to experiencing disruptions throughout the night and sleeping far too much. The relationship between poor sleep and elevated uric acid is so strong that sleep researchers are now calling elevated uric acid an *independent risk factor* for sleep disorders such as obstructive sleep apnea. And we know that this is a two-way street, because poor sleep's negative effects on metabolism and inflammatory processes mean that it also directly increases the risk of elevated uric acid. In fact, sleep is so dialed into our metabolism—and vice versa—that improving one automatically boosts the other.

Did your sleep improve at all during week 1? It might have without your doing anything at all in the slumber department other than tweaking your diet. But if you usually get fewer than six hours of sleep per night, you can start increasing that period of time to at least seven hours. This is the bare minimum if you want to have normal, healthful levels of the fluctuating hormones in your body that control metabolism. If you've been getting by on, say, five or six hours, then work your way up to seven in fifteen- or thirty-minute intervals (more on this below).

Although there are a few rare individuals who are short sleepers, meaning they can get by on fewer than six hours of sleep—some as little as four—without any health consequences, that doesn't describe the vast majority of people. You're fooling yourself if you think you can get away with sleeping like Leonardo da Vinci, who allegedly slept for a total of two hours per day in the form of twenty-minute naps roughly every four hours. You know you need more than what you're banking. Don't dismiss the value of sleep in your life. It's free medicine.

As you put the focus on sleep this week, make sure you're doing all you can to maximize high-quality, restful sleep. Consistent, high-quality sleep can be tough to come by, and there will be days when daily life simply gets in the way of a good night. That's okay. Remember, we're aiming for progress, not perfection. It might also take time to settle into a new sleep routine if your sleep patterns in the past have been erratic and unpredictable. The body loves predictability—it's how it keeps its *homeo-stasis,* or equilibrium. And there's no better way to support that homeo-stasis than to optimize your sleep. Don't expect to get a perfect night's rest right off the bat, but keep in mind that even a slightly higher quality of sleep will work wonders for your health and metabolism.

Below are some tips for establishing good sleep hygiene.

Maintain consistent sleep habits that match your rhythms: Go to bed and get up at roughly the same time seven days a week, every single day of the year—holidays and weekends included. Everyone has different sleep needs and personal circadian rhythms that are partly hardwired. It's true that there are such things as night owls and early risers. And sleep needs do change with age (most teenagers, for example, love to stay up late and sleep in because their adolescent physiology matches that pattern). Most of us need seven to nine hours of sleep, but more than a third of us report sleeping fewer than seven hours. As a general rule, aim to be in bed before midnight to make sure you reap enough restorative, non-rapid-eye-movement (non-REM) sleep, which dominates the early part of the night. And be as strict as possible about your wake time. Sleep quality is best improved by making sure you get up at the same time no matter what. This ensures that your circadian rhythm stays on cue and attuned to your body's needs.

Send the body signals of sleep: Keep your bedtime routine consistent and incorporate calming activities that tell your body it's time for sleep. These activities might include reading, a warm bath, writing in a journal, listening to music, drinking herbal tea, light stretching, deep breathing, meditating, or whatever you need to do to wind down. If anxieties run high at night and you find yourself ruminating in bed while trying to fall asleep, a good strategy is to spend time before bed writing down your worries on the left side of a piece of paper and coming up with at least one action item for addressing each worry on the right side. But don't take the worry to bed with you. When the worrisome thoughts intrude as you lie there, try to see them as floating above you and tell yourself they are not helpful. You'll deal with them tomorrow.

We're strict with our children at bedtime when they are young, but we often forget about our own bedtime rituals in the wake of adult life's distractions and competing demands. Bedtime rituals work wonders in helping us feel primed for slumber. It should come as no surprise that keeping brain- and eye-stimulating electronics in the bedroom is a bad idea. But people still break this most basic rule. You'll especially want to limit your exposure to blue light before bed by minimizing screen time (or by wearing blue-light-blocking glasses if you must be in front of a screen). The goal is to keep your bedroom a quiet, peaceful sanctuary free of bright lights, clutter, and rousing hardware (e.g., TVs, computers, tablets, phones, and so on). Maintain dim lighting. Cultivate a mood for sleep. When you set the right tone for sleep, you send your body the right signals for easy slumber.

LIGHT THERAPY: TIMING IS EVERYTHING

While you'll want to avoid bright lights before bedtime, especially blue light from screens, it helps to let natural sunlight (which does contain blue light) shine in first thing in the morning. Early morning light will reset your body's clock naturally by traveling through your eyes to the suprachiasmatic nucleus, a tiny part of your brain that serves as the central pacemaker for your circadian rhythm.

Be cool and comfortable: Anyone who has tried to sleep well in a hot and stuffy room knows from the experience that it doesn't work. If possible, set the bedroom temperature between sixty-five and seventy degrees. This is the ideal range for sleep, though it may vary by a few degrees from person to person. Our bodies are programmed to experience a slight dip in core temperature in the evening, promoting sleep. The temperature drop starts around two hours before you go to sleep and coincides with the release of the sleep-inducing hormone melatonin. So turning the thermostat down at night may help with temperature regulation and your body's internal needs, thereby supporting a "tight" night. Also think about your mattress, sheets, pillows, and sleepwear: you want them to maximize your comfort and keep you cool. You don't have to go out and buy all new goods, but invest in the best sleep products you can afford. Plenty of companies today sell high-quality sleep products that won't break the bank.

Work your way up to at least seven hours: Telling someone to go from a habit of sleeping five or six hours a night to seven or eight can be an unrealistic directive. It won't happen overnight (pun intended), and that's okay. Baby steps, baby steps—even in the sleep department. Here's what to do: make adjustments in fifteen- or thirty-minute increments over a series of days or weeks. Choose which side of the cycle—bedtime or wake time—you want to adjust. For most people, wake times are set in stone and pretty consistent, but bedtimes are more flexible. If that's the case for you, dial back your bedtime by fifteen minutes for a few days, then dial it back another fifteen minutes for a total of thirty minutes from your original bedtime. Maintain that routine for another several days until you feel ready to trim back another fifteen minutes. Do that until repeatedly you reach a fully blocked sleep time of seven or eight hours. This may take days or weeks to achieve, but the goal is worth the effort.

Avoid self-medicating with sleep aids: The occasional sleep aid won't kill you. But chronic use of them can become a problem. The goal is to arrive at sound sleep on a routine basis without extra help. I'm not referring to earplugs or eye masks here, both of which I approve of as sleep aids; I'm talking about over-the-counter and prescription drugs that artificially induce sleep—for example, "p.m." formulas that include sedating antihistamines such as diphenhydramine and doxylamine. Even if they claim to be nonaddictive, they can still create a psychological dependency. Better to regulate your sleep naturally.

No sleep aid, whether an over-the-counter formula or a prescription, induces natural sleep. Sedation is not the same as sleep. Granted, there may be a benefit to taking a short-term prescription sleep aid under the guidance of a doctor, and there may be a time and place for what I call sleep-promoting supplements such as melatonin and valerian root, which is derived from an herb. Cannabidiol (CBD) supplements formulated for sleep that do not contain the psychoactive compound tetrahydrocannabinol (THC) can also serve a sleep-supporting role on occasion when used correctly.[1] Although sleep-promoting supplements fall under the sleep-aid category, they are unique in their actions because they can help induce natural sleep. But in general, pill-free strategies to improve your sleep hygiene will likely outperform everything else in the long term.

I will add one caveat: sometimes deficiencies in certain nutrients and vitamins can aggravate sleep troubles. Although melatonin, the hormone that helps us fall asleep at night, is commonly talked about in sleep circles, most people don't actually have deficits in melatonin. According to my friend and colleague Dr. Michael Breus, a clinical psychologist and one of few doctors board-certified in sleep medicine, deficiencies in vitamin D and magnesium can be culprits in poor sleep. You may want to try adding those supplements to your regimen if sleep continues to escape you.

Identify and manage substances hostile to sleep: Any number of things—from prescription medicine to caffeine, alcohol, and nicotine—can disrupt your sleep. Both caffeine and nicotine are stimulants. Anyone who still smokes should adopt a plan to quit, for smoking alone will increase your risk of everything under the sun. As I recommended above, when it comes to caffeine, try to avoid it after 2:00 p.m. This will give your body time to process it so it doesn't affect sleep. The half-life of caffeine, or the time it takes for the body to break it down to half its original quantity and eventually clear it from the system, varies widely among people. It could range anywhere between 1.5 and 9.5 hours, but the average is approximately five to six hours. (Pregnancy, which places a huge demand on metabolism, can increase the half-life of caffeine by as much as fifteen hours, making pregnant women extra sensitive to it!) If you're super sensitive to caffeine and seem to metabolize it very slowly, you may want to back up this cutoff time to noon and move to drinks lower in caffeine.

Ask your doctor or pharmacist about the potential sleep repercussions of medications you take routinely. In fact, I'd also suggest that you revisit the list of drugs that can raise uric acid (see page 124) and make those part of your conversation, too. See if you can develop a plan of action to wean yourself from pharmaceuticals that could be contributing to metabolic problems. Of course, you don't want to stop taking any medically necessary drug, but you may find that as you move through this program, you'll ameliorate many symptoms and might not need to be as strongly medicated. Be aware that lots of over-the-counter medications can contain sleep-disrupting ingredients. Popular headache remedies, for example, often include caffeine.

Alcohol, while creating a sedative effect immediately upon consumption, can disrupt sleep while it's being processed by the body; one of the enzymes needed to break down alcohol has stimulating effects. Alcohol also causes the release of adrenaline and disrupts the production of serotonin, an important brain chemical that initiates sleep. Avoid alcohol within three hours of bedtime, a good cutoff time for meals, too, as noted below.

Time your dinner appropriately: No one likes to go to bed on a full or empty stomach. Find your sweet spot, leaving approximately three hours between dinnertime and bedtime. Also be aware of foods that can be difficult to digest easily before going to bed, such as fatty, cheesy, spicy, and fried foods. Everyone's experience with meal timing will be different. As a general rule, eat on a regular schedule throughout the day (ideally, as you'll soon read, within an eight-to-twelve-hour window). Erratic eating will disturb your circadian rhythm and throw important hormones, including those related to appetite and hunger, out of balance. If you've ever struggled with late-night cravings and eating, you can likely blame poor sleep habits that affect hormones related to hunger cues.

If you suffer from insomnia-causing nocturnal hypoglycemia (low nighttime blood glucose levels), try a bedtime snack. Nocturnal hypoglycemia is common among people with diabetes and other metabolic conditions. If your blood sugar drops too low, it causes the release of hormones that stimulate the brain and tell you to eat. Good bedtime snacks include those high in the amino acid tryptophan, which is a natural promoter of sleep. Foods high in tryptophan that won't raise uric acid include cottage cheese, eggs, and nuts (especially almonds). Just watch your portion size, however. A handful of nuts might be perfect, but a bagful is too many. Bedtime snacks often entail eating outside your optimal eating window, but once in a while, it's perfectly fine.

Use technology: The number of devices and products hitting the multibillion-dollar sleep-aid market is dizzying. From high-tech smartwatches and rings that can track the quality and quantity of your sleep to apps that offer a wide selection of stories and meditations for bedtime, there's no shortage of sleep-enhancing supplies.

One popular device that I've grown to love is the Ōura ring, created by Finnish inventor Petteri Lahtela, whom I've had the pleasure of interviewing on my podcast. He explained how important restorative sleep is for maintaining health and how the Ōura ring helps people truly understand the quality of their sleep and make changes to improve it.

I have found this device to be extremely helpful, though it's not the only product on the market for tracking your sleep. You can find other devices and apps that provide detailed information about the time you spend each night in light sleep, deep sleep, and REM sleep. You can learn how long it takes for you to fall sleep (sleep latency) and obtain a 360-degree picture of your sleep quality. You can then use the data to tweak certain things the next day—caffeine cutoff time, for example—in preparation for another night's sleep. It's real-time experimentation! You'll find more ideas on my curated list online at DrPerlmutter.com.

ACTIVATE TO DROP ACID

We intuitively know that exercise, like sleep, does a body good. But now we have an interesting new perspective to consider as to why exercise is so good for us: it helps us drop uric acid and avoid elevating it to abnormal levels. Exercise's forceful effects on supporting the healthy metabolism of sugar (including both glucose and fructose), reducing inflammation, fostering balanced hormones, boosting endothelial function in blood vessels (think nitric oxide and insulin signaling), and activating antioxidant processes and fat-burning switches such as the AMPK pathway are what define the magic of movement. All these positive outcomes act as a backstop to increased uric acid production. Some tips follow.

Start somewhere and get moving: Aim to engage in aerobic physical activity if you're not already doing so for a minimum of twenty minutes a day. Use this week to establish a routine you enjoy that gets your heart rate up by at least 50 percent of your resting baseline. Remember, you are creating new habits for a lifetime, and you don't want to get burned out easily by overdoing it and then quitting (or worse, getting injured). But you also don't want to become too comfortable and shy away from challenging your body in ways that boost health and increase longevity.

Ideally, and as I've advised in the past, a comprehensive workout should encompass a mix of cardio, strength training, and stretching. But if you're starting from scratch, begin slowly with cardio and then add strength training and stretching over time. Strength training can be done with classic gym equipment, free weights, or your own body weight in classes geared toward this activity. These activities often entail lots of stretching, too, but you don't need a formal class to work on maintaining your flexibility. You can perform many stretching exercises on your own—no guided instruction necessary.

Remember, in addition to all the cardiovascular and weight-management benefits you'll gain from exercise, studies show that people who, in addition to eating well, exercise regularly, compete in sports, or just walk at a good clip daily manage uric acid, maximize the health of their metabolisms, protect their brains from decline, and minimize major risk factors for virtually every chronic preventable disease.

If you've been leading a sedentary lifestyle, then simply go for a twenty-minute walk daily and add more minutes as you acclimate to your routine. Be realistic about your starting point: if you haven't exercised in a long time, you shouldn't run out the door and go for ten miles. The goal is sustainable movement!

Remove barriers to regular exercise: Plan how and when you will work out. Don't *find* time; *make* time. To that end, have your exercise clothes and shoes ready the night before no matter what time you choose to exercise. And prioritize the element of fun: forcing yourself through the motions will be a lot less effective in the long run than finding activities that excite and energize you. Switch up your routine if it isn't working for you. You can always add intensity to your workouts by increasing their speed and/or duration. If you're an avid hiker, for example, tackle more hills or carry a three- or five-pound free weight in each hand and perform some bicep curls as you walk. I have found the Apple watch helpful in setting and achieving goals for endurance, distance, heart rate, and so on.

Amp it up: For those of you who already maintain a fitness regimen, see if you can increase your workouts to a minimum of thirty minutes a day, at least five days a week, with the goal of eventually reaching sixty minutes daily. This might also be the week you try something different, such as joining a group exercise class or dusting off an old bicycle in the garage. These days, opportunities to exercise are everywhere, so there's really no excuse. The pandemic forced many of us to desert the gym and find ways to move within the confines of home. And I know plenty of people, loyal gym rats before the pandemic, who actually got fitter and leaner after devising workouts at home. The pandemic sparked an explosion of online programming. You can stream videos and exercise classes in the comfort of your own home. On-demand and live-streamed classes offered by companies such as Peloton, Daily Burn, and Alo Moves gained considerable popularity, even among people who don't own any equipment. You can complete a successful sweat session without any tools other than a water bottle, a towel, ample space in which to move, and a screen on which you can follow a set of moves with an instructor, either live or prerecorded. Do what speaks to you, your body, and your interests.

Don't underestimate the power of a group: Engaging in physical activity with other people helps keep you motivated and moving. Try drafting a friend into your exercise routine for one day each week. Consider joining a running or walking group. Ask a coworker if he or she would be interested in going for a walk at lunchtime. Active.com has a great assortment of local groups and activities — 5Ks, hikes, century rides (bicycle rides of one hundred miles or more), family-friendly sports, and other suggestions — as well as a variety of helpful articles for people starting an exercise plan. The site also offers a directory of virtual programs in your geographic area. Meetup.com provides a list of nearby group meetings, including walks and hikes.

Mix it up: Once you've found the routines you enjoy, you can schedule your daily routines around various types of exercise. For example, on Mondays, Wednesdays, and Fridays you might take a cardio class online or in a studio; on Tuesdays and Thursdays you might stream a yoga class from your living room. On Saturday, you might go for a hike with friends or swim laps in a pool, and you might take Sunday off to rest. I recommend getting out your calendar and scheduling physical activity: write down what you're going to do and when. If it's not formally scheduled, it's not likely to happen. Make the commitment to reach a point where you're moving at least an hour a day.

Make room for motionless days: If you have a day during which there's absolutely no time to devote to a continuous segment of formal exercise, which is bound to happen, think about the ways you can sneak in minutes of physical activity. All the research indicates that you can get the same health benefits from three ten-minute bouts of exercise as you can from a single thirty-minute workout. So if you're short on time on any given day, just break up your routine into bite-size chunks. And think of ways to combine exercise with other tasks: for example, make work calls while walking outside or watch your favorite show while completing a set of stretching exercises or yoga moves. If you own a bicycle but never find time to ride it, invest in a trainer, hook the back wheel into it, and you've got yourself a spin bike; you can cycle in the garage while multi-tasking on your smartphone.

If possible, limit the minutes you spend sitting down. If your job is relatively sedentary, get up and walk around for at least two minutes every hour; don't be caught sitting for hours on end. Remember, a mere two minutes of movement per hour can dramatically reduce the risk of premature death. The more you move throughout the day, the more your body stands to gain.

As I said in part 1, research shows that high-intensity exercise is associated with high levels of uric acid, at least in the acute phase. This is to be expected, because high-intensity exercise will increase muscle breakdown, which leads to elevated purines and ultimately elevated uric acid. However, the benefits exercise confers to metabolism, not to mention weight management, make exercise a true offset to elevated uric acid in the long term. And the vast majority of people are not going to overdo exercise to the point where they harm their bodies by having chronically elevated uric acid. If you're someone who enjoys intense forms of exercise, just be sure you're balancing your workouts with resting days and enough recovery periods in between high-intensity sessions.

NURTURE YOUR NATURE

It's human nature to enjoy the great outdoors. Shakespeare was right: "One touch of nature makes the whole world kin." Science has long documented nature's effects on physiology, from helping us regulate our emotions and combat stress to physically lowering inflammation, reducing blood pressure, and supporting immune function through a variety of mechanisms, one of which comes purely from the boost in vitamin D production that occurs when the sun hits our skin. One of the ways nature can be so influential on our stress levels is that it activates the relaxation-promoting parasympathetic nervous system, dampening the stress-promoting sympathetic nervous system and fostering a positive outlook. Studies show that being in nature lowers cortisol levels and helps us stay more even-keeled mentally. It also helps us become more focused, more empathic, and less impulsive. Other demonstrated benefits to immersing oneself in nature include improved sleep and reduced blood glucose — two key aspects of the overall goal of dropping uric acid. Studies directly tying nature therapy to lowering uric acid have yet to be completed: clinical trials are currently under way in patients with metabolic syndrome and cardiovascular risk factors whose uric acid levels are tracked as an important parameter.

The Japanese even have a name for the practice of spending time in nature in order to benefit from its healing effects: *Shinrin-yoku*, which translates as "taking in the forest atmosphere" or "forest bathing." I wrote about this at length in *Brain Wash*, citing a rich library of scientific data proving the power of Mother Nature in our health. Plan to spend more time in nature and see if you can commit to a thirty-minute walk in the woods — or in nature of some sort — at least once weekly. Mother Nature is one of our most accessible free companions to better health.

Obviously, not all of us live near the woods, but you can find plenty of substitutes wherever you are: nearby parks, mountainous regions, the beach or a lake, your backyard. Don't worry too much about accomplishing a specific goal while immersing yourself in nature. Instead, just try to take in the sounds, sights, and smells of the living things around you, using all your senses. Go barefoot if you can for some part of the experience! You can also combine your time in nature with other acid-dropping activities such as exercise. If you take a walk around your neighborhood first thing in the morning, for example, you'll reset your circadian rhythm with exposure to that early light.

PRACTICE TIME-RESTRICTED EATING

As I said in chapter 6, research on time-restricted eating (TRE) and metabolism indicates that limiting your meals to a twelve-hour window can improve insulin sensitivity, blood pressure, and immune function. It can also help lower inflammation and support the body's healthy circadian rhythm. The effects will help you maintain healthful uric acid levels.

Below are three options for TRE to choose from. If you've never fasted before, take the beginner's route and work your way up to the advanced version by the third week.

- **Beginner:** Consume all your meals within a twelve-hour window—say, between 8:00 a.m. and 8:00 p.m.—and do not eat outside that time frame.

- **Intermediate:** See if you can push breakfast to midmorning (e.g., 10:00 a.m.) and then stop eating by 8:00 p.m. Remember: every hour after the twelve-hour fasting mark moves you toward better metabolic health.

- **Advanced:** Skip breakfast and have your first meal of the day at noon, then eat your last meal by 8:00 p.m. This is sometimes called the 16:8 split.

- **Extreme:** Try a twenty-four- or forty-eight-hour fast. I don't recommend taking it to the forty-eight-hour level, however, until you've fine-tuned your metabolism on the LUV program and have established healthful new baseline measurements of metabolic health.

Outside the eating window, you can drink water and, if you're delaying or skipping breakfast, you can drink coffee and tea, but do not add any calories in the form of milk or cream. Outside the eating window, keep your beverages totally calorie-free.

Feel free to mix and match your TRE window. Maybe you'll maintain a 12:12 split on Monday, Wednesday, Friday, and Sunday and switch to the 16:8 split on the other days—or vice versa. Getting used to TRE is like getting used to regular exercise. It might be challenging at first, but with time and practice as your body acclimates to a new metabolism, it will get easier—and you will one day look forward to timing your meals, just as you time most everything else important in your life.

CHAPTER 10

Week 3: A Sweet Opportunity

Learn to LUV and Live High

Healing is a matter of time, but it is sometimes also a matter of opportunity.

— HIPPOCRATES

I'VE STATED IT BEFORE, and I'll state it again: what you choose to eat and drink is one of the most important decisions you make each day. It may even be *the* most important decision. Food is a gateway to exquisitely managing uric acid and, in turn, remodeling your body. It is a ticket to a life of vibrant health and well-being. Now that you're in the third week, I trust you're in a better place than you were just a couple of weeks ago. You're choosing to eat better, move more, and focus on achieving restful sleep. Now what?

This is the week to streamline your new routine and pay special attention to the weak spots in your life. As you move forward, think about what else you could be doing to improve your life and take your health to greater heights.

ESTABLISH YOUR RHYTHM

What was most challenging over the past two weeks? Did you miss having your favorite meals? Are you having difficulty getting to bed on time? Is it hard to carve out time for workout sessions or walks in nature? Are you feeling overwhelmed? If so, use this week to find a rhythm in your new routine. Identify areas in your life where you struggle to maintain the protocol, and see what you can do to rectify that. Below are a few tips that you might find helpful in your transformation.

Spot your flaws and focus on them: Be honest with yourself—what is your biggest weakness? We all have at least one. Is your addiction to processed sugar- and carb-heavy foods hard to nix? Is insomnia disrupting your best efforts? Do you lack the willpower for regular exercise? Write down what, exactly, continues to be difficult and see what you can do to defuse those bombs in your life. Don't be afraid of them, but do something about them. Establish at least three nonnegotiables you think you can realistically stick to—e.g., abstinence from soda pop and sweetened beverages, keeping your smartphone out of the bedroom at night, making sure to move at least two minutes per hour and get outside to soak in Mother Nature at least once weekly, even if it's just in your backyard or a local park. Hold yourself accountable.

Articulate your goals and values in writing: Write a letter to yourself describing your immediate and long-term goals along with the reasons why you want to transform your life. Read it aloud each morning and evening and post it wherever you'll see it regularly—by your desk, for example. Find what most drives you and remind yourself repeatedly why you've made this investment in your future. Maybe you want to keep up with your active children, alleviate a serious health condition, lose significant weight, have a more intimate relationship with your partner, feel more energized and rested, or be more efficient and productive at work. When you write out your intentions and articulate them, you're more likely to maintain the habits that will ultimately help you realize your goals. Be specific: for example, "I want to feel vibrant all day long"; "I want to trek Glacier National Park with my kids next year"; "I want to lose thirty pounds"; or "I don't want to die the way my parents did." Keep the big picture in plain sight. This will help you not only maintain a healthful lifestyle but also get back on track if you slip up occasionally.

Plan every week in advance in as much detail and as precisely as possible: It's amazing how much careful planning can help us stick to our resolutions and reach our goals. We don't plan big road trips or exotic vacations abroad without mapping everything out, and the same should be true of our day-to-day habits. It helps to set aside a few minutes over the weekend to plan the upcoming week and take into consideration your agenda, appointments, and commitments. Map out your meals and grocery list, noting when you'll shop and where. On days when you need to eat away from home, plan what you will eat on the go and aim to take along meals you've prepared at home so you're not stuck grabbing food prepared elsewhere (more on eating out below).

Schedule your workouts, and if you anticipate a day when a single full session will not be possible, get creative. For example, move a lunch meeting to the afternoon and use your midday break to at least go for a brisk walk. Block out your sleeping hours every night, and be sure to maintain the same bedtime; be religious about it. Find opportunities to combine exercise with being outside in nature (e.g., scenic walks, hikes, runs, bicycle rides). Be on the lookout for those days when you know you'll get home late and won't have the energy or time to cook. Have a contingency plan in place. This is especially helpful if you have children to feed. Remember, this transformation is as much about the people around you as it is about you.

In chapter 8, I recommended keeping a food journal, but you could expand that to include a calendar and record as many details as possible. Take cues from professional athletes and Olympians: they rigorously plan every minute of their days, from waking time to workouts to meals to engagements with other people to downtime to bedtime. It's how they are able to perform at their very best. You can, too.

Tackle toxic stress: If it's simply psychological stress you feel, and you've tried your usual coping skills, see about finding a therapist to help you tailor mental strategies that work for you. We all carry a certain level of stress, but sometimes it helps to seek professional support. It's never been easier to find a therapist, given that the pandemic helped promote telemedicine; you don't even have to go anywhere to seek help 24-7. Plenty of apps are on the market (with likely more coming) that connect you securely and privately with mental health professionals through a smartphone, tablet, or other device.

A lot of our stress today comes from too much exposure to the unceasing cycle of negative news. Try going on a media diet and being strict with the news you expose yourself to. Limit your screen time each day. We tend to underestimate how much the news can literally make us sick. The media we watch and listen to daily has an impact on our thinking, behavior, emotions, and even our body chemistry, because stress changes our eating and sleeping patterns while triggering unhealthful levels of stress hormones and further stoking fear and worry. Be especially sure to avoid the news before bedtime. Create boundaries, even if that means unfollowing someone on social media who continually posts content that rattles you. Be as judicious with your media consumption as you are with your nutrition. Find ways to destress through mindful practices; again, you can download apps to help you do just that and let technology act as a pocket therapist.

Be consistent but open to flexibility: Each of us slips away from good habits once in a while, and that's what makes us human. We're all bound to have days when we stay sedentary, eat poorly, and toss health-promoting strategies out the window. After sticking to the program as closely as possible for three weeks, aim to live by this book's guidelines at least 80 percent of the time, and know that you'll veer off track the remaining 20 percent of the time. Between vacations, holidays, special occasions, and dinners out, you'll fill up that 20 percent and be fine. Just don't let a small slip derail you forever.

To that end, remember to find consistency in your daily patterns. Consistency is not about rigidity. It's about behaving in ways that serve you without making you feel like you're going to extremes or forcing yourself to do something you don't like. Finding your own unique version of consistency will be key to success. You'll figure out what works best for you and what doesn't. Practice may make perfect, but let's go with practice makes progress.

EATING OUT SMARTLY

On most days of the week, commit to eating meals that you prepare yourself. Eventually you will brave eating out at a restaurant and enjoy meals prepared by others. As you navigate menus, focus on dishes that are clean, simple, and abide by the LUV Diet rules (the ten guidelines on page 175). See if you can return to your favorite restaurants and order off the menu while still following the protocol. If you find it too challenging, try new restaurants that might cater to your needs.

It's not that hard to make any menu work as long as you're savvy about your decisions. Watch out for elaborate dishes made with a plethora of ingredients and sauces that are likely loaded with added sugar and salt. Prioritize fresh vegetables and salads with sides of healthful, low-purine protein, but be careful about ingredients you wouldn't use at home, such as commercial vegetable oils, dressings, and condiments. Forget fried items and stick with steamed or baked selections. Replace starchy sides such as bread and potatoes with green salads topped simply with extra virgin olive oil, or bring one of my acid-lowering vinaigrettes to the restaurant. When in doubt, ask about the dishes, and don't be afraid to speak directly with the head cook or chef so you know what's really on the menu. Like someone with a serious food allergy, in whom a misstep could result in a trip to the ER, you deserve to know what's in the food you're ordering.

ESTABLISH YOUR GO-TO STAPLES

People who maintain lean, fit bodies with high metabolisms often rely on the same everyday wholesome meals and do not veer too far afield (or depend on meals with a lot of ingredients). They have their mainstay dishes they can trust to keep them nourished. You'll find plenty of original recipes in chapter 11 as well as online at DrPerlmutter.com. Following are some simple meals that you can repeat day after day. Don't underestimate the power of leftovers—you can always whip up something for lunch or dinner using some of the cooked vegetables or proteins from the day before!

Staple Breakfast Ideas (with Coffee)

* Two pasture-raised eggs any style, with a side of seasonal vegetables pan-fried with extra virgin olive oil or butter, plus two slices of avocado (one-fourth of the whole fruit)

* One serving (about one cup) of plain unsweetened full-fat Greek-style yogurt (with active live cultures), topped with chia or flax seeds, chopped walnuts, fresh berries, a sprinkle of cinnamon or cardamom, and an optional drizzle of honey

* A simple smoothie, made from a quarter cup of canned unsweetened coconut milk, a quarter cup of water (or more for desired consistency), a quarter cup of frozen berries, a quarter of a ripe avocado, a tablespoon of raw unsalted sunflower seeds or almonds, a tablespoon of hemp hearts (hulled hemp seeds), a tablespoon of organic no-sugar-added

sunflower-seed butter or almond butter, a half-inch piece of peeled and chopped ginger root, and half a teaspoon of ground cinnamon—or try my Raspberry Tahini Smoothie or Apple Pie Smoothie (both on page 269).

Staple Lunch and Dinner Ideas

- A large salad made with mixed baby greens, raw cut vegetables (e.g., broccoli, green bell peppers, celery, and cucumber), pomegranate seeds, chopped raw unsalted nuts, chopped red onion, cherry tomatoes, a tablespoon each of fresh thyme and rosemary, and three to four ounces of diced cooked chicken breast or turkey, dressed with Tart-Cherry Vinaigrette (page 252) or simply extra virgin olive oil and the juice of one lemon

- Three to five ounces of baked or roasted chicken or grilled wild-caught fish with a side of steamed above-ground vegetables and half a cup of wild or brown rice mixed with a tablespoon of raw pine nuts or sliced almonds

- Mixed vegetables (e.g., broccoli, red onion, green beans, bell peppers, asparagus, brussels sprouts, mushrooms) stir-fried in avocado oil, with three to five ounces of grilled chicken, cold-water wild-caught fish, or grass-fed steak and an optional side of half a cup of gluten-free grain

- Vegetable and protein "tacos" made with grilled or roasted vegetables and canned wild-caught salmon or cubed cooked chicken or pork served inside lettuce cups and topped with one of my vinaigrettes or simply extra virgin olive oil

As you can likely guess from these suggestions, you should try to include at least one acid-lowering ingredient in each meal. Make large batches of acid-dropping salad dressings—Tart-Cherry Vinaigrette (page 252), Lemon Broccoli-Seed Tahini Dressing (page 248), Green Tahini Dressing (page 247)—and those can be your mainstay toppings for salad greens and steamed or roasted vegetables.

Never run out of vegetables to complete a meal: flash-frozen vegetables and berries you keep stocked in the freezer are perfectly fine if you're unable to buy fresh produce for whatever reason. Keep tart or Bing cherries on hand for snacking if you love cherries. Have some reliable portable nutrition, too. If you know me, you know I usually travel with avocados, nuts, and canned sockeye salmon.

Canned foods can be excellent sources of nutrition, as long as you're careful about which canned products you're buying and you steer clear of added sugar and sodium. My top canned picks include tomatoes, spinach (contains more vitamin C per serving than its fresh counterpart), beans (e.g., kidney, navy, black, pinto), chickpeas, olives, green beans, artichoke hearts, and hearts of palm. Cartons of organic soups (e.g., lentil, roasted tomato) that are low in sodium and contain no added sugar can also be good choices. Just be sure to read your labels. You can make a meal with these soups by tossing in more vegetables and a handful of healthful protein, such as diced cooked chicken or a leftover piece of fish from the night before. Watch out for canned fruit that is labeled "packed in its own juice." That could be a euphemism for fruit juice concentrate, which you do not want.

THE POWER OF FOOD PAIRING

What you eat and when you eat matter. But so does what *order* you eat your foods in. Never eat what Dr. Casey Means calls naked carbohydrates—carbs without any accompanying fat, protein, or fiber. Research has shown that when carbohydrates are eaten first in the meal, before any protein or fat, the glucose response is often higher than it is when those carbohydrates are eaten later in the meal. One study showed that when vegetables and chicken are consumed fifteen minutes before carbohydrates (in this study, ciabatta and orange juice), glucose levels after the meal were decreased by 27 percent after thirty minutes and almost 37 percent after sixty minutes.[1] Moreover, insulin levels one and two hours after the meal were significantly lower when protein and vegetables were eaten before the carbohydrates. Combining fat and carbs can also help offset the glucose spike from the carbs. The simple toss of a few raw nuts into a carb-heavy meal can have dramatic effects on the way your body responds.

Although I should hope you won't be eating white bread again anytime soon, it's worth noting that in a study in which people were given white bread with almonds, their glucose spikes afterward were significantly lower than they were when the white bread was eaten alone. In addition, the more almonds the participants ate, the more their glucose was reduced.[2] And in insulin-resistant individuals, high amounts of fiber are shown to be associated not only with reduced post-meal glucose spikes and insulin levels but also with reduced glycemic variability. Glycemic variability, you'll recall, is a real deal breaker for our metabolism. Great sources of fiber include legumes, above-ground vegetables, whole fruits, nuts, and seeds such as flax, chia, pumpkin, and sesame. Try to eat a minimum of thirty-five grams of fiber per day.

GAIN A NEW PERSPECTIVE AND FIND YOUR OPPORTUNITIES

My final lesson to you in this third week is to start to view health and, conversely, illness, as sweet *opportunities*. You have an opportunity that you may never have seen coming until the pandemic hit. Let me explain.

As I crossed the finish line with this manuscript, the COVID-19 pandemic was surging across many parts of the United States, and the Delta variant was spreading ferociously, claiming even more lives. We've all just been through an extremely difficult, trying, and exhausting couple of years, and I hope they will not repeat themselves anytime soon. We are learning to live with the threat of this new virus, which will seemingly last forever in our environment, at least for now. But there's a sweet silver lining to embrace in this endeavor: when there's an existential threat to manage daily, we have a powerful motivating force to do everything we can to stay healthy, sane, and safe. And that includes keeping our bodies as fit as possible—fit in our organs, systems, minds, and sense of well-being.

The virus that causes COVID-19, SARS-CoV-2, does not discriminate—it will infect whomever it can and start replicating. Every human is a potential host. That's simply what viruses do to survive. But we've witnessed stark contrasts in way the resulting disease progresses in various people. While the virus doesn't discriminate in terms of who gets infected, it does discriminate in how it manifests itself. Perhaps no other infectious agent that humans have encountered has been as wily and unpredictable as this menace. COVID exposed all our preexisting issues, ranging from social inequality to each individual's true underlying state of health. While we like to think we're a healthy nation, with the best health care in the world, COVID has taught us otherwise.

When my son, Dr. Austin Perlmutter, an internal medicine physician, penned an article for *Medium* that addressed the ways in which COVID is an opportunistic infection, it got me thinking.[3] What he meant was that COVID takes advantage of patients whose immune systems are not functioning optimally. In the past we would have considered less-than-optimal immune function to be a characteristic of people who have had, for example, chemotherapy or radiation treatment, exposure to immune-suppressing medications after organ transplantation, or a diagnosed autoimmune disease. But as Austin poignantly pointed out, we now need to broaden our scope and accept the notion that so many of our most common degenerative conditions, from diabetes and obesity to dementias, compromise immune function and allow the SARS-CoV-2 virus the opportunity to do its dirty work. As my son wrote, "Our chronic health conditions have created a foundation of unhealthy immunity. They represent a major susceptibility to infections, and COVID-19 has proven itself capable of exploiting this weakness...The difference between infections and chronic diseases may not be as significant as we once believed. Instead, our risk for severe complications from an infection may be more about our underlying immunity than the pathogen itself."

We are living in an age of degenerative and man-made diseases— ailments we bring on ourselves that are almost entirely avoidable. Just as we can each choose to smoke and live with a greatly increased risk of death, we can also choose to be metabolically sick and live with those consequences. If you live in an industrialized nation, you're not likely to die from malnutrition, starvation, or even from an infection if you're healthy. But worldwide, high blood pressure, obesity, hypertension, and smoking are four of the top five risk factors for death—all predominantly preventable risk factors.[4] As this book has shown, at the heart of our health challenges today is a long-standing and deep-rooted problem with our metabolism, which directly translates to immune dysfunction.

While it may have taken a pandemic to shine a light on the fact that our underlying conditions don't play well with COVID, scientists have long demonstrated that everything from heart disease to cancer can be understood through mechanisms of faulty immunity. And faulty immunity has everything to do with faulty metabolism. More to the point, as you've now learned, central to the threat to metabolism and therefore stable immune function is a persistent elevation of uric acid—now common in developed nations around the world. Metabolic issues are an acquired immunocompromised state, and managing levels of uric acid is turning out to be an incredibly powerful tool in keeping us metabolically intact—and physiologically sound. When we measure abnormal elevations of uric acid, we are receiving information that's equal parts a warning and an opportunity to intervene. And now that we know the value of optimizing immunity in the wake of a prolonged clash with COVID, there's no better time to rein in an unhealthy metabolism and keep close tabs on uric acid along the way.

To this end, I encourage you to go back to your written goals and values and add that word: *opportunity*. Then add a list of things you want to change, reverse, or ameliorate. Go ahead and write down all the "bad" things you hope to improve. Be as specific or general as you like. Examples: low energy, type 2 diabetes, depression, severe anxiety, OCD, bipolar disorder, weight gain, chronic pain, arthritis, headaches, migraines, digestive issues, brain fog, binge eating, psoriasis, kidney disease, gout, coronary artery disease, premature aging—whatever you write down, add the word *opportunity*. And think about that for a moment. Take it in. Own it. Embrace this new perspective.

And remember that you control your health destiny. When you learn to LUV, you can live high.

CHAPTER 11

Recipes to LUV

AT DAILY DOSE (DAILYDOSELIFE.COM), the founder and CEO, Tricia Williams, lives by the motto "Reach for the kitchen cabinet before the medicine cabinet." No doubt it's a dictum I can most definitely stand behind and preach myself. Tricia's mission is to help people find better health through food, and, like me, she understands that the future of health care lies in prevention. After a decade of creating custom meal programs for professional athletes, celebrities, and high performers, she founded Daily Dose to make healthful, easy-to-prepare, and delicious meals accessible to anyone. And she knows the science and art of culinary genius. She earned a food therapy certification from Annemarie Colbin at the Natural Gourmet Institute, where she learned to use the kitchen as a pharmacy.

It was a joy to collaborate with her on original recipes that meet the LUV guidelines while being easy to prepare and outrageously delicious, packed with flavor and nutrition. In addition to these recipes, you'll find an assortment of others at DrPerlmutter.com. Most of my recipes only take minutes to prepare as everyday meals, but you'll want to devote time to a choice few for a weekend feast with friends and family. For unusual ingredients, I've made a few extra notes for you in various recipes so there's no confusion about where to find unfamiliar items. The good news is that between the bounty of foods now found in our everyday markets and online destinations, there's ample access to these ingredients. Local farmers markets can also offer the freshest seasonal food around. Whenever possible, choose organic and non-GMO ingredients; seek wild-caught fish and pasture-raised eggs.

If there are any ingredients you don't like, find smart substitutions. Onions, for example, are used in many of these recipes because they contain uric acid–lowering compounds (e.g., quercetin), but you can choose another vegetable, such as celery or fennel, as a replacement. Shallots are in the onion family but don't have the same sharp flavor and intense heat as your typical red or white onion; many people find them to be an excellent alternative. Broccoli seeds are great to toss into a variety of dishes, and you can buy one- or two-pound bags to have at the ready or keep a spice grinder filled with them for easy crushing and dispensing during meal prep. (Sometimes broccoli seeds are used whole in baked recipes for texture, and other times they are ground or cracked and used as a garnish or as an addition to salads and such.)

A quick note about salt: given the lessons you've learned, please use it judiciously and sparingly. Most of these recipes allow for a "pinch of sea salt, or to taste," but if you're managing any metabolic issues, you would do well to avoid it entirely. Salt intake can be expertly controlled when you prepare meals from scratch and don't use processed or prepackaged products. These recipes will help you learn how to assemble delicious, nutrient-dense meals without added ingredients that will sabotage your health. I hope you experiment with these recipes and tailor them to your liking using the main guidelines of the LUV Diet.

Bon appétit!

BREAKFAST

Coconut Pudding

Yield: 4 servings
Prep time: About 18 minutes

For the pudding

> 1 pound fresh or thawed frozen young Thai coconut meat (see Note)
>
> ¼ cup water
>
> 1 tablespoon granulated allulose, or to taste
>
> 1 teaspoon vanilla extract

For the topping

> ¼ cup raw unsalted cashews, chopped
>
> ½ teaspoon nigella seeds
>
> 1 teaspoon hemp hearts
>
> ½ cup pitted and halved fresh or thawed frozen tart cherries
>
> ½ cup fresh or thawed frozen blueberries
>
> ½ cup fresh or thawed frozen raspberries

Place the coconut meat, water, allulose, and vanilla in a blender. Blend until smooth and creamy. Refrigerate for 1 hour.

In a small bowl, mix together cashews, nigella seeds, and hemp hearts.

Spoon the pudding into four serving bowls. Top with the cherries and berries and sprinkle with the nut-and-seed mixture.

NOTE: Fresh young Thai coconut meat can be found refrigerated and/or frozen in most grocery stores.

Yogurt with Ginger Carrot Marmalade

Yield: 2 servings
Prep time: About 30 minutes

For the crunch

1 teaspoon hemp hearts

1 teaspoon nigella seeds

For the marmalade

2 cups peeled and grated carrots

2 unpeeled Granny Smith apples, cored and grated

2 cups water

2 teaspoons orange zest

¼ cup freshly squeezed lemon juice

1 teaspoon peeled and grated fresh ginger

½ teaspoon ground cardamom

½ cup granulated allulose

12 ounces plain unsweetened full-fat Greek-style or regular yogurt

Combine the hemp hearts and nigella seeds in a small bowl. Set aside.

Combine the carrots, apples, water, and orange zest in a medium saucepan. Bring to a boil over medium-high heat.

Reduce the heat to medium. Add the lemon juice, ginger, cardamom, and allulose. Continue to cook for 20 minutes, or until thickened. Remove from the heat and allow the mixture to cool to room temperature.

Spoon the yogurt into two serving bowls. Top with the ginger carrot marmalade and sprinkle with the reserved seed mixture.

Poached Apples and Yogurt

Yield: 4 servings
Prep time: About 30 minutes

4 unpeeled apples, cored (see Note)

½ cup granulated allulose

2 cups fruity red wine

1 cup water

1 tablespoon tart cherry extract (see Note)

1 teaspoon freshly squeezed lemon juice

1 cinnamon stick

2 cardamom pods

12 ounces plain unsweetened full-fat labneh or yogurt (see Note)

2 tablespoons sliced raw unsalted almonds

2 tablespoons chopped raw unsalted cashews

Quarter the apples and set aside.

Combine the allulose, red wine, water, tart cherry extract, lemon juice, cinnamon stick, and cardamom in a medium saucepan and bring to a boil over medium-high heat. Reduce the heat to a simmer and add the apples. Cook for 25 minutes, or until the apples are soft.

Remove the apples with a slotted spoon and set aside. Return the poaching liquid to medium heat and reduce by three-quarters, around 25 to 30 minutes. Remove from the heat and allow the liquid to cool until it's just slightly warm or at room temperature.

Divide the reserved apple quarters among four serving bowls. Spoon the labneh over the apples, sprinkle with the almonds and cashews, and spoon some poaching liquid over the yogurt.

NOTE: Braeburn and Pink Lady apples are ideal choices for their sweetness, but you can choose other apples so long as you avoid sour varieties such as Granny Smith. Do not peel them, because there's quercetin in the skin. Labneh is a Middle Eastern cheese made from strained yogurt that's tangier, thicker, and creamier than traditional yogurt. If you can't find it in your local market, any plain unsweetened full-fat yogurt will do. Tart cherry extract can be found in health food stores or online.

Chocolate, Almond Butter, and Chia Pudding

Yield: 2 servings
Prep time: About 12 minutes

½ cup canned unsweetened coconut milk

½ cup water

2 tablespoons raw cacao powder

1 tablespoon granulated allulose

1 teaspoon vanilla extract

Pinch of sea salt, or to taste

¼ cup chia seeds

2 tablespoons unsalted raw almond butter

¾ cup fresh or thawed frozen raspberries

Whisk the coconut milk, water, cacao, allulose, vanilla, and salt together in a medium bowl. Stir in the chia seeds. Cover the mixture and set aside for 1 hour, allowing the seeds to bloom. Refrigerate, covered, for at least two hours.

Spoon the pudding into two serving bowls, top with the almond butter and raspberries, and serve.

Sprouted Quinoa Porridge

Yield: 2 *servings*
Prep time: About 18 minutes

- 1 cup uncooked quinoa
- 1 cup water
- 1 cup unsweetened almond milk
- 2 teaspoons ground ginger
- 2 teaspoons ground cinnamon
- Pinch of sea salt, or to taste
- ¼ cup fresh or thawed frozen blueberries
- ¼ cup fresh or thawed frozen raspberries
- ¼ cup crushed raw unsalted walnuts

Place the quinoa and water in a bowl and allow to soak overnight at room temperature. In the morning, drain and rinse the quinoa.

Combine the quinoa, almond milk, ginger, cinnamon, and salt in a medium saucepan. Bring to a boil, then reduce the heat and simmer for about 10 minutes. Remove the pan from the heat, spoon the porridge into serving bowls, and top with the berries and walnuts.

LUV Pancakes

Yield: 4 *servings (about 16 pancakes)*
Prep time: About 20 minutes

For the cherry berry compote

- 1 cup fresh or thawed frozen tart cherries, pitted
- 1 cup fresh or thawed frozen raspberries
- 1 cup fresh or thawed frozen blueberries

2 tablespoons granulated allulose

¼ cup water

For the pancakes

3 large eggs

2 tablespoons granulated allulose

1½ cups almond flour

Pinch of sea salt, or to taste

¼ teaspoon ground cinnamon

Pinch of ground cardamom

¼ teaspoon baking soda

1 tablespoon cracked broccoli seeds (see Note)

Unsalted butter or extra virgin olive oil for cooking

Combine the cherries, berries, allulose, and water in a medium saucepan over medium heat. Stir occasionally until thickened, about 10 minutes. Set aside.

In a large bowl, whisk together the eggs, allulose, almond flour, salt, cinnamon, cardamom, baking soda, and broccoli seeds. Let stand for 10 minutes.

Heat the butter or oil in a medium skillet over medium heat. Drop a tablespoon of the batter into the skillet for each pancake, filling the skillet with a few pancakes at a time and repeating the process until the batter is all used up. Wait for little air bubbles to form, then flip the pancakes over so they are evenly browned on both sides. Remove from the heat and top with the reserved compote.

NOTE: Broccoli seeds are easy to find both in supermarkets and online. You can crack them with the back of a knife, in a spice grinder, or in a pepper mill.

Cherry Almond Loaf

Yield: 6 *servings*
Prep time: About 45 minutes

> 2½ cups almond flour
>
> ½ teaspoon baking soda
>
> 1 teaspoon ground cinnamon
>
> ½ cup granulated allulose
>
> 3 large eggs
>
> 1 teaspoon vanilla extract
>
> ¼ cup (4 tablespoons) unsalted butter, melted and cooled
>
> ½ cup pitted and halved fresh or thawed frozen tart cherries

Preheat the oven to 350°F.

Combine the almond flour, baking soda, cinnamon, and allulose in a large bowl. In a separate medium bowl, whisk together the eggs, vanilla, and butter. Stir the wet mixture into the flour mixture until thoroughly combined. Fold in the cherries.

Pour the batter into a nonstick 9-inch loaf pan and bake for 30–35 minutes, or until a toothpick or cake tester inserted in the middle comes out clean.

Broccoli Sprout, Green Pepper, and Red Onion Frittata

Yield: 2 *servings*
Prep time: About 18 minutes

> 6 large eggs
>
> Pinch of sea salt, or to taste
>
> 2 tablespoons extra virgin olive oil
>
> ¼ cup peeled and chopped red onion

¼ cup chopped green bell pepper

1 cup broccoli sprouts

½ teaspoon cracked broccoli seeds (see Note on page 237)

Preheat the oven to 300°F.

Whisk the eggs and salt together in a medium bowl. Set aside.

Heat the olive oil over medium heat in an 8-inch nonstick ovenproof skillet. Sauté the onions and peppers until the onions are translucent, about 6 minutes. Scatter the broccoli sprouts evenly over the top. Pour the eggs into the pan, making sure to cover the sprouts.

Transfer the pan to the oven and bake for 20 minutes, or until the eggs are set.

Allow to cool slightly, then sprinkle with the cracked broccoli seeds and serve.

Greek Farm Egg Cups

Yield: 2 servings
Prep time: About 25 minutes

6 large eggs

Pinch of sea salt, or to taste

1 tablespoon extra virgin olive oil

¼ cup peeled and chopped red onion

1 bunch Tuscan kale leaves, stemmed and sliced into ribbons

3 ounces feta cheese, crumbled

Preheat the oven to 300°F.

Whisk the eggs and salt together in a medium bowl. Set aside.

Heat the olive oil in a small sauté pan over medium heat. Add the onions and sauté until translucent, about 4 minutes. Add the kale and sauté for 2 more minutes, or until the leaves are soft.

Divide the vegetable mixture evenly among four nonstick muffin cups. Pour the eggs evenly into the cups. Top each cup with crumbled feta. Bake for 18 minutes, or until the egg mixture is set.

Everything Biscuits with Smoked Salmon and Sour Cream

Yield: 4 servings
Prep time: About 25 minutes

For the everything spice mix

  1 teaspoon sesame seeds

  1 teaspoon broccoli seeds (see Note on page 237)

  ½ teaspoon dried onion flakes

  ½ teaspoon granulated garlic

  ½ teaspoon sea salt

For the biscuits

  2½ cups almond flour

  ¼ teaspoon sea salt

  ½ teaspoon baking soda

  ¼ cup (4 tablespoons) unsalted butter, melted and cooled

  2 large eggs

For the filling

  4 tablespoons full-fat sour cream

  4 ounces smoked salmon, sliced (8 slices)

  1 scallion, chopped

Preheat the oven to 350°F.

To make the spice mix, combine the sesame seeds, broccoli seeds, dried onion flakes, granulated garlic, and salt in a small bowl. Set aside.

To make the biscuits, combine the almond flour, salt, and baking soda in a medium bowl. In a separate bowl, whisk together the butter and eggs. Stir the eggs into the flour mixture until a dough forms.

Roll out the dough to a ¾-inch thickness. Using a 3-inch biscuit cutter, cut four biscuits out of the rolled-out dough. Transfer the biscuits to a parchment-lined baking sheet. Sprinkle with the reserved spice mixture and bake for 15 minutes, or until the biscuits are golden brown.

Let the biscuits cool, then slice them in half horizontally using a serrated knife and serve each with a tablespoon of sour cream, two slices of smoked salmon, and chopped scallion.

LUNCH

Chicken Salad with Broccoli-Sprout Pesto

Yield: 2 servings
Prep time: About 18 minutes

For the pesto

2 cups broccoli sprouts

2 cups baby spinach leaves

½ cup chopped raw unsalted walnuts

1 tablespoon white miso paste

½ teaspoon sea salt

¼ teaspoon red pepper flakes

¾ cup extra virgin olive oil

For the chicken salad

10 ounces boneless skinless chicken breast, cooked and diced

¼ cup finely diced green bell pepper

¼ cup peeled and finely diced red onion

For the salad

4 cups baby spinach leaves

½ avocado, diced

1 tablespoon extra virgin olive oil

Freshly squeezed juice of ½ lemon

Sea salt to taste

To make the pesto, combine the broccoli sprouts, spinach, walnuts, miso, salt, red pepper flakes, and olive oil in a food processor and blend until smooth.

To make the chicken salad, combine the chicken, bell peppers, and onions in a medium bowl. Add 4 tablespoons of pesto, or more to taste. Stir to combine well. (The remaining pesto can be stored in an airtight container in the refrigerator for up to two weeks.)

To make the salad, combine the spinach and avocado in a medium bowl. Toss with olive oil, lemon juice, and salt. Spoon the chicken salad on top and serve.

Turkey Patties with Leek and Mint

Yield: 2 servings
Prep time: About 18 minutes

For the dressing

½ cup raw unsalted cashews

2 cups warm water

½ cup unsweetened almond milk

2½ tablespoons apple cider vinegar

2 tablespoons dulse flakes (see Note)

1 tablespoon white miso paste

2 tablespoons Dijon mustard

Freshly squeezed juice of ½ lemon

Pinch of sea salt and freshly ground black pepper, or to taste

For the patties

2 tablespoons extra virgin olive oil

½ cup thinly sliced leeks

12 ounces lean ground turkey

5 fresh mint leaves, sliced in ribbons

Pinch of sea salt, or to taste

For the salad

1 bunch Tuscan kale leaves, stemmed and chopped

¼ red onion, peeled and thinly sliced

To make the dressing, soak the cashews in the warm water for 1 hour. Drain and discard the soaking water. Place the cashews in a blender with the almond milk, vinegar, dulse flakes, miso, mustard, lemon juice, salt, and pepper and blend until smooth and creamy.

To make the patties, heat the olive oil in a medium skillet over medium heat. Add the leeks and sauté until golden, about 5 minutes. Set aside to cool for a few minutes.

In a medium bowl, combine the cooled leeks, turkey, mint, and salt. Form into four patties.

Return the skillet to medium heat. Cook the patties for about 3 minutes on each side, then remove from the heat.

To make the salad, combine the kale and red onions in a medium bowl, then transfer to a serving plate. Arrange the patties over the kale and onions and spoon on the desired amount of dressing. (The remaining dressing can be stored in an airtight container in the refrigerator for up to two weeks.)

NOTE: Dulse flakes are made from an edible red seaweed that grows wild in the cold ocean waters of the Pacific Northwest and the North Atlantic. Like all edible seaweed, dulse provides fiber and protein and is rich in vitamins, trace minerals, healthful fatty acids, and antioxidants (when it's pan-fried, some people say it tastes like bacon). It can be found in most well-stocked grocery stores and online.

Chopped Salad

Yield: 2 servings
Prep time: About 10 minutes

   3 heads gem lettuce, quartered

   1 medium heirloom or beefsteak tomato, diced

   1 avocado, diced

   1 green bell pepper, diced

   1 8-ounce can lentils, rinsed and drained

   2 tablespoons Green Tahini Dressing (page 247), or to taste

Place the lettuce in serving bowl. Top with the tomato, avocado, bell pepper, and lentils. Drizzle with Green Tahini Dressing.

Grilled Zucchini Steaks with Pesto

Yield: 2 servings
Prep time: About 14 minutes

   1 bunch Tuscan kale leaves, stemmed and chopped

   3 tablespoons extra virgin olive oil, divided

   2 medium zucchini

   Pinch of sea salt, or to taste

   2 tablespoons Broccoli-Sprout Pesto (page 242)

   ³/₄ cup halved Sun Gold tomatoes

Preheat a grill to medium-high. In a medium bowl, massage the kale leaves with 1½ tablespoons of the olive oil. Set aside.

Cut the zucchini in half lengthwise. Brush both sides with the remaining olive oil and season with salt. Grill for 3 minutes per side. Remove from the heat and spread the pesto evenly over the cut side of the zucchini. Serve on a bed of kale and top with the tomatoes.

Soft-Boiled Eggs and Shaved Brussels Sprouts Salad with Parmesan

Yield: 2 servings
Prep time: About 20 minutes

For the dressing

½ cup raw unsalted cashews

2 cups warm water

1 tablespoon Dijon mustard

2 tablespoons freshly squeezed lemon juice

¼ teaspoon sea salt

½ cup water

For the eggs

3 cups shaved brussels sprouts

½ red onion, peeled and thinly sliced

4 large eggs in the shell

2 ounces shaved Parmesan cheese

To make the dressing, soak the cashews in the warm water for 1 hour. Drain and discard the soaking water. Place the cashews in a blender with the mustard, lemon juice, salt, and water. Blend until smooth and creamy.

Toss the brussels sprouts and onions with the desired amount of dressing in a medium bowl. (The remaining dressing can be stored in an airtight container in the refrigerator for up to two weeks.) Divide the salad between two serving bowls and set aside.

Bring a small pot of water to a boil. Reduce the heat to medium and carefully add the eggs. Cook for 5 minutes. Place the eggs into a bowl of ice water for 2 minutes. Peel off the shells and cut the eggs in half. Top the brussels sprouts with the eggs and shaved Parmesan.

Whole Roasted Cauliflower with Green Tahini Dressing

Yield: 2 servings
Prep time: About 1 hour

For the dressing

¼ cup tahini

1 bunch fresh Italian parsley leaves

Freshly squeezed juice of 2 limes

1 clove garlic, peeled

½ teaspoon sea salt

1 teaspoon broccoli seeds (see Note on page 237)

¼ cup cold water

¼ cup extra virgin olive oil

For the cauliflower

1 small head cauliflower

5 tablespoons extra virgin olive oil, divided

Pinch of sea salt, or to taste

⅓ cup raw unsalted pistachios, crushed

⅓ cup fresh pomegranate seeds

¼ red onion, peeled and thinly sliced

Preheat the oven to 325°F.

Combine the tahini, parsley, lime juice, garlic, salt, broccoli seeds, water, and olive oil in a blender and blend until smooth and creamy. Set aside.

Place the cauliflower on a parchment-lined baking sheet. Brush with 3 tablespoons of the olive oil and season with salt. Roast for 40 minutes. Remove from the oven and brush with the remaining olive oil. Increase the temperature to 400°F and cook for an additional 15 minutes, or until golden brown.

Spoon the desired amount of dressing over the cauliflower. (The remaining dressing can be stored in an airtight container in the refrigerator for up to two weeks.) Cut in wedges to serve. Garnish with pistachios, pomegranate seeds, and onions.

Za'atar Chickpea Salad with Lemon Broccoli-Seed Tahini Dressing

Yield: 2 servings
Prep time: About 15 minutes

For the chickpeas

1 15-ounce can chickpeas, drained and rinsed

2 tablespoons extra virgin olive oil

2 tablespoons za'atar seasoning

Freshly squeezed juice of ½ lemon

Sea salt to taste

For the dressing

¼ cup tahini

1 teaspoon grated lemon zest

Freshly squeezed juice of 1 lemon

1 clove garlic, peeled

½ teaspoon sea salt

1 teaspoon broccoli seeds (see Note on page 237)

¼ cup cold water

¼ cup extra virgin olive oil

For the salad

4 cups arugula

½ cup halved grape tomatoes

¼ red onion, peeled and thinly sliced

To make the chickpeas, combine the chickpeas, olive oil, za'atar, lemon juice, and salt in a bowl. Let marinate in the refrigerator for at least 1 hour.

To make the dressing, combine the tahini, lemon zest, lemon juice, garlic, salt, broccoli seeds, water, and olive oil in a blender. Blend until smooth and creamy.

To make the salad, toss the arugula, tomatoes, and onions with the desired amount of dressing in a large bowl. (The remaining dressing can be stored in an airtight container in the refrigerator for up to two weeks.) Top with the chickpeas and serve.

Jackfruit Lettuce Tacos

Yield: 2 servings
Prep time: About 12 minutes

For the jackfruit

1 14-ounce can or pouch jackfruit, drained and rinsed (see Note)

1½ tablespoons extra virgin olive oil

1 teaspoon ground cumin

1 teaspoon chopped cilantro leaves

1 fresh serrano chili pepper, seeded and sliced

Freshly squeezed juice of ½ lime

Pinch of sea salt, or to taste

For the tacos

6 large gem or romaine lettuce leaves

1 cup shredded red or green cabbage

1 cup diced avocado

¼ cup thinly sliced radishes

In a medium bowl, combine the jackfruit, olive oil, cumin, cilantro, chili, lime juice, and salt.

Fill each lettuce leaf with cabbage, top with the jackfruit mixture, and garnish with the avocado and radishes.

NOTE: Jackfruit comes from a tropical tree grown in Asia, Africa, and South America; it's the largest tree-borne fruit in the world and is related to figs. Its shredded-meat-like texture makes it a common protein substitute for vegans and vegetarians. It's sold in many markets and online and is ready to use out of the bag.

DINNER

Thyme-Roasted Pork Tenderloin

Yield: 2 servings

Prep time: About 25 minutes

For the pork

  1 tablespoon extra virgin olive oil

  1 12-ounce pork tenderloin

  Pinch of sea salt, or to taste

  6 sprigs fresh thyme

For the broccoli

  1 tablespoon sea salt

  2 cups broccoli florets

  1½ tablespoons extra virgin olive oil

For the apples

  ¾ cup Poached Apples (page 234)

Preheat the oven to 400°F.

To make the pork, heat the olive oil in a large skillet over medium-high heat. Season the pork with the salt and sear it for 2 minutes on each side. Transfer to a roasting pan, cover with the thyme sprigs, and bake for 12–15 minutes, or until the internal temperature reaches 145°F. Discard the thyme sprigs and allow to rest for 20 minutes before slicing.

Meanwhile, make the broccoli. Bring 6 cups of water and the salt to a rolling boil. Add the broccoli and boil for 3 minutes. Drain and toss with the olive oil.

Slice the pork and serve with the broccoli and apples.

Za'atar-Crusted Rack of Lamb with Arugula and Tart-Cherry Vinaigrette

Yield: 2 *servings*

Prep time: About 40 minutes

For the lamb

1 rack of baby lamb, about 1 pound, trimmed of fat and bones frenched

Pinch of sea salt, or to taste

1 tablespoon extra virgin olive oil

3 tablespoons za'atar seasoning

1 small lemon, sliced into rounds

For the vinaigrette

¼ cup fresh or thawed frozen tart cherries, pitted

2 cardamom pods

1½ tablespoons apple cider vinegar

1½ teaspoons Dijon mustard

¼ cup extra virgin olive oil

Sea salt and freshly ground black pepper to taste

For the salad

4 cups arugula or other dark leafy greens

¼ cup fresh pomegranate seeds

¼ red onion, peeled and thinly sliced

Allow the lamb to rest at room temperature for 30 minutes. Preheat the oven to 450°F.

Season the lamb with the salt. Coat it evenly with the olive oil, then rub in the za'atar. Place the lamb on a baking sheet and cover with the lemon slices. Bake for 15 minutes, or until the internal temperature reaches 145°F. Let the meat rest for 20 minutes, then slice it into chops.

Meanwhile, combine the cherries, cardamom, vinegar, and mustard in a blender and pulse until chunky. With the blender on low, stream in the olive oil. Season with salt and pepper.

Toss the arugula with the desired amount of salad dressing. (The remaining dressing can be stored in an airtight container in the refrigerator for up to two weeks.) Divide the salad between two serving plates, top with the lamb chops, then garnish with pomegranate seeds and onions.

Instant Pot Steak Shawarma Stew

Yield: 4 servings

Prep time: About 2 hours (plus at least 4 hours of marinating time)

- 1 tablespoon sea salt
- 1 tablespoon ground cumin
- 1 teaspoon ground turmeric
- ½ teaspoon ground allspice
- ½ teaspoon ground cinnamon
- ½ teaspoon ground ginger
- ¼ teaspoon ground cloves
- ¼ teaspoon cayenne pepper
- ¼ cup extra virgin olive oil
- 3 tablespoons apple cider vinegar
- 2 pounds boneless grass-fed beef chuck, cut in half
- 1 head garlic, unpeeled, top removed
- 1 cup water
- 1 shallot, peeled and thinly sliced
- 1 red bell pepper, thinly sliced
- 1 green bell pepper, thinly sliced
- ¼ cup thinly sliced radishes

In a large bowl, combine the salt, cumin, turmeric, allspice, cinnamon, ginger, cloves, cayenne, olive oil, and vinegar. Add the beef and garlic, making sure they are both generously coated. Cover and marinate in the refrigerator for at least 4 hours or overnight.

Transfer the beef and garlic to an Instant Pot. Add the water, seal the lid, and cook on high for 90 minutes. Allow the pressure to release for 10 minutes.

Transfer the beef to a serving bowl and shred it with two forks. Remove the garlic and discard. Add half the braising liquid, then garnish with the shallots, peppers, and radishes.

Pressure Cooker Chicken, Tart Cherries, and Green Olives

Yield: 4 servings
Prep time: About 30 minutes

- 8 bone-in, skin-on chicken thighs
- 1 teaspoon sea salt
- 2 tablespoons extra virgin olive oil, divided
- ½ cup dry white wine
- 1 large lemon, sliced into rounds
- 4 cloves garlic, peeled and smashed
- 2 shallots, peeled and thinly sliced
- 4 sprigs fresh thyme
- 1 cup pitted and halved Castelvetrano olives
- 1 cup pitted and halved fresh or thawed frozen tart cherries

Season the chicken with the salt and set aside.

Set a pressure cooker to medium sauté mode. Add 1 tablespoon of the olive oil. Once hot, add the chicken. Brown for 2½ minutes on each side, then transfer the chicken to a plate.

Add the wine to the pot and scrape the bottom with a spatula to deglaze. Return the chicken to the pot, then add the lemon, garlic, shallots, and thyme. Cook on medium pressure for 10 minutes. Allow the pressure to release for an additional 10 minutes. Discard the thyme sprigs.

Transfer the chicken, shallots, and lemon to a serving platter. Top with the olives and cherries, then drizzle with the remaining olive oil.

Grilled Halibut with Tomatoes and Hearts of Palm

Yield: 2 servings
Prep time: About 15 minutes

    2 6-ounce halibut fillets
    3 tablespoons extra virgin olive oil, divided
    Pinch of sea salt, or to taste
    2 heirloom or beefsteak tomatoes, sliced
    4 canned hearts of palm, sliced
    3 scallions, chopped
    8 fresh basil leaves, torn
    ½ teaspoon grated lemon zest
    ½ teaspoon cracked broccoli seeds (see Note on page 237)

Preheat the grill to medium-high.

Brush the halibut on both sides with 1½ tablespoons of the olive oil. Season with the salt. Grill the halibut until cooked through, about 4 minutes on each side.

Arrange the tomatoes, hearts of palm, scallions, and basil on each of two serving plates. Top with the halibut. Drizzle the remaining olive oil over the fish, then sprinkle with the lemon zest and broccoli seeds.

Harissa-Roasted Halibut with Roasted Zucchini, Tomatoes, Peppers, and Blistered Red Onions

Yield: 2 servings
Prep time: About 25 minutes

For the halibut

> 1 teaspoon sea salt
>
> 1 teaspoon ground cardamom
>
> ½ teaspoon ground cumin
>
> ½ teaspoon ground turmeric
>
> 2 tablespoons harissa
>
> 1 clove garlic, peeled and minced
>
> 2 teaspoons extra virgin olive oil
>
> 2 6-ounce halibut fillets

For the vegetables

> 2 tablespoons extra virgin olive oil
>
> ¼ red onion, peeled and thinly sliced
>
> 1 medium zucchini, cut into ¼-inch rounds
>
> ½ green bell pepper, cut into ½-inch dice
>
> ½ cup halved grape tomatoes
>
> Pinch of sea salt, or to taste

Preheat the oven to 350°F.

To make the fish, whisk the salt, cardamom, cumin, turmeric, harissa, garlic, and olive oil in a small bowl. Place the halibut fillets on a parchment-lined baking sheet. Coat the fillets evenly with the spice mixture. Roast for 15–18 minutes, or until the fillets are cooked through. Transfer to two serving plates and let rest for 10 minutes.

Meanwhile, to make the vegetables, heat the olive oil in a large sauté pan over medium heat. Add the onions and sauté until slightly crispy, about 10 minutes. Add the zucchini and green peppers and cook, stirring frequently, about 4 minutes. Add the tomatoes and continue cooking an additional 2 minutes. Season with salt and serve alongside the fish.

Roasted Fluke with Crushed Walnuts and Chives

Yield: 2 servings
Prep time: About 25 minutes

For the fluke

  2 6-ounce fluke fillets

  Pinch of sea salt, or to taste

  1 tablespoon extra virgin olive oil

  ½ cup crushed raw unsalted walnuts

  2 teaspoons chopped fresh chives

For the salad

  2 tablespoons Tart Cherry Vinaigrette (page 252), or to taste

  1 large bunch Tuscan kale, stemmed and chopped

  ³⁄₄ cup fresh or thawed frozen raspberries

  1 Persian cucumber, thinly sliced

Preheat the oven to 325°F.

Place the fluke fillets on a parchment-lined baking sheet. Season with the salt and drizzle with the olive oil. Top evenly with the crushed walnuts. Bake for 12–15 minutes, or until the fillets are cooked through. Transfer to two serving plates and let cool for 10 minutes. Sprinkle with the chives.

In a medium bowl, massage the desired amount of dressing into the kale. Toss in the raspberries and cucumbers and serve alongside the fluke.

Sheet Pan Shrimp with Asparagus and Lemon Salsa

Yield: 2 servings
Prep time: About 18 minutes

For the salsa

> 2 lemons
>
> 2 tablespoons sliced raw unsalted almonds
>
> 2 tablespoons chopped fresh Italian parsley leaves

For the shrimp

> 1½ tablespoons melted unsalted butter
>
> 1½ tablespoons extra virgin olive oil
>
> 1 bunch fresh asparagus, trimmed
>
> Pinch of sea salt, or to taste
>
> 1 pound medium wild-caught uncooked shrimp, peeled and deveined

Preheat the oven to 400°F.

Peel and chop the lemons and remove the seeds. Combine the lemons, almonds, and parsley in a small bowl. Set aside.

Whisk together the butter and olive oil in a small bowl.

Arrange the asparagus evenly on one side of a baking sheet lined with parchment and drizzle with half the butter-oil mixture. Season with salt. Arrange the shrimp evenly on the other side of the sheet and drizzle with the remaining butter-oil mixture. Season with salt. Roast for 8–10 minutes, or until the shrimp are pink.

Divide the asparagus between two serving plates and top with the shrimp and lemon salsa.

Roasted Cod with Broccolini

Yield: 2 servings
Prep time: About 18 minutes

    2 cups chopped broccolini
    ½ red onion, peeled and sliced
    1 green bell pepper, sliced
    3 tablespoons extra virgin olive oil, divided
    Pinch of sea salt, or to taste
    1 tablespoon finely chopped fresh chives
    ½ cup pitted and halved Castelvetrano olives
    2 6-ounce cod fillets

Preheat the oven to 400°F.

Toss the broccolini, onion, and green pepper with 2 tablespoons of the olive oil in a large bowl. Season with salt. Spread evenly on a parchment-lined baking sheet. Roast for 12–15 minutes. Return the vegetables to the mixing bowl and toss with the chives and olives.

Reduce the oven temperature to 375°F. Season the cod fillets with salt. Heat the remaining olive oil in a large oven-safe skillet over medium-high heat. Sear the cod for 3 minutes on each side, then transfer the skillet to the oven and roast for 8 minutes, or until the fillets are cooked through. Divide the broccolini mixture between two serving plates and top with the cod.

Jerk Jackfruit Chili

Yield: 6 servings
Prep time: About 30 minutes

    2 tablespoons extra virgin olive oil
    1 small red onion, peeled and diced
    1 tablespoon jerk seasoning

2 large fresh heirloom or beefsteak tomatoes, diced

1 14-ounce can or pouch jackfruit, drained and rinsed (see Note on page 250)

1 15-ounce can black beans, drained and rinsed

1 15-ounce can aduki (also called azduki or azuki) beans, drained and rinsed

1 cup canned unsweetened coconut milk

Pinch of sea salt, or to taste

2 cups baby spinach leaves

Heat the olive oil in a large pot over medium heat. Add the onions and cook until translucent, about 3 minutes. Stir in the jerk seasoning and continue cooking for 1 minute. Add the tomatoes, jackfruit, black beans, aduki beans, and coconut milk. Season with salt. Bring to a boil, then reduce heat and simmer for 20 minutes, stirring occasionally.

Stir in the spinach just before serving.

Rainbow Vegetable-Noodle Salad

Yield: 2 servings
Prep time: About 15 minutes

For the sauce

3 tablespoons unsalted raw almond butter

1 tablespoon white miso paste

1 teaspoon peeled and chopped fresh ginger

2 tablespoons apple cider vinegar

1 tablespoon freshly squeezed lime juice

Pinch of cayenne pepper

Pinch of sea salt, or to taste

3 tablespoons extra virgin olive oil

For the salad

> 1 cup zucchini noodles
>
> 1 cup butternut squash noodles
>
> ¼ red onion, peeled and thinly sliced
>
> 1 green bell pepper, thinly sliced
>
> ½ cup shredded carrots
>
> 1 teaspoon chopped fresh cilantro leaves
>
> ¼ cup chopped raw unsalted cashews
>
> 1 teaspoon sesame seeds

Combine the almond butter, miso, ginger, vinegar, lime juice, cayenne, and salt in a blender and blend until smooth. With the blender on low speed, stream in the olive oil until the sauce is smooth and creamy.

In a large bowl, combine the zucchini noodles, squash noodles, onion, bell pepper, and carrots. Mix in the desired amount of sauce. (The remaining sauce can be stored in an airtight container in the refrigerator for up to two weeks; it makes a great topping for crudités.) Garnish with the cilantro, cashews, and sesame seeds.

Roasted Spaghetti Squash with Broccoli-Sprout Pesto

Yield: 2 servings

Prep time: About 45 minutes

> 1 medium spaghetti squash
>
> 2 tablespoons extra virgin olive oil
>
> Pinch of sea salt, or to taste
>
> ½ cup Broccoli-Sprout Pesto (page 261)
>
> ½ cup halved grape tomatoes
>
> ½ cup halved Sun Gold tomatoes
>
> 1 teaspoon broccoli seeds, cracked (see Note on page 237)

Preheat the oven to 400°F.

Cut the spaghetti squash in half lengthwise. Scrape out the seeds. Drizzle the insides with the olive oil and season with the salt. Place the squash cut side down on a parchment-lined baking sheet. Using a fork, poke a few holes on the skin side of the squash halves. Roast for 35–40 minutes, or until the squash is soft. Cool for 10 minutes.

Using a fork, scrape the squash out of the skin and place it in a medium bowl. Toss with the pesto and garnish with the tomatoes and broccoli seeds.

Roasted Cauliflower "Wings" with Broccoli-Sprout Romesco Dip

Yield: 2 servings
Prep time: About 30 minutes

For the romesco

  2 green bell peppers
  2 cups broccoli sprouts
  ½ cup raw unsalted almonds
  1 tablespoon white miso paste
  Pinch of sea salt, or to taste
  ¾ cup extra virgin olive oil
  Freshly squeezed juice of ½ lemon

For the cauliflower

  4 cups cauliflower florets
  4 tablespoons extra virgin olive oil
  Pinch of sea salt, or to taste

Preheat the oven to 375°F.

To make the sauce, roast the peppers over a medium open flame, rotating occasionally until all sides are blackened. Remove from the heat and let cool. Remove the skins, stems, and seeds.

Combine the peppers, broccoli sprouts, almonds, miso, salt, olive oil, and lemon juice in a food processor and pulse until creamy.

To prepare the cauliflower, toss the florets, olive oil, and salt in a large bowl. Spread out evenly on a parchment-lined baking sheet. Roast for 20–25 minutes, turning once halfway through cooking time, until florets are browned. Serve with romesco dip.

Mushroom "Bolognese"

Yield: 4 servings
Prep time: About 40 minutes

- 2 tablespoons extra virgin olive oil
- 2 tablespoons unsalted butter
- ¼ cup peeled and finely chopped shallots
- ½ cup finely diced celery
- 2 cloves garlic, peeled and smashed
- 1 sprig fresh rosemary
- 1 pound cremini mushrooms, finely diced
- ½ pound shiitake mushrooms, sliced
- Pinch of sea salt, or to taste
- 1 cup vegetable stock
- 1 cup crushed canned or fresh tomatoes
- 1 recipe Roasted Spaghetti Squash (without pesto; see page 261) or 4 cups cooked vegetable noodles

In a large pot, heat the olive oil and butter over medium heat. Add the shallots and celery and cook until translucent, about 3 minutes. Add the garlic, rosemary, and mushrooms. Cook until the mushrooms are slightly caramelized, stirring occasionally, about 15 minutes. Season with the salt.

Add the vegetable stock and crushed tomatoes. Bring to a boil, then reduce the heat and simmer for 15–20 minutes. Serve over spaghetti squash or your favorite vegetable noodles.

SNACKS

Coconut Chia Pudding

Yield: 4 *servings*
Prep time: About 10 minutes

2 cups canned unsweetened coconut milk

1 teaspoon vanilla extract

1 tablespoon granulated allulose

Pinch of sea salt, or to taste

¼ cup chia seeds

Fresh or thawed frozen raspberries, tart cherries, or blueberries for garnish

Shaved dark chocolate for garnish

Whisk the coconut milk, vanilla, allulose, and salt in a medium bowl. Stir in the chia seeds and allow to bloom for 1 hour at room temperature, covered. Refrigerate, covered, for 2 hours before serving. Top with berries, cherries, or shaved chocolate.

Turmeric-Fermented Hard-Boiled Eggs

Yield: 4 *servings*
Prep time: About 25 minutes

2 cups apple cider vinegar

½ cup water

1 teaspoon granulated allulose

1 teaspoon sea salt

2 teaspoons ground turmeric

8 hard-boiled eggs, peeled

3 shallots, peeled and thinly sliced

2 sprigs fresh thyme

1 tablespoon black peppercorns

Bring the vinegar, water, allulose, salt, and turmeric to a simmer in a medium saucepan. Let cool to room temperature.

Place the eggs in a large (16-ounce) mason jar with the shallots, thyme, and peppercorns. Pour the vinegar mixture over the eggs. Cover the jar and refrigerate for at least three days. (The eggs will keep in the refrigerator for up to fourteen days.)

Cinnamon Turmeric Yogurt

Yield: 2 servings
Prep time: About 10 minutes

12 ounces plain unsweetened full-fat Greek-style yogurt

$^3/_4$ teaspoon ground turmeric

$^3/_4$ teaspoon ground cinnamon

Pinch of ground cardamom

Pinch of freshly ground black pepper

1 teaspoon granulated allulose

Fresh or thawed frozen blueberries for garnish

Chopped raw unsalted walnuts for garnish

Combine the Greek yogurt, turmeric, cinnamon, cardamom, black pepper, and allulose in a medium bowl. Mix thoroughly. Enjoy plain or topped with blueberries and walnuts.

Crudités with Cashew Sriracha Mayo

Yield: 4 servings

Prep time: About 12 minutes

For the crudités

2 Persian cucumbers

2 carrots, peeled

1 green bell pepper

1 cup fresh cherry tomatoes

For the mayo

½ cup raw unsalted cashews

1 cup warm water

⅓ cup water

1 tablespoon freshly squeezed lime juice

Pinch of sea salt, or to taste

1 teaspoon wheat-free tamari

1 tablespoon sriracha

Cut the cucumbers, carrots, and bell pepper into julienne strips. Cut the cherry tomatoes in half lengthwise.

To make the mayo, soak the cashews in the warm water for 1 hour. Drain and discard the soaking water. Place the cashews in a blender with ⅓ cup water, lime juice, salt, tamari, and sriracha. Blend until smooth and creamy. Serve with the crudités.

Brussels Sprouts Kimchi

Yield: *4 servings*

Prep time: *About 15 minutes*

> 2 teaspoons sea salt
>
> 1 quart water
>
> ½ red onion, peeled and sliced
>
> 4 cloves garlic, peeled
>
> 1 teaspoon peeled and chopped fresh ginger
>
> 1 teaspoon fennel seeds
>
> 1 teaspoon coriander seeds
>
> 1 tablespoon wheat-free tamari
>
> 2 teaspoons gochugaru (see Note)
>
> 2 teaspoons sriracha
>
> 1 pound brussels sprouts, trimmed and quartered

Dissolve the salt in the water and set aside. Pulse the onion, garlic, ginger, fennel, coriander, tamari, gochugaru, and sriracha in a food processor until smooth. Stir the paste thoroughly into the salted water.

Place the brussels sprouts into two large (16-ounce) sterilized mason jars. Cover with the brine. Make sure the brussels sprouts are fully submerged. Leave 1 inch of headspace in the jars. Cover with the lids and let sit at room temperature for three to five days, or until the mixture is releasing bubbles.

The kimchi can be stored in the refrigerator for up to six weeks.

NOTE: Gochugaru is a Korean red chili powder you can buy online, in Asian markets, or in regular supermarkets that have a section devoted to Asian ingredients. If you cannot find gochugaru, you can substitute with crushed red pepper flakes, cayenne pepper, or even paprika.

DRINKS

Raspberry Tahini Smoothie

Yield: 2 servings
Prep time: About 10 minutes

  1 cup frozen raspberries

  2 fresh figs

  2 tablespoons tahini

  1 teaspoon granulated allulose, or to taste

  1 cup canned unsweetened coconut milk

  1 cup water

  1 cup ice

Place the raspberries, figs, tahini, allulose, coconut milk, water, and ice in a blender. Blend on high speed until smooth and creamy.

Apple Pie Smoothie

Yield: 2 servings
Prep time: About 10 minutes

  1 unpeeled McIntosh or other red apple, seeded and cubed

  1 cup unsweetened almond milk

  1 cup plain unsweetened full-fat Greek-style yogurt

  2 tablespoons unsalted raw almond butter

  1 teaspoon ground cinnamon

  ½ teaspoon vanilla extract

  Pinch of ground nutmeg

  Pinch of ground ginger

  1 teaspoon granulated allulose, or to taste

1 teaspoon broccoli seeds (see Note on page 237)

1 cup ice

Combine the apple, almond milk, yogurt, almond butter, cinnamon, vanilla, nutmeg, ginger, allulose, broccoli seeds, and ice in a blender. Blend until smooth and creamy.

Tart Cherry Lime Mocktail

Yield: 2 servings
Prep time: About 10 minutes

2 tablespoons tart cherry extract (see Note on page 235)

16 ounces sparkling water

2 lime wedges

Place the cherry extract in a serving pitcher. Pour in the sparkling water and serve over ice, garnished with lime wedges.

Raw Cacao Almond Cold Brew Coffee

Yield: 2 servings
Prep time: About 10 minutes

¾ cup unsweetened almond milk

1 tablespoon raw cacao powder

½ teaspoon ground cinnamon

¼ teaspoon ground cardamom

Pinch of sea salt

1 teaspoon granulated allulose, or to taste

16 ounces cold brew coffee

Whisk the almond milk, cacao, cinnamon, cardamom, salt, and allulose together in a small bowl. Pour the coffee into a serving pitcher and add the almond-milk mixture. Stir and serve over ice.

Raspberry Mint Lemonade

Yield: 4 servings
Prep time: About 10 minutes

1 tablespoon tart cherry extract (see Note on page 235)

1 cup fresh or thawed frozen raspberries, muddled

1 cup water

¼ cup freshly squeezed lemon juice

⅓ cup granulated allulose

4 sprigs fresh mint

Combine the cherry extract, raspberries, water, lemon juice, and allulose in a serving pitcher. Stir well and serve over ice, garnished with mint sprigs.

Epilogue

If you don't like the road you're walking, start paving another one.

— DOLLY PARTON

IF YOU HAD TO NAME the best medical advancements in the history of humankind—those that have changed the world and allowed people to live longer and better—what comes to mind? Once you start to really think about it, an endless list of discoveries and developments emerges, some pretty basic and others high-tech: anesthesia, vaccines, antibiotics, hand washing, insulin for type 1 diabetics, organ transplantation, genomic sequencing, medical imaging (X-rays, CT scans, and MRIs), stem cell therapy, immunotherapy, artificial intelligence…the list goes on. It would be hard to rank these quantum leaps in medicine.

One of my favorites, however, is the discovery that smoking tobacco causes lung cancer. As rudimentary and incontrovertible as it sounds now, making the connection between smoking cigarettes and cancer, particularly lung cancer, has been hailed as one of our greatest achievements in medicine. It helped direct serious attention to the behaviors and environmental factors that affect health, and subsequently, antismoking campaigns took secondhand smoke into consideration, too. There are analogies to be drawn between this important breakthrough and the discovery of the dangers of elevated uric acid, which I'll get to in a moment. But first, some brief backstory.

The cigarette has been called "the deadliest artifact in the history of human civilization."[1] Until smoking gained popularity, toward the end of the nineteenth century, lung cancer was so rare as to be unheard of. In 1929, Fritz Lickint, a German physician who'd been obsessed with studying the health effects of smoking, published the first formal statistical evidence linking tobacco smoking with lung cancer. Although other scientists had previously shown an association between tobacco use and lung cancer, including the American physician Dr. Isaac Adler, who suggested more than a decade previously that smoking was behind increasing rates of lung cancer, no one had reported studies backed by such huge amounts of rigorous data. The evidence was so clear and obvious to Lickint that he believed no additional studies were necessary and that the solution was to ban smoking. He doggedly proclaimed that prevention is better than cure. Too bad preventive medicine had yet to be fully understood and embraced; at that time, medicine remained primarily focused on treating disease.

As they say, timing is everything. Lickint's findings went largely unnoticed because they appeared during the period of unrest in Germany that preceded World War II. He would go down in history as "one of the great unsung heroes of 20th-century medical science."[2] The man who would take more credit for the cigarette–lung cancer link was Richard Doll, a British doctor who, in 1950, tried to sound the alarm that smoking was triggering an epidemic of lung cancer in the postwar United Kingdom. In 1951, Doll proved the connection unequivocally by starting a fifty-year longitudinal study that showed that half of all smokers died from their addiction and that quitting significantly reduced or eliminated that risk. But Doll's warnings were muted by the powerful tobacco industry, which continued to relentlessly promote the health benefits of its product: "More doctors smoke Camels than any other cigarette" and "Smoke a Lucky to feel your level best!" were among the advertisements going around; companies even claimed that cigarettes improved digestion and helped one keep a slender figure.

We all know otherwise now, but it was not until 1964, when the US surgeon general issued the first report educating Americans on the incredibly toxic effects of smoking, that people finally registered the truth. By the late 1960s, polls showed that the majority of people believed smoking might cause cancer. Incredibly, though, only one-third of all US doctors believed that the case against cigarettes had been established (and lots of doctors smoked).

The reason I bring up this little piece of history is because we can draw parallels between the story of smoking and tobacco awareness and understanding the damage that long-term elevated uric acid can have. To consider the comparison from another angle, we can view elevated uric acid as a kind of smoke, though I hope it doesn't take another half a century for people to get the message. As I like to say—and pardon the cliché—where there's smoke, there's fire. Just as smoke precedes fire, elevated uric acid precedes many unwanted outcomes and has a direct connection to biological pandemonium. We can no longer ignore the data telling us about this other buried truth—another exposure we can indeed control in our lives. Living with chronically high uric acid is mostly a choice, given how much we know about the lifestyle factors that trigger dangerous elevations.

For all living things, life is an ongoing cycle of destruction and construction. And we want the balance of those two forces to be correct within us. Striking that balance begins with a balanced body—a direct result of the lifestyle choices we make daily. As I've said throughout this book, chronic elevation in uric acid is one clear and obvious sign that something is amiss in the body that needs to be addressed before symptoms of a more serious condition set in. The good news is that dropping acid is as easy as taking the baby steps I've outlined, and it really does start with what you put in your mouth.

Throughout my work as a doctor, lecturer, and author, I've fielded a lot of questions on every subject imaginable when it comes to health and wellness (you can read my list of top Q&As online at DrPerlmutter.com under the "Learn" tab). One of my favorites is this: If I had fifteen minutes to educate another doctor about anything, what would it be and why?

That's easy to answer. Quite simply, nutrition matters more than you could imagine. Food is our most important health ally. I believe that if we all make one small change today to improve our diets, whether by eliminating added refined sugars or by turning a meat- and carb-centric diet into a plant-based one, we would experience dramatic improvements in our health—and swiftly. When seeking a better, fitter, and more fulfilling life, you have to start somewhere, and nutrition is an entryway. Not drugs; not painful crash diets or unrealistic exercise protocols. Just my favorite four-letter word: *food*. I'm glad to see a movement finally taking shape in the health-care community toward appreciating and proselytizing about the power of food in medicine.

If one of every five deaths across the globe is now attributable to a suboptimal diet—more than are attributable to any other risk factor, including tobacco—is that not the writing on the wall? We're all aware of the dangers of smoking. Now we must accept the dangers of a poor diet, which results in metabolic dysfunction, the manifestations of which include uric acid dysregulation. And now that we've tagged uric acid as a "master conductor in the worldwide symphony" of chronic disease, an expression you'll remember from chapter 1, we must do what we can to bring this important metabolite into balance.

I applaud the scientists who now push for more research into using "food is medicine" interventions to prevent, manage, treat, and perhaps reverse illness. Imagine a future in which we encounter medically tailored meals prescribed by doctors. The integration of "food is medicine" into health care will require radical shifts in medical training and education as well as sustainable funding to promote programs that support this movement. This would of course include addressing food insecurity, which is a problem not only in underdeveloped areas of the world but also throughout the wealthiest of nations.

The global COVID-19 pandemic has not only brought the fragility of health-care systems across the world into sharp relief, it's also cast a bright light on the fragility of food systems, including the skyrocketing rates of food insecurity and the lack of access to healthful food for people who struggle with diet-related illnesses. Ending this crisis starts with incorporating the "food is medicine" approach into health-care systems. Which also means making a heroic shift away from subsidizing corn, soy, and sugar (the "candy-coated cartel," as the Cato Institute has called our nation's sugar program) and instead propping up farmers who harvest an array of healthful foods.[3] The payoffs could be huge. Researchers in the United States found, for example, that over a lifetime, a 30 percent subsidy on fruits and vegetables would prevent 1.93 million cardiovascular disease events and save approximately $40 billion in health-care costs.[4]

In Massachusetts and California, "food is medicine" interventions are already under way with high-risk populations — individuals who have mental or other complex health conditions, people who struggle with the basic activities of daily living, and people who frequently land in the emergency room.[5] In Massachusetts, for example, a program was launched in 2019 to provide home-delivered meals, groceries, cooking tools, nutrition education, and transportation to people who need access to good food. Results from the experiment, which is being paid for by the government's health-care system, will start to roll out in 2022. And in California, the Food Is Medicine Coalition is a program that coordinates an effort among state agencies to provide nutrition services and medically tailored meals that benefit vulnerable people. Their work is paying off: studies in recent years have shown dramatic reductions in health-care costs and hospitalizations among patients who receive complete medical nutrition for six months.[6] That term alone — *medical nutrition* — is one we should increasingly embrace in our consciousness and lexicon.

I predict we'll see more of these kinds of positive results, which will further encourage such programs across the country and in other parts of the world. The other good news is that the US government has appropriated millions of dollars of agriculture funding in order to establish "produce prescription programs" in eight states around the country. These

programs provide vouchers or debit cards, distributed by health-care providers, that are redeemable for free or discounted produce at various loca-
tions. Programs are also under way at major research universities, hospitals,
and institutions to assist and educate people in their communities about
food as medicine.

I praise these campaigns, which can help pave new roads to better
health for everyone regardless of age, race, socioeconomic status, and
geographic location. But until these programs roll out on a massive scale,
and until we can reengineer the food and beverage industry, each of us
needs to play our part, starting with our own individual lives. As it's said,
think globally, act locally (and personally).

My hope is that I've given you information you can use to create
incremental positive change in your life. The goal is to live in harmony
with your body's natural processes, a system developed over millions of
years of evolution.

Today we are starving for proper nourishment to support health. We
are starving for more movement and refreshing sleep. And we are eager
to usher in this revolution in our evolution. In the fifty-odd years since
antitobacco efforts began following the surgeon general's report, more
than eight million American lives have been saved. How many millions
of lives could have been saved since then had we known about uric acid's
role in fomenting fires in the body?

Go do your part. Pave your new path forward.

Find your sweet spot, where you can abide by the LUV protocol and
make a difference, starting with yourself. Then share your experience.

I'll keep doing my part.

Join me.

Acknowledgments

BOOKS OF THIS NATURE ARISE from the collective force of many creative and diversely talented people focused on one goal. I am deeply grateful to the following people who made it all happen.

Thanks to my dear friend and literary agent, Bonnie Solow. Years ago, your enthusiasm for *Grain Brain* catalyzed all that has followed. My gratitude for your leadership, attention to detail, and constant source of publishing wisdom is beyond measure.

Thanks to the tireless team at Little, Brown Spark, who have championed my work through the years. A special thanks goes to Tracy Behar, my editor, who has an unparalleled gift for making sure the message remains clear, succinct, and practical. From first to final draft, your editorial genius made this a much better book. Thanks also to Michael Pietsch, Bruce Nichols, Ian Straus, Jessica Chun, Juliana Horbachevsky, Craig Young, Sabrina Callahan, Julianna Lee, Barbara Clark, Pat Jalbert-Levine, and Melissa Mathlin. It's always a pleasure to work with such a dedicated, professional group.

Thanks to Amy Stanton and Rebecca Reinbold of Stanton & Company for your forward-looking creative efforts in the marketing of this work and your wonderful ability to work so seamlessly with the Little, Brown Spark team. And to Jonathan Jacobs and Accelerate360 for your incredibly knowledgeable approach to enhancing our social media exposure.

Thanks to Tricia Williams at Daily Dose, who crafted incredible recipes to match the LUV Diet guidelines and make cooking fun.

Additional thanks are due to Kate Workman, our director of operations, for being so circumspect in every aspect of all our projects.

Thanks also to Jerry Adams Jr. and Ellyne Lonergan for your diligence and creativity on manifesting the PBS special to accompany this book.

I am grateful to my wife, Leize, and to my children, Austin and Reisha, who have never ceased to encourage and support me on my journey.

And finally, a very special and heartfelt thanks goes to my cowriter, Kristin Loberg, for our friendship, our fishing stories, and the honor, yet again, of being able to share in the great adventure—creating such an important book.

Notes

The following is a partial list of scientific papers, books, articles, and online resources that you might find helpful in learning more about some of the ideas and concepts expressed in this book. This is by no means an exhaustive list, but it will get you started in taking a new perspective and living up to the principles of *Drop Acid*. Many of these citations relate to studies briefly mentioned or described in detail in the text. These materials can also open doors for further research and inquiry. If you do not see a reference listed here that was mentioned in the book, please visit DrPerlmutter.com, where you can access more studies and an ongoing updated list of references.

Introduction: The Acid Test

1. See https://peterattiamd.com/.
2. See the Centers for Disease Control and Prevention, at www.cdc.gov, and the American Heart Association, at www.heart.org.
3. See "Hidden in Plain Sight," SugarScience, University of California at San Francisco, https://sugarscience.ucsf.edu/hidden-in-plain-sight/.
4. Alexander Haig, *Uric Acid as a Factor in the Causation of Disease: A Contribution to the Pathology of High Arterial Tension, Headache, Epilepsy, Mental Depression, Paroxysmal Hæmoglobinuria and Anæmia, Bright's Disease, Diabetes, Gout, Rheumatism, and Other Disorders* (London: Franklin Classics, 2018). Also see Alexander Haig, "Uric Acid as a Factor in the Causation of Disease — A Contribution to the Pathology of High Blood Pressure, Headache, Epilepsy, Mental Depression, Paroxysmal Hemoglobinuria and Anemia, Bright's Disease, Gout, Rheumatism and other Disorders," JAMA 31, no. 3 (1898): 139, https://doi.org/10.1001/jama.1898 .02450030041022.

5. Theodora Fragkou, Konstantina Goula, and Ourania Drakoulogkona, "The History of Gout Through Centuries," *Nephrology Dialysis Transplantation* 30, supplement 3 (May 2015): iii377–80, https://doi.org/10.1093/ndt/gfv186.05.

6. *Oxford English Dictionary*, 2nd ed. (Oxford, UK: Oxford University Press, 2004).

7. George Nuki and Peter A. Simkin, "A Concise History of Gout and Hyperuricemia and Their Treatment," *Arthritis Research & Therapy* 8, supplement 1 (2006): S1, https://doi.org/10.1186/ar1906.

8. Julie Maurer, "Early Gout Is Bad for the Heart: Recent Research Context," *MedPage Today*, November 28, 2019, https://www.medpagetoday.com/reading-room /acrr/generalrheumatology/83581. Also see Yan Li et al., "Clinical Characteristics of Early-Onset Gout in Outpatient Setting," *ACR Open Rheumatology* 1, no. 7 (2019): 397–402, https://doi.org/10.1002/acr2.11057.

9. Jasvinder A. Singh, "Gout: Will the 'King of Diseases' Be the First Rheumatic Disease to Be Cured?," *BMC Medicine* 14 (2016): 180, https://doi.org/10.1186 /s12916-016-0732-1.

10. Christina George and David A. Minter, "Hyperuricemia," *StatPearls* (Treasure Island, FL: 2021), https://www.ncbi.nlm.nih.gov/books/NBK459218/.

11. Jiunn-Horng Chen et al., "Serum Uric Acid Level as an Independent Risk Factor for All-Cause, Cardiovascular, and Ischemic Stroke Mortality: A Chinese Cohort Study," *Arthritis & Rheumatology* 61, no. 2 (February 2009): 225–32, https://doi .org/10.1002/art.24164. Also see Erick Prado de Oliveira and Roberto Carlos Burini, "High Plasma Uric Acid Concentration: Causes and Consequences," *Diabetology & Metabolic Syndrome* 4 (April 2012): 12, https://doi.org/10.1186/1758-5996-4-12.

12. Rashika El Ridi and Hatem Tallima, "Physiological Functions and Pathogenic Potential of Uric Acid: A Review," *Journal of Advanced Research* 8, no. 5 (September 2017): 487–93, https://doi.org/10.1016/j.jare.2017.03.003.

13. El Ridi and Tallima, "Physiological Functions and Pathogenic Potential of Uric Acid."

14. James J. DiNicolantonio, James H. O'Keefe, and Sean C. Lucan, "Added Fructose: A Principal Driver of Type 2 Diabetes Mellitus and Its Consequences," *Mayo Clinic Proceedings* 90, no. 3 (March 2015): 372–81, https://doi.org/10.1016/j.mayocp.2014 .12.019.

15. Fiorenzo Stirpe et al., "Fructose-induced Hyperuricaemia," *The Lancet* 296, no. 7686 (December 1970): 1310–11, https://doi.org/10.1016/s0140-6736(70)92269-5.

16. Michael I. Goran et al., "The Obesogenic Effect of High Fructose Exposure During Early Development," *Nature Reviews Endocrinology* 9, no. 8 (August 2013): 494–500.

17. Christopher Rivard et al., "Sack and Sugar, and the Aetiology of Gout in England Between 1650 and 1900," *Rheumatology* 52, no. 3 (March 2013): 421–26, https:// doi.org/10.1093/rheumatology/kes297.

18. Lina Zgaga et al., "The Association of Dietary Intake of Purine-Rich Vegetables, Sugar-Sweetened Beverages and Dairy with Plasma Urate, in a Cross-Sectional

Study," *PLOS ONE* 7, no. 6 (2012): e38123, https://doi.org/10.1371/journal .pone.0038123.

19. Jasvinder A. Singh, Supriya G. Reddy, and Joseph Kundukulam, "Risk Factors for Gout and Prevention: A Systematic Review of the Literature," *Current Opinion in Rheumatology* 23, no. 2 (March 2011): 192–202, https://doi.org/10.1097/BOR.0b013 e3283438e13.

20. Christian Enzinger et al., "Risk Factors for Progression of Brain Atrophy in Aging: Six-Year Follow-Up of Normal Subjects," *Neurology* 64, no. 10 (May 24, 2005): 1704–11, https://doi.org/10.1212/01.WNL.0000161871.83614.BB.

21. Paul K. Crane et al., "Glucose Levels and Risk of Dementia," *New England Journal of Medicine* 369, no. 6 (August 2013): 540–48, https://doi.org/10.1056/NEJMoa1215740.

Chapter 1: U Defined

1. Gertrude W. Van Pelt, "A Study of Haig's Uric Acid Theory," *Boston Medical and Surgical Journal* 134, no. 6 (1896): 129–34, https://doi.org/10.1056/NEJM1896020 61340601.

2. Richard J. Johnson et al., "Lessons from Comparative Physiology: Could Uric Acid Represent a Physiologic Alarm Signal Gone Awry in Western Society?," *Journal of Comparative Physiology B: Biochemical, Systemic, and Environmental Physiology* 179, no. 1 (January 2009): 67–76, https://doi.org/10.1007/s00360-008-0291-7.

3. See Framingham Heart Study, http://www.framinghamheartstudy.org.

4. Bruce F. Culleton et al., "Serum Uric Acid and Risk for Cardiovascular Disease and Death: The Framingham Heart Study," *Annals of Internal Medicine* 131, no. 1 (July 1999): 7–13, https://doi.org/10.7326/0003-4819-131-1-199907060-00003.

5. To access a partial list of Dr. Richard J. Johnson's research papers, go to his Google Scholar page at https://scholar.google.com/citations?user=dTgECeMAA AAJ&hl=en.

6. Richard J. Johnson and Peter Andrews, "The Fat Gene," *Scientific American* 313, no. 4 (October 2015): 64–69, https://doi.org/10.1038/scientificamerican1015-64.

7. Johnson and Andrews, "The Fat Gene."

8. Johnson and Andrews, "The Fat Gene."

9. Daniel I. Feig, Beth Soletsky, and Richard J. Johnson, "Effect of Allopurinol on Blood Pressure of Adolescents with Newly Diagnosed Essential Hypertension: A Randomized Trial," *JAMA* 300, no. 8 (August 2008): 924–32, https://doi .org/10.1001/jama.300.8.924.

10. Mehmet Kanbay et al., "A Randomized Study of Allopurinol on Endothelial Function and Estimated Glomular Filtration Rate in Asymptomatic Hyperuricemic Subjects with Normal Renal Function," *Clinical Journal of the American Society of Nephrology* 6, no. 8 (August 2011): 1887–94, https://doi.org/10.2215/CJN.11451210. Also see Jacob George and Allan D. Struthers, "Role of Urate, Xanthine Oxidase

and the Effects of Allopurinol in Vascular Oxidative Stress," *Vascular Health and Risk Management* 5, no. 1 (2009): 265–72, https://doi.org/10.2147/vhrm.s4265; Scott W. Muir et al., "Allopurinol Use Yields Potentially Beneficial Effects on Inflammatory Indices in Those with Recent Ischemic Stroke: A Randomized, Double-Blind, Placebo-Controlled Trial," *Stroke* 39, no. 12 (December 2008): 3303–7, https://doi.org/10.1161/STROKEAHA.108.519793; Jesse Dawson et al., "The Effect of Allopurinol on the Cerebral Vasculature of Patients with Subcortical Stroke; a Randomized Trial," *British Journal of Clinical Pharmacology* 68, no. 5 (November 2009): 662–68, https://doi.org/10.1111/j.1365-2125.2009.03497.x; Fernando E García-Arroyo et al., "Allopurinol Prevents the Lipogenic Response Induced by an Acute Oral Fructose Challenge in Short-Term Fructose Fed Rats," *Biomolecules* 9, no. 10 (October 2019): 601, https://doi.org/10.3390/biom9100601; Jasvinder A. Singh and Shaohua Yu, "Allopurinol and the Risk of Stroke in Older Adults Receiving Medicare," *BMC Neurology* 16, no. 1 (September 2016): 164, https://doi.org/10.1186/s12883-016-0692-2; Marilisa Bove et al., "An Evidence-Based Review on Urate-Lowering Treatments: Implications for Optimal Treatment of Chronic Hyperuricemia," *Vascular Health and Risk Management* 13 (February 2017): 23–28, https://doi.org/10.2147/VHRM.S115080.

11. Federica Piani, Arrigo F. G. Cicero, and Claudio Borghi, "Uric Acid and Hypertension: Prognostic Role and Guide for Treatment," *Journal of Clinical Medicine* 10, no. 3 (January 2021): 448, https://doi.org/10.3390/jcm10030448. Also see Qing Xiong, Jie Liu, and Yancheng Xu, "Effects of Uric Acid on Diabetes Mellitus and Its Chronic Complications," *International Journal of Endocrinology* 2019, article ID 9691345 (October 2019), https://doi.org/10.1155/2019/9691345; Anju Gill et al., "Correlation of the Serum Insulin and the Serum Uric Acid Levels with the Glycated Haemoglobin Levels in the Patients of Type 2 Diabetes Mellitus," *Journal of Clinical and Diagnostic Research* 7, no. 7 (July 2013): 1295–97, https://doi.org/10.7860/JCDR/2013/6017.3121; Zohreh Soltani et al., "Potential Role of Uric Acid in Metabolic Syndrome, Hypertension, Kidney Injury, and Cardiovascular Diseases: Is It Time for Reappraisal?," *Current Hypertension Reports* 15, no. 3 (June 2013): 175–81, https://doi.org/10.1007/s11906-013-0344-5; Magdalena Madero et al., "A Pilot Study on the Impact of a Low Fructose Diet and Allopurinol on Clinic Blood Pressure Among Overweight and Prehypertensive Subjects: A Randomized Placebo Controlled Trial," *Journal of the American Society of Hypertension* 9, no. 11 (November 2015): 837–44, https://doi.org/10.1016/j.jash.2015.07.008.

12. James T. Kratzer et al., "Evolutionary History and Metabolic Insights of Ancient Mammalian Uricases," *Proceedings of the National Academy of Sciences* (USA) 111, no. 10 (March 2014): 3763–68, https://doi.org/10.1073/pnas.1320393111.

13. Catarina Rendeiro et al., "Fructose Decreases Physical Activity and Increases Body Fat Without Affecting Hippocampal Neurogenesis and Learning Relative to an Isocaloric Glucose Diet," *Scientific Reports* 5 (2015): 9589, https://doi.org/10.1038

/srep09589. Also see Beckman Institute for Advanced Science and Technology, "Fructose Contributes to Weight Gain, Physical Inactivity, and Body Fat, Researchers Find," *ScienceDaily*, June 1, 2015, www.sciencedaily.com/releases/2015/06/150 601122540.htm.

14. Dianne P. Figlewicz et al., "Effect of Moderate Intake of Sweeteners on Metabolic Health in the Rat," *Physiology & Behavior* 98, no. 5 (December 2009): 618–24, https://doi.org/10.1016/j.physbeh.2009.09.016. Also see Isabelle Aeberli et al., "Moderate Amounts of Fructose Consumption Impair Insulin Sensitivity in Healthy Young Men: A Randomized Controlled Trial," *Diabetes Care* 36, no. 1 (January 2013): 150–56, https://doi.org/10.2337/dc12-0540.

15. Mehmet Kanbay et al., "Uric Acid in Metabolic Syndrome: From an Innocent Bystander to a Central Player," *European Journal of Internal Medicine* 29 (April 2016): 3–8, https://doi.org/10.1016/j.ejim.2015.11.026.

16. Tsuneo Konta et al., "Association Between Serum Uric Acid Levels and Mortality: A Nationwide Community-Based Cohort Study," *Scientific Reports* 10, no. 1 (April 2020): 6066, https://doi.org/10.1038/s41598-020-63134-0.

17. Jiunn-Horng Chen et al., "Serum Uric Acid Level as an Independent Risk Factor for All-Cause, Cardiovascular, and Ischemic Stroke Mortality: A Chinese Cohort Study," *Arthritis & Rheumatology* 61, no. 2 (February 2009): 225–32, https://doi .org/10.1002/art.24164.

18. Yan-Ci Zhao et al., "Nonalcoholic Fatty Liver Disease: An Emerging Driver of Hypertension," *Hypertension* 75, no. 2 (February 2020): 275–84, https://doi .org/10.1161/HYPERTENSIONAHA.119.13419. Also see Philipp Kasper et al., "NAFLD and Cardiovascular Diseases: A Clinical Review," *Clinical Research in Cardiology* 110, no. 7 (July 2021): 921–37, https://doi.org/10.1007/s00392-020-01709-7.

19. Zobair M. Younossi, "Non-alcoholic Fatty Liver Disease — A Global Public Health Perspective," *Journal of Hepatology* 70, no. 3 (March 2019): 531–44, https://doi .org/10.1016/j.jhep.2018.10.033.

20. Guntur Darmawan, Laniyati Hamijoyo, and Irsan Hasan, "Association Between Serum Uric Acid and Non-alcoholic Fatty Liver Disease: A Meta-Analysis," *Acta Medica Indonesiana* 49, no. 2 (April 2017): 136–47. Also see Ekaterini Margariti et al., "Non-alcoholic Fatty Liver Disease May Develop in Individuals with Normal Body Mass Index," *Annals of Gastroenterology* 25, no. 1 (2012): 45–51; Alihan Oral et al., "Relationship Between Serum Uric Acid Levels and Nonalcoholic Fatty Liver Disease in Non-obese Patients," *Medicina* 55, no. 9 (September 2019): 600, https://doi.org/10.3390/medicina55090600.

21. Paschalis Paschos et al., "Can Serum Uric Acid Lowering Therapy Contribute to the Prevention or Treatment of Nonalcoholic Fatty Liver Disease?," *Current Vascular Pharmacology* 16, no. 3 (2018): 269–75, https://doi.org/10.2174/157016111566617 0621082237.

22. Rosangela Spiga et al., "Uric Acid Is Associated with Inflammatory Biomarkers

and Induces Inflammation via Activating the NF-κB Signaling Pathway in HepG2 Cells," *Arteriosclerosis, Thrombosis, and Vascular Biology* 37, no. 6 (June 2017): 1241–49, https://doi.org/10.1161/ATVBAHA.117.309128. Also see Toshiko Tanaka et al., "A Double Blind Placebo Controlled Randomized Trial of the Effect of Acute Uric Acid Changes on Inflammatory Markers in Humans: A Pilot Study," *PLOS ONE* 12, no. 8 (August 2017): e0181100, https://doi.org/10.1371/journal.pone.0181100; Carmelinda Ruggiero et al., "Uric Acid and Inflammatory Markers," *European Heart Journal* 27, no. 10 (May 2006): 1174–81, https://doi.org/10.1093/eurheartj /ehi879.

23. Christine Gorman, Alice Park, and Kristina Dell, "Health: The Fires Within," *Time* 163, no. 8 (February 23, 2004).

24. Gorman, Park, and Dell, "Health."

25. Gorman, Park, and Dell, "Health."

26. See my January 3, 2016, podcast recording with Dr. Ludwig at https://www.drperl mutter.com/. For more about Dr. Ludwig and his work, see https://www.drdavidlud wig.com/.

27. Carmelinda Ruggiero et al., "Usefulness of Uric Acid to Predict Changes in C-Reactive Protein and Interleukin-6 in 3-Year Period in Italians Aged 21 to 98 Years," *American Journal of Cardiology* 100, no. 1 (July 2007): 115–21, https://doi .org/10.1016/j.amjcard.2007.02.065.

28. Dietrich Rothenbacher et al., "Relationship Between Inflammatory Cytokines and Uric Acid Levels with Adverse Cardiovascular Outcomes in Patients with Stable Coronary Heart Disease," *PLOS ONE* 7, no. 9 (2012): e45907, https://doi .org/10.1371/journal.pone.0045907.

29. Norman K. Pollock et al., "Greater Fructose Consumption Is Associated with Cardiometabolic Risk Markers and Visceral Adiposity in Adolescents," *Journal of Nutrition* 142, no. 2 (February 2012): 251–57, https://doi.org/10.3945/jn.111.150219. Also see Lucia Pacifico et al., "Pediatric Nonalcoholic Fatty Liver Disease, Metabolic Syndrome and Cardiovascular Risk," *World Journal of Gastroenterology* 17, no. 26 (July 2011): 3082–91; Jia Zheng et al., "Early Life Fructose Exposure and Its Implications for Long-Term Cardiometabolic Health in Offspring," *Nutrients* 8, no. 11 (November 2016): 685, https://doi.org/10.3390/nu8110685; Sarah C. Couch et al., "Fructose Intake and Cardiovascular Risk Factors in Youth with Type 1 Diabetes: SEARCH for Diabetes in Youth Study," *Diabetes Research and Clinical Practice* 100, no. 2 (May 2013): 265–71, https://doi.org/10.1016/j.diabres.2013.03.013; Bohyun Park et al., "Association Between Serum Levels of Uric Acid and Blood Pressure Tracking in Childhood," *American Journal of Hypertension* 30, no. 7 (July 2017): 713–18, https://doi.org/10.1093/ajh/hpx037.

30. Arnold B. Alper Jr. et al., "Childhood Uric Acid Predicts Adult Blood Pressure: The Bogalusa Heart Study," *Hypertension* 45, no. 1 (January 2005): 34–38, https:// doi.org/10.1161/01.HYP.0000150783.79172.bb. Also see "Increased Uric Acid Levels

in Early Life May Lead to High Blood Pressure Later On," News-Medical.Net, March 15, 2017, https://www.news-medical.net/news/20170315/Increased-uric-acid -levels-in-early-life-may-lead-to-high-blood-pressure-later-on.aspx.

31. Darlle Santos Araujo et al., "Salivary Uric Acid Is a Predictive Marker of Body Fat Percentage in Adolescents," *Nutrition Research* 74 (February 2020): 62–70, https:// doi.org/10.1016/j.nutres.2019.11.007.

32. See "Obesity and Overweight," National Center for Health Statistics, https://www .cdc.gov/nchs/fastats/obesity-overweight.htm.

33. "Obesity and Overweight."

34. Zachary J. Ward et al., "Projected U.S. State-Level Prevalence of Adult Obesity and Severe Obesity," *New England Journal of Medicine* 381 (December 2019): 2440–50, https://doi.org/10.1056/NEJMsa1909301.

35. "Obesity and Overweight."

36. "Obesity and Overweight."

37. Grishma Hirode and Robert J. Wong, "Trends in the Prevalence of Metabolic Syndrome in the United States, 2011–2016," *JAMA* 323, no. 24 (June 2020): 2526–28, https://doi.org/10.1001/jama.2020.4501.

38. Ting Huai Shi, Binhuan Wang, and Sundar Natarajan, "The Influence of Metabolic Syndrome in Predicting Mortality Risk Among US Adults: Importance of Metabolic Syndrome Even in Adults with Normal Weight," *Preventing Chronic Disease* 17 (May 2020): E36, https://doi.org/10.5888/pcd17.200020.

39. Richard J. Johnson et al., "Redefining Metabolic Syndrome as a Fat Storage Condition Based on Studies of Comparative Physiology," *Obesity* 21, no. 4 (April 2013): 659–64, https://doi.org/10.1002/oby.20026.

40. Shreyasi Chatterjee and Amritpal Mudher, "Alzheimer's Disease and Type 2 Diabetes: A Critical Assessment of the Shared Pathological Traits," *Frontiers in Neuroscience* 12 (June 2018): 383, https://doi.org/10.3389/fnins.2018.00383. Also see Sujung Yoon et al., "Brain Changes in Overweight/Obese and Normal-Weight Adults with Type 2 Diabetes Mellitus," *Diabetologia* 60, no. 7 (2017): 1207–17, https://doi.org/10.1007/s00125-017-4266-7.

41. Claudio Barbiellini Amidei et al., "Association Between Age at Diabetes Onset and Subsequent Risk of Dementia," *JAMA* 325, no. 16 (April 2021): 1640–49, https://doi.org/10.1001/jama.2021.4001.

42. Fanfan Zheng et al., "HbA$_{1c}$, Diabetes and Cognitive Decline: the English Longitudinal Study of Ageing," *Diabetologia* 61, no. 4 (April 2018): 839–48, https://doi .org/10.1007/s00125-017-4541-7.

43. Richard J. Johnson et al., "Cerebral Fructose Metabolism as a Potential Mechanism Driving Alzheimer's Disease," *Frontiers in Aging Neuroscience* 12 (September 2020): 560865, https://doi.org/10.3389/fnagi.2020.560865.

44. Prateek Lohia et al., "Metabolic Syndrome and Clinical Outcomes in Patients Infected with COVID-19: Does Age, Sex, and Race of the Patient with Metabolic

Syndrome Matter?," *Journal of Diabetes* 13, no. 5 (January 2021): 420–29, https://doi.org/10.1111/1753-0407.13157.

45. Bo Chen et al., "Serum Uric Acid Concentrations and Risk of Adverse Outcomes in Patients With COVID-19," *Frontiers in Endocrinology* 12 (May 2021): 633767, https://doi.org/10.3389/fendo.2021.633767.

46. Maxime Taquet et al., "6-month Neurological and Psychiatric Outcomes in 236 379 Survivors of COVID-19: A Retrospective Cohort Study Using Electronic Health Records," *Lancet Psychiatry* 8, no. 5 (May 2021): 416–27, https://doi.org/10.1016/S2215-0366(21)00084-5.

47. Barry M. Popkin et al., "Individuals with Obesity and COVID-19: A Global Perspective on the Epidemiology and Biological Relationships," *Obesity Reviews* 21, no. 11 (November 2020): e13128, https://doi.org/10.1111/obr.13128.

48. Firoozeh Hosseini-Esfahani et al., "Dietary Fructose and Risk of Metabolic Syndrome in Adults: Tehran Lipid and Glucose Study," *Nutrition & Metabolism* 8, no. 1 (July 2011): 50, https://doi.org/10.1186/1743-7075-8-50.

49. Laura Billiet et al., "Review of Hyperuricemia as New Marker for Metabolic Syndrome," *ISRN Rheumatology* 2014, article ID 852954 (February 2014), https://doi.org/10.1155/2014/852954. Also see Christopher King et al., "Uric Acid as a Cause of the Metabolic Syndrome," *Contributions to Nephrology* 192 (2018): 88–102, https://doi.org/10.1159/000484283; Marek Kretowicz et al., "The Impact of Fructose on Renal Function and Blood Pressure," *International Journal of Nephrology* 2011, article ID 315879 (2011), https://doi.org/10.4061/2011/315879; Clive M. Brown et al., "Fructose Ingestion Acutely Elevates Blood Pressure in Healthy Young Humans," *American Journal of Physiology — Regulatory, Integrative and Comparative Physiology* 294, no. 3 (March 2008): R730–37, https://doi.org/10.1152/ajpregu.00680.2007; Alice Victoria Klein and Hosen Kiat, "The Mechanisms Underlying Fructose-Induced Hypertension: A Review," *Journal of Hypertension* 33, no. 5 (May 2015): 912–20, https://doi.org/10.1097/HJH.0000000000000551.

50. Kanbay et al., "Uric Acid in Metabolic Syndrome."

51. Usama A. A. Sharaf El Din, Mona M. Salem, and Dina O. Abdulazim, "Uric Acid in the Pathogenesis of Metabolic, Renal, and Cardiovascular Diseases: A Review," *Journal of Advanced Research* 8, no. 5 (September 2017): 537–48, https://doi.org/10.1016/j.jare.2016.11.004. Also see Seung Jae Lee, Byeong Kil Oh, and Ki-Chul Sung, "Uric Acid and Cardiometabolic Diseases," *Clinical Hypertension* 26, article no. 13 (June 2020), https://doi.org/10.1186/s40885-020-00146-y; Takahiko Nakagawa et al., "Unearthing Uric Acid: An Ancient Factor with Recently Found Significance in Renal and Cardiovascular Disease," *Kidney International* 69, no. 10 (May 2006): 1722–25, https://doi.org/10.1038/sj.ki.5000391; Takahiko Nakagawa et al., "The Conundrum of Hyperuricemia, Metabolic Syndrome, and Renal Disease," *Internal and Emergency Medicine* 3, no. 4 (December 2008): 313–18, https://doi.org/10.1007/s11739-008-0141-3.

52. Zahra Bahadoran et al., "Hyperuricemia-Induced Endothelial Insulin Resistance: The Nitric Oxide Connection," *Pflügers Archiv: European Journal of Physiology* (July 2021), https://doi.org/10.1007/s00424-021-02606-2.

53. Hong Wang et al., "Nitric Oxide Directly Promotes Vascular Endothelial Insulin Transport," *Diabetes* 62, no. 12 (December 2013): 4030–42, https://doi.org/10.2337/db13-0627.

54. Christine Gersch et al., "Inactivation of Nitric Oxide by Uric Acid," *Nucleosides, Nucleotides & Nucleic Acids* 27, no. 8 (August 2008): 967–78, https://doi.org/10.1080/15257770802257952. Also see Giuseppe Mercuro et al., "Effect of Hyperuricemia Upon Endothelial Function in Patients at Increased Cardiovascular Risk," *American Journal of Cardiology* 94, no. 7 (October 2004): 932–35, https://doi.org/10.1016/j.amjcard.2004.06.032.

55. Anju Gill et al., "Correlation of the Serum Insulin and the Serum Uric Acid Levels with the Glycated Haemoglobin Levels in the Patients of Type 2 Diabetes Mellitus," *Journal of Clinical and Diagnostic Research* 7, no. 7 (July 2013): 1295–97, https://doi.org/10.7860/JCDR/2013/6017.3121.

56. Sepehr Salem et al., "Serum Uric Acid as a Risk Predictor for Erectile Dysfunction," *Journal of Sexual Medicine* 11, no. 5 (May 2014): 1118–24, https://doi.org/10.1111/jsm.12495. Also see Yalcin Solak et al., "Uric Acid Level and Erectile Dysfunction in Patients with Coronary Artery Disease," *Journal of Sexual Medicine* 11, no. 1 (January 2014): 165–72, https://doi.org/10.1111/jsm.12332; Alessandra Barassi et al., "Levels of Uric Acid in Erectile Dysfunction of Different Aetiology," *Aging Male* 21, no. 3 (September 2018): 200–205, https://doi.org/10.1080/13685538.2017.1420158.

57. Jan Adamowicz and Tomasz Drewa, "Is There a Link Between Soft Drinks and Erectile Dysfunction?," *Central European Journal of Urology* 64, no. 3 (2011): 140–43, https://doi.org/10.5173/ceju.2011.03.art8.

58. Leo A. B. Joosten et al., "Asymptomatic Hyperuricaemia: A Silent Activator of the Innate Immune System," *Nature Reviews Rheumatology* 16, no. 2 (February 2020): 75–86, https://doi.org/10.1038/s41584-019-0334-3. Also see Georgiana Cabău et al., "Urate-Induced Immune Programming: Consequences for Gouty Arthritis and Hyperuricemia," *Immunological Reviews* 294, no. 1 (March 2020): 92–105, https://doi.org/10.1111/imr.12833.

59. Sung Kweon Cho et al., "U-Shaped Association Between Serum Uric Acid Level and Risk of Mortality: A Cohort Study," *Arthritis & Rheumatology* 70, no. 7 (July 2018): 1122–32, https://doi.org/10.1002/art.40472.

Chapter 2: Survival of the Fattest

1. Malcolm W. Browne, "Pity a Tyrannosaur? Sue Had Gout," *New York Times*, May 22, 1997.

2. James V. Neel, "Diabetes Mellitus: A 'Thrifty' Genotype Rendered Detrimental by 'Progress'?," *American Journal of Human Genetics* 14, no. 4 (December 1962): 353–62.

3. Loren Cordain et al., "Origins and Evolution of the Western Diet: Health Implications for the 21st Century," *American Journal of Clinical Nutrition* 81, no. 2 (February 2005): 341–54, https://doi.org/10.1093/ajcn.81.2.341.

4. Pedro Carrera-Bastos et al., "The Western Diet and Lifestyle and Diseases of Civilization," *Research Reports in Clinical Cardiology* 2 (2011): 15–35, https://doi.org/10.2147/RRCC.S16919.

5. Herman Pontzer, Brian M. Wood, and David A. Raichlen, "Hunter-Gatherers as Models in Public Health," *Obesity Reviews* 19, Supplement 1 (December 2018): 24–35, https://doi.org/10.1111/obr.12785.

6. Johnson and Andrews, "The Fat Gene."

7. Johnson and Andrews, "The Fat Gene."

8. A multitude of studies covers this phenomenon; see Christina Cicerchi et al., "Uric Acid-Dependent Inhibition of AMP Kinase Induces Hepatic Glucose Production in Diabetes and Starvation: Evolutionary Implications of the Uricase Loss in Hominids," *FASEB Journal* 28, no. 8 (August 2014): 3339–50, https://doi.org/10.1096/fj.13-243634. Also see Richard J. Johnson et al., "Uric Acid, Evolution and Primitive Cultures," *Seminars in Nephrology* 25, no. 1 (January 2005): 3–8, https://doi.org/10.1016/j.semnephrol.2004.09.002.

9. Belinda S. W. Chan, "Ancient Insights into Uric Acid Metabolism in Primates," *Proceedings of the National Academy of Sciences* (USA) 111, no. 10 (March 2014): 3657–58, https://doi.org/10.1073/pnas.1401037111.

10. Richard J. Johnson et al., "Metabolic and Kidney Diseases in the Setting of Climate Change, Water Shortage, and Survival Factors," *Journal of the American Society of Nephrology* 27, no. 8 (August 2016): 2247–56, https://doi.org/10.1681/ASN.2015121314. Also see Elza Muscelli et al., "Effect of Insulin on Renal Sodium and Uric Acid Handling in Essential Hypertension," *American Journal of Hypertension* 9, no. 8 (August 1996): 746–52, https://doi.org/10.1016/0895-7061(96)00098-2.

11. Richard J. Johnson et al., "Fructose Metabolism as a Common Evolutionary Pathway of Survival Associated with Climate Change, Food Shortage and Droughts," *Journal of Internal Medicine* 287, no. 3 (March 2020): 252–62, https://doi.org/10.1111/joim.12993.

12. The research abounds with literature dating back decades implicating fructose in hyperuricemia and the development of many other pathologies. Here are some gems: Jaakko Perheentupa and Kari Raivio, "Fructose-Induced Hyperuricaemia," *The Lancet* 290, no. 7515 (September 1967): 528–31, https://doi.org/10.1016/s0140-6736(67)90494-1; Takahiko Nakagawa et al., "A Causal Role for Uric Acid in Fructose-Induced Metabolic Syndrome," *American Journal of Physiology—Renal Physiology* 290, no. 3 (March 2006): F625–31, https://doi.org/10.1152/ajprenal.00140.2005; Sally Robertson, "High Uric Acid Precursor of Obesity, Metabolic Syndrome," News-Medical.Net, September 20, 2012, https://www.news-medical.net/news/20120920/High-uric-acid-precursor-of-obesity-metabolic-syndrome.aspx;

Geoffrey Livesey and Richard Taylor, "Fructose Consumption and Consequences for Glycation, Plasma Triacylglycerol, and Body Weight: Meta-analyses and Meta-regression Models of Intervention Studies," *American Journal of Clinical Nutrition* 88, no. 5 (November 2008): 1419–37; Food Insight, "Questions and Answers About Fructose," September 29, 2009, International Food Information Council Foundation, https://foodinsight.org/questions-and-answers-about-fructose/; Masanari Kuwabara et al., "Asymptomatic Hyperuricemia Without Comorbidities Predicts Cardiometabolic Diseases: Five-Year Japanese Cohort Study," *Hypertension* 69, no. 6 (June 2017): 1036–44, https://doi.org/10.1161/HYPERTENSIONAHA .116.08998; Magdalena Madero et al., "The Effect of Two Energy-Restricted Diets, a Low-Fructose Diet Versus a Moderate Natural Fructose Diet, on Weight Loss and Metabolic Syndrome Parameters: A Randomized Controlled Trial," *Metabolism* 60, no. 11 (November 2011): 1551–59, https://doi.org/10.1016/j.metabol.2011.04.001; Vivian L. Choo et al., "Food Sources of Fructose-Containing Sugars and Glycaemic Control: Systematic Review and Meta-analysis of Controlled Intervention Studies," *The BMJ* 363 (November 2018): k4644, https://doi.org/10.1136/bmj .k4644; Isao Muraki et al., "Fruit Consumption and Risk of Type 2 Diabetes: Results from Three Prospective Longitudinal Cohort Studies," *The BMJ* 347 (August 2013): f5001, https://doi.org/10.1136/bmj.f5001; Ravi Dhingra et al., "Soft Drink Consumption and Risk of Developing Cardiometabolic Risk Factors and the Metabolic Syndrome in Middle-Aged Adults in the Community," *Circulation* 116, no. 5 (July 2007): 480–88, https://doi.org/10.1161/CIRCULATIONAHA .107.689935; Zhila Semnani-Azad et al., "Association of Major Food Sources of Fructose-Containing Sugars with Incident Metabolic Syndrome: A Systematic Review and Meta-analysis," *JAMA Network Open* 3, no. 7 (July 2020): e209993, https://doi.org/10.1001/jamanetworkopen.2020.9993; William Nseir, Fares Nassar, and Nimer Assy, "Soft Drinks Consumption and Nonalcoholic Fatty Liver Disease," *World Journal of Gastroenterology* 16, no. 21 (June 2010): 2579–88, https:// doi.org/10.3748/wjg.v16.i21.2579; Manoocher Soleimani and Pooneh Alborzi, "The Role of Salt in the Pathogenesis of Fructose-Induced Hypertension," *International Journal of Nephrology* 2011, article ID 392708 (2011), https://doi.org/10.4061/2011 /392708; James J. DiNicolantonio and Sean C. Lucan, "The Wrong White Crystals: Not Salt but Sugar as Aetiological in Hypertension and Cardiometabolic Disease," *Open Heart* 1, no. 1 (November 2014): e000167, https://doi.org/10.1136 /openhrt-2014-000167; Jonathan Q. Purnell et al., "Brain Functional Magnetic Resonance Imaging Response to Glucose and Fructose Infusions in Humans," *Diabetes, Obesity and Metabolism* 13, no. 3 (March 2011): 229–34, https://doi.org/10 .1111/j.1463-1326.2010.01340.x.

13. Sanjay Basu et al., "The Relationship of Sugar to Population-Level Diabetes Prevalence: An Econometric Analysis of Repeated Cross-Sectional Data," *PLOS ONE* 8, no. 2 (2013): e57873, https://doi.org/10.1371/journal.pone.0057873.

14. See SugarScience, "How Much Is Too Much? The Growing Concern over Too Much Added Sugar in Our Diets," University of San Francisco, https://sugar science.ucsf.edu/the-growing-concern-of-overconsumption.html#.YShIyVNKjX0.

15. Ryan W. Walker, Kelly A. Dumke, and Michael I. Goran, "Fructose Content in Popular Beverages Made with and Without High-Fructose Corn Syrup," *Nutrition* 30, nos. 7–8 (July–August 2014): 928–35, https://doi.org/10.1016/j.nut.2014.04.003.

16. James P. Casey, "High Fructose Corn Syrup—A Case History of Innovation," *Research Management* 19, no. 5 (September 1976): 27–32, https://doi.org/10.1080/0 0345334.1976.11756374. Also see Kara Newman, *The Secret Financial Life of Food: From Commodities Markets to Supermarkets* (New York: Columbia University Press, 2013).

17. James M. Rippe, ed., *Fructose, High Fructose Corn Syrup, Sucrose and Health* (New York: Springer, 2014). Also see Mark S. Segal, Elizabeth Gollub, and Richard J. Johnson, "Is the Fructose Index More Relevant with Regards to Cardiovascular Disease Than the Glycemic Index?," *European Journal of Nutrition* 46, no. 7 (October 2007): 406–17, https://doi.org/10.1007/s00394-007-0680-9.

18. Anna L. Gosling, Elizabeth Matisoo-Smith, and Tony R. Merriman, "Hyperuricaemia in the Pacific: Why the Elevated Serum Urate Levels?," *Rheumatology International* 34, no. 6 (June 2014): 743–57, https://doi.org/10.1007/s00296-013-2922-x.

19. Meera Senthilingam, "How Paradise Became the Fattest Place in the World," CNN.com, May 1, 2015, https://www.cnn.com/2015/05/01/health/pacific-islands -obesity/index.html.

20. Senthilingham, "How Paradise Became the Fattest Place in the World."

21. See the World Health Organization's report *Overweight and Obesity in the Western Pacific Region: An Equity Perspective* (Manila: World Health Organization Regional Office for the Western Pacific, 2017).

22. Barry S. Rose, "Gout in the Maoris," *Seminars in Arthritis and Rheumatism* 5, no. 2 (November 1975): 121–45, https://doi.org/10.1016/0049-0172(75)90002-5.

23. Rose, "Gout in the Maoris."

24. Hanxiao Sun et al., "The Impact of Global and Local Polynesian Genetic Ancestry on Complex Traits in Native Hawaiians," *PLOS Genetics* 17, no. 2 (February 2021): e1009273, https://doi.org/10.1371/journal.pgen.1009273. Also see Liufu Cui et al., "Prevalence and Risk Factors of Hyperuricemia: Results of the Kailuan Cohort Study," *Modern Rheumatology* 27, no. 6 (November 2017): 1066–71, https://doi.org /10.1080/14397595.2017.1300117.

25. Veronica Hackethal, "Samoan 'Obesity' Gene Found in Half of Population There," *Medscape Medical News*, August 3, 2016, https://www.medscape.com/viewarticle /866987.

26. Tony R. Merriman and Nicola Dalbeth, "The Genetic Basis of Hyperuricaemia and Gout," *Joint Bone Spine* 78, no. 1 (January 2011): 35–40, https://doi.org /10.1016/j.jbspin.2010.02.027.

27. Robert G. Hughes and Mark A. Lawrence, "Globalization, Food and Health in Pacific Island Countries," *Asia Pacific Journal of Clinical Nutrition* 14, no. 4 (April 2005): 298–306.

28. Nurshad Ali et al., "Prevalence of Hyperuricemia and the Relationship Between Serum Uric Acid and Obesity: A Study on Bangladeshi Adults," *PLOS ONE* 13, no. 11 (November 2018): e0206850, https://doi.org/10.1371/journal.pone.0206850. Also see Mahantesh I. Biradar et al., "The Causal Role of Elevated Uric Acid and Waist Circumference on the Risk of Metabolic Syndrome Components," *International Journal of Obesity* 44, no. 4 (April 2020): 865–74, https://doi.org/10.1038/s41366-019-0487-9.

29. Miguel A. Lanaspa et al., "Opposing Activity Changes in AMP Deaminase and AMP-Activated Protein Kinase in the Hibernating Ground Squirrel," *PLOS ONE* 10, no. 4 (April 2015): e0123509, https://doi.org/10.1371/journal.pone.0123509.

30. Miguel A. Lanaspa et al., "Counteracting Roles of AMP Deaminase and AMP Kinase in the Development of Fatty Liver," *PLOS ONE* 7, no. 11 (2012): e48801, https://doi.org/10.1371/journal.pone.0048801.

31. Qiulan Lv et al., "Association of Hyperuricemia with Immune Disorders and Intestinal Barrier Dysfunction," *Frontiers in Physiology* 11 (November 2020): 524236, https://doi.org/10.3389/fphys.2020.524236.

32. Zhuang Guo et al., "Intestinal Microbiota Distinguish Gout Patients from Healthy Humans," *Scientific Reports* 6 (February 2016): 20602, https://doi.org/10.1038/srep20602.

Chapter 3: The Fallacy of Fructose

1. Brian Melley, "Sugar and Corn Syrup Industries Square Off in Court Over Ad Claims," NBC News, November 2, 2015, https://www.nbcnews.com/business/business-news/sugar-corn-syrup-industries-square-court-over-ad-claims-n455951. Also see Lisa McLaughlin, "Is High-Fructose Corn Syrup Really Good for You?" *Time*, September 17, 2008, http://content.time.com/time/health/article/0,8599,1841910,00.html.

2. For a narrative summary of the lawsuit, see Eric Lipton, "Rival Industries Sweet-Talk the Public," *New York Times*, February 11, 2014.

3. Sarah N. Heiss and Benjamin R. Bates, "When a Spoonful of Fallacies Helps the Sweetener Go Down: The Corn Refiner Association's Use of Straw-Person Arguments in Health Debates Surrounding High-Fructose Corn Syrup," *Health Communication* 31, no. 8 (August 2016): 1029–35, https://doi.org/10.1080/10410236.2015.1027988.

4. Sarah N. Heiss, "'Healthy' Discussions About Risk: The Corn Refiners Association's Strategic Negotiation of Authority in the Debate Over High Fructose Corn Syrup," *Public Understanding of Science* 22, no. 2 (February 2013): 219–35, https://doi.org/10.1177/0963662511402281.

5. Jeff Gelski, "Sweet Ending: Sugar Groups, Corn Refiners Settle Lawsuit," *Food Business News*, November 20, 2015, https://www.foodbusinessnews.net/articles /5376-sweet-ending-sugar-groups-corn-refiners-settle-lawsuit.

6. "Abundance of Fructose Not Good for the Liver, Heart," Harvard Health Publishing, Harvard Medical School, September 1, 2011, https://www.health.harvard.edu /heart-health/abundance-of-fructose-not-good-for-the-liver-heart.

7. Miriam B. Vos et al., "Dietary Fructose Consumption Among US Children and Adults: The Third National Health and Nutrition Examination Survey," *Medscape Journal of Medicine* 10, no. 7 (July 2008): 160.

8. Emily E. Ventura, Jaimie N. Davis, and Michael I. Goran, "Sugar Content of Popular Sweetened Beverages Based on Objective Laboratory Analysis: Focus on Fructose Content," *Obesity* 19, no. 4 (April 2011): 868–74, https://doi.org/10.1038 /oby.2010.255.

9. Kristen Domonell, "Just How Bad Is Sugar for You, Really?," *Right as Rain*, University of Washington School of Medicine, October 30, 2017, https://rightas rain.uwmedicine.org/body/food/just-how-bad-sugar-you-really. Also see Associated Press, "Just How Much Sugar Do Americans Consume? It's Complicated," *STAT*, September 20, 2016, https://www.statnews.com/2016/09/20/sugar-consumption-ame ricans/.

10. Sabrina Ayoub-Charette et al., "Important Food Sources of Fructose-Containing Sugars and Incident Gout: A Systematic Review and Meta-analysis of Prospective Cohort Studies," *BMJ Open* 9, no. 5 (May 2019): e024171, https://doi.org/10.1136 /bmjopen-2018-024171. Also see Nicola Dalbeth et al., "Body Mass Index Modulates the Relationship of Sugar-Sweetened Beverage Intake with Serum Urate Concentrations and Gout," *Arthritis Research & Therapy* 17, no. 1 (September 2015): 263, https://doi.org/10.1186/s13075-015-0781-4.

11. Robert H. Lustig, "The Fructose Epidemic," *The Bariatrician* (Spring 2009): 10–19, http://dustinmaherfitness.com/wp-content/uploads/2011/04/Bariatrician-Fruc tose.pdf.

12. Richard O. Marshall and Earl R. Kooi, "Enzymatic Conversion of D-Glucose to D-Fructose," *Science* 125, no. 3249 (April 1957): 648–49, https://doi.org/10.1126 /science.125.3249.648.

13. "High Fructose Corn Syrup Production Industry in the US—Market Research Report," IBISWorld.com (updated December 2020). Also see Barry M. Popkin and Corinna Hawkes, "Sweetening of the Global Diet, Particularly Beverages: Patterns, Trends, and Policy Responses," *Lancet Diabetes Endocrinology* 4, no. 2 (February 2016): 174–86, https://doi.org/10.1016/S2213-8587(15)00419-2.

14. Jean-Pierre Després and Susan Jebb, "Sugar-Sweetened Beverages: One Piece of the Obesity Puzzle?," *Journal of Cardiovascular Magnetic Resonance* 3, no. 3 (December 2010): 2–4. Also see Dong-Mei Zhang, Rui-Qing Jiao, and Ling-Dong Kong, "High Dietary Fructose: Direct or Indirect Dangerous Factors Disturbing Tissue and

Organ Functions," *Nutrients* 9, no. 4 (March 2017): 335, https://doi.org/10.3390/nu9040335.

15. Drew DeSilver, "What's on Your Table? How America's Diet Has Changed Over the Decades," Pew Research Center, December 13, 2016, https://www.pewresearch.org/fact-tank/2016/12/13/whats-on-your-table-how-americas-diet-has-changed-over-the-decades/.

16. Michael I. Goran, Stanley J. Ulijaszek, and Emily E. Ventura, "High Fructose Corn Syrup and Diabetes Prevalence: A Global Perspective," *Global Public Health* 8, no. 1 (2013): 55–64, https://doi.org/10.1080/17441692.2012.736257.

17. Jonathan E. Shaw, Richard A. Sicree, and Paul Z. Zimmet, "Global Estimates of the Prevalence of Diabetes for 2010 and 2030," *Diabetes Research and Clinical Practice* 87, no. 1 (January 2010): 4–14, https://doi.org/10.1016/j.diabres.2009.10.007.

18. Veronique Douard and Ronaldo P. Ferraris, "The Role of Fructose Transporters in Diseases Linked to Excessive Fructose Intake," *Journal of Physiology* 591, no. 2 (January 2013): 401–14, https://doi.org/10.1113/jphysiol.2011.215731. Also see Manal F. Abdelmalek et al., "Higher Dietary Fructose Is Associated with Impaired Hepatic Adenosine Triphosphate Homeostasis in Obese Individuals with Type 2 Diabetes," *Hepatology* 56, no. 3 (2012): 952–60, https://doi.org/10.1002/hep.25741.

19. Miguel A. Lanaspa et al., "Uric Acid Stimulates Fructokinase and Accelerates Fructose Metabolism in the Development of Fatty Liver," *PLOS ONE* 7, no. 10 (2012): e47948, https://doi.org/10.1371/journal.pone.0047948.

20. I amassed volumes of studies on the effects of fructose in the body. Here are some citations to get you started: Kimber L. Stanhope et al., "Consumption of Fructose and High Fructose Corn Syrup Increase Postprandial Triglycerides, LDL-Cholesterol, and Apolipoprotein-B in Young Men and Women," *Journal of Clinical Endocrinology and Metabolism* 96, no. 10 (October 2011): E1596–605, https://doi.org/10.1210/jc.2011-1251; Karen W. Della Corte et al., "Effect of Dietary Sugar Intake on Biomarkers of Subclinical Inflammation: A Systematic Review and Meta-analysis of Intervention Studies," *Nutrients* 10, no. 5 (May 2018): 606, https://doi.org/10.3390/nu10050606; Reza Rezvani et al., "Effects of Sugar-Sweetened Beverages on Plasma Acylation Stimulating Protein, Leptin and Adiponectin: Relationships with Metabolic Outcomes," *Obesity* 21, no. 12 (December 2013): 2471–80, https://doi.org/10.1002/oby.20437; Xiaosen Ouyang et al., "Fructose Consumption as a Risk Factor for Non-alcoholic Fatty Liver Disease," *Journal of Hepatology* 48, no. 6 (June 2008): 993–99, https://doi.org/10.1016/j.jhep.2008.02.011; Sharon S. Elliott et al., "Fructose, Weight Gain, and the Insulin Resistance Syndrome," *American Journal of Clinical Nutrition* 76, no. 5 (November 2002): 911–22, https://doi.org/10.1093/ajcn/76.5.911; Gjin Ndrepepa, "Uric Acid and Cardiovascular Disease," *Clinica Chimica Acta* 484 (September 2018): 150–63, https://doi.org/10.1016/j.cca.2018.05.046; Ali Abid et al., "Soft Drink Consumption Is Associated with Fatty Liver Disease Independent of Metabolic Syndrome," *Journal of Hepatology* 51,

no. 5 (November 2009): 918–24, https://doi.org/10.1016/j.jhep.2009.05.033; Roya Kelishadi, Marjan Mansourian, and Motahar Heidari-Beni, "Association of Fructose Consumption and Components of Metabolic Syndrome in Human Studies: A Systematic Review and Meta-analysis," *Nutrition* 30, no. 5 (May 2014): 503–10, https://doi.org/10.1016/j.nut.2013.08.014; Olena Glushakova et al., "Fructose Induces the Inflammatory Molecule ICAM-1 in Endothelial Cells," *Journal of the American Society of Nephrology* 19, no. 9 (September 2008): 1712–20, https://doi.org/10.1681/ASN.2007121304; Zeid Khitan and Dong Hyun Kim, "Fructose: A Key Factor in the Development of Metabolic Syndrome and Hypertension," *Journal of Nutrition and Metabolism* 2013, article ID 682673 (2013), https://doi.org/10.1155/2013/682673; Richard J. Johnson et al., "Hypothesis: Could Excessive Fructose Intake and Uric Acid Cause Type 2 Diabetes?" *Endocrine Reviews* 30, no. 1 (February 2009): 96–116, https://doi.org/10.1210/er.2008-0033; Richard J. Johnson et al., "Potential Role of Sugar (Fructose) in the Epidemic of Hypertension, Obesity and the Metabolic Syndrome, Diabetes, Kidney Disease, and Cardiovascular Disease," *American Journal of Clinical Nutrition* 86, no. 4 (October 2007): 899–906; Miguel A. Lanaspa et al., "Uric Acid Induces Hepatic Steatosis by Generation of Mitochondrial Oxidative Stress: Potential Role in Fructose-Dependent and -Independent Fatty Liver," *Journal of Biological Chemistry* 287, no. 48 (November 2012): 40732–44, https://doi.org/10.1074/jbc.M112.399899; Young Hee Rho, Yanyan Zhu, and Hyon K. Choi, "The Epidemiology of Uric Acid and Fructose," *Seminars in Nephrology* 31, no. 5 (September 2011): 410–19, https://doi.org/10.1016/j.semnephrol.2011.08.004; Richard J. Johnson et al., "Sugar, Uric Acid, and the Etiology of Diabetes and Obesity," *Diabetes* 62, no. 10 (October 2013): 3307–15, https://doi.org/10.2337/db12-1814.

21. Amy J. Bidwell, "Chronic Fructose Ingestion as a Major Health Concern: Is a Sedentary Lifestyle Making It Worse? A Review," *Nutrients* 9, no. 6 (May 2017): 549, https://doi.org/10.3390/nu9060549.

22. Kimber L. Stanhope et al., "Consuming Fructose-Sweetened, Not Glucose-Sweetened, Beverages Increases Visceral Adiposity and Lipids and Decreases Insulin Sensitivity in Overweight/Obese Humans," *Journal of Clinical Investigation* 119, no. 5 (May 2009): 1322–34, https://doi.org/10.1172/JCI37385. Also see Kimber L. Stanhope and Peter J. Havel, "Endocrine and Metabolic Effects of Consuming Beverages Sweetened with Fructose, Glucose, Sucrose, or High-Fructose Corn Syrup," *American Journal of Clinical Nutrition* 88, no. 6 (December 2008): 1733S–37S, https://doi.org/10.3945/ajcn.2008.25825D; Chad L. Cox et al., "Circulating Concentrations of Monocyte Chemoattractant Protein-1, Plasminogen Activator Inhibitor-1, and Soluble Leukocyte Adhesion Molecule-1 in Overweight/Obese Men and Women Consuming Fructose- or Glucose-Sweetened Beverages for 10 weeks," *Journal of Clinical Endocrinology and Metabolism* 96, no. 12 (December 2011): E2034–38, https://doi.org/10.1210/jc.2011-1050.

23. Michael M. Swarbrick et al., "Consumption of Fructose-Sweetened Beverages for 10 weeks Increases Postprandial Triacylglycerol and Apolipoprotein-B Concentrations in Overweight and Obese Women," *British Journal of Nutrition* 100, no. 5 (November 2008): 947–52, https://doi.org/10.1017/S0007114508968252.

24. D. David Wang et al., "Effect of Fructose on Postprandial Triglycerides: A Systematic Review and Meta-analysis of Controlled Feeding Trials," *Atherosclerosis* 232, no. 1 (January 2014): 125–33, https://doi.org/10.1016/j.atherosclerosis.2013.10.019.

25. Blossom C. M. Stephan et al., "Increased Fructose Intake as a Risk Factor for Dementia," *Journals of Gerontology, Series A* 65A, no. 8 (August 2010): 809–14, https://doi.org/10.1093/gerona/glq079. Also see Mario Siervo et al., "Reemphasizing the Role of Fructose Intake as a Risk Factor for Dementia," *Journals of Gerontology, Series A* 66A, no. 5 (May 2011): 534–36, https://doi.org/10.1093/gerona/glq222.

26. University of Chicago Medical Center, "Sleep Loss Boosts Appetite, May Encourage Weight Gain," *ScienceDaily*, December 7, 2004, www.sciencedaily.com/releases/2004/12/041206210355.htm.

27. Alexandra Shapiro et al., "Fructose-Induced Leptin Resistance Exacerbates Weight Gain in Response to Subsequent High-Fat Feeding," *American Journal of Physiology—Regulatory, Integrative and Comparative Physiology* 295, no. 5 (November 2008): R1370–75, https://doi.org/10.1152/ajpregu.00195.2008.

28. Karen L. Teff, "Dietary Fructose Reduces Circulating Insulin and Leptin, Attenuates Postprandial Suppression of Ghrelin, and Increases Triglycerides in Women," *Journal of Clinical Endocrinology and Metabolism* 89, no. 6 (June 2004): 2963–72, https://doi.org/10.1210/jc.2003-031855.

29. Miguel A. Lanaspa et al., "High Salt Intake Causes Leptin Resistance and Obesity in Mice by Stimulating Endogenous Fructose Production and Metabolism," *Proceedings of the National Academy of Sciences* (USA) 115, no. 12 (March 2018): 3138–43, https://doi.org/10.1073/pnas.1713837115.

30. Takahiko Nakagawa et al., "A Causal Role for Uric Acid in Fructose-Induced Metabolic Syndrome," *American Journal of Physiology—Renal Physiology* 290, no. 3 (March 2006): F625–31, https://doi.org/10.1152/ajprenal.00140.2005.

31. The following papers offer a review of the science: Daniel I. Feig, Beth Soletsky, and Richard J. Johnson, "Effect of Allopurinol on Blood Pressure of Adolescents with Newly Diagnosed Essential Hypertension: A Randomized Trial," *JAMA* 300, no. 8 (August 2008): 924–32, https://doi.org/10.1001/jama.300.8.924; Beth Soletsky and Daniel I. Feig, "Uric Acid Reduction Rectifies Prehypertension in Obese Adolescents," *Hypertension* 60, no. 5 (November 2012): 1148–56, https://doi.org/10.1161/HYPERTENSIONAHA.112.196980; Daniel I. Feig, Duk-Hee Kang, and Richard J. Johnson, "Uric Acid and Cardiovascular Risk," *New England Journal of Medicine* 359, no. 17 (October 2008): 1811–21, https://doi.org/10.1056/NEJMra0800885; Cristiana Caliceti et al., "Fructose Intake, Serum Uric Acid, and Cardiometabolic Disorders: A Critical Review," *Nutrients* 9, no. 4 (April 2017): 395, https://doi.org/10.3390/nu9040395; Marek

Kretowicz et al., "The Impact of Fructose on Renal Function and Blood Pressure," *International Journal of Nephrology* 2011, article ID 315879 (2011), https://doi.org/10.4061/2011/315879; Zeid Khitan and Dong Hyun Kim, "Fructose: A Key Factor in the Development of Metabolic Syndrome and Hypertension," *Journal of Nutrition and Metabolism* 2013, article ID 682673 (2013), https://doi.org/10.1155/2013/682673.

32. Allison M. Meyers, Devry Mourra, and Jeff A. Beeler, "High Fructose Corn Syrup Induces Metabolic Dysregulation and Altered Dopamine Signaling in the Absence of Obesity," *PLOS ONE* 12, no. 12 (December 2017): e0190206, https://doi.org/10.1371/journal.pone.0190206.

33. See "Data and Statistics About ADHD" on the CDC website, https://www.cdc.gov/ncbddd/adhd/data.html.

34. National Institutes of Health, "Prescribed Stimulant Use for ADHD Continues to Rise Steadily," September 28, 2011, https://www.nih.gov/news-events/news-releases/prescribed-stimulant-use-adhd-continues-rise-steadily.

35. Richard J. Johnson et al., "Attention-Deficit/Hyperactivity Disorder: Is It Time to Reappraise the Role of Sugar Consumption?," *Postgraduate Medical Journal* 123, no. 5 (September 2011): 39–49, https://doi.org/10.3810/pgm.2011.09.2458.

36. Carlos M. Barrera, Robert E. Hunter, and William P. Dunlap, "Hyperuricemia and Locomotor Activity in Developing Rats," *Pharmacology Biochemistry and Behavior* 33, no. 2 (June 1989): 367–69, https://doi.org/10.1016/0091-3057(89)90515-7.

37. Angelina R. Sutin et al., "Impulsivity Is Associated with Uric Acid: Evidence from Humans and Mice," *Biological Psychiatry* 75, no. 1 (January 2014): 31–37, https://doi.org/10.1016/j.biopsych.2013.02.024.

38. Paul Manowitz et al., "Uric Acid Level Increases in Humans Engaged in Gambling: A Preliminary Report," *Biological Psychology* 36, no. 3 (September 1993): 223–29, https://doi.org/10.1016/0301-0511(93)90019-5.

39. Amaal Alruwaily et al., "Child Social Media Influencers and Unhealthy Food Product Placement," *Pediatrics* 146, no. 5 (November 2020): e20194057, https://doi.org/10.1542/peds.2019-4057.

40. Norman K. Pollock et al., "Greater Fructose Consumption Is Associated with Cardiometabolic Risk Markers and Visceral Adiposity in Adolescents," *Journal of Nutrition* 142, no. 2 (February 2012): 251–57, https://doi.org/10.3945/jn.111.150219. Also see Josiane Aparecida de Miranda et al., "The Role of Uric Acid in the Insulin Resistance in Children and Adolescents with Obesity," *Revista Paulista de Pediatria* 33, no. 4 (December 2015): 431–36, https://doi.org/10.1016/j.rpped.2015.03.009; Michael I. Goran et al., "The Obesogenic Effect of High Fructose Exposure During Early Development," *Nature Reviews Endocrinology* 9, no. 8 (August 2013): 494–500, https://doi.org/10.1038/nrendo.2013.108.

41. David Perlmutter and Casey Means, "Op-Ed: The Bitter Truth of USDA's Sugar Guidelines," *MedPage Today*, February 21, 2021, https://www.medpagetoday.com/primarycare/dietnutrition/91281.

Chapter 4: The U-bomb in Your Brain

1. For updated facts and figures on Alzheimer's disease, go to the Alzheimer's Association website at www.alz.org. Also see the National Institute on Aging's page dedicated to the facts at https://www.nia.nih.gov/health/alzheimers-disease-fact-sheet.
2. Dan J. Stein and Ilina Singh, eds., *Global Mental Health and Neuroethics*, Global Mental Health in Practice 1 (Cambridge, MA: Academic Press, 2020), 229.
3. Rachel A. Whitmer et al., "Obesity in Middle Age and Future Risk of Dementia: A 27 Year Longitudinal Population Based Study," *The BMJ* 330, no. 7504 (June 2005): 1360, https://doi.org/10.1136/bmj.38446.466238.E0.
4. Kazushi Suzuki et al., "Elevated Serum Uric Acid Levels Are Related to Cognitive Deterioration in an Elderly Japanese Population," *Dementia and Geriatric Cognitive Disorders Extra* 6, no. 3 (September–December 2016): 580–88, https://doi.org/10.1159/000454660.
5. Sjoerd M. Euser et al., "Serum Uric Acid and Cognitive Function and Dementia," *Brain* 132, no. 2 (February 2009): 377–82, https://doi.org/10.1093/brain/awn316. Also see Aamir A. Khan et al., "Serum Uric Acid Level and Association with Cognitive Impairment and Dementia: Systematic Review and Meta-analysis," *Age* 38, no. 1 (February 2016): 16, https://doi.org/10.1007/s11357-016-9871-8; Augustin Latourte et al., "Uric Acid and Incident Dementia Over 12 Years of Follow-Up: A Population-Based Cohort Study," *Annals of the Rheumatic Diseases* 77, no. 3 (March 2018): 328–35, https://doi.org/10.1136/annrheumdis-2016-210767; Giovambattista Desideri et al., "Uric Acid Amplifies Aβ Amyloid Effects Involved in the Cognitive Dysfunction/Dementia: Evidences from an Experimental Model in Vitro," *Journal of Cellular Physiology* 232, no. 5 (May 2017): 1069–78, https://doi.org/10.1002/jcp.25509; May A. Beydoun et al., "Serum Uric Acid and Its Association with Longitudinal Cognitive Change Among Urban Adults," *Journal of Alzheimer's Disease* 52, no. 4 (April 2016): 1415–30, https://doi.org/10.3233/JAD-160028.
6. "Mini-Strokes Linked to Uric Acid Levels," *ScienceDaily*, October 5, 2007, https://www.sciencedaily.com/releases/2007/10/071001172809.htm. Also see "Mini Strokes Linked to Uric Acid Levels," Johns Hopkins Medicine, https://www.hopkinsmedicine.org/news/media/releases/mini_strokes_linked_to_uric_acid_levels.
7. Baris Afsar et al., "Relationship Between Uric Acid and Subtle Cognitive Dysfunction in Chronic Kidney Disease," *American Journal of Nephrology* 34, no. 1 (2011): 49–54, https://doi.org/10.1159/000329097.
8. Shaheen E. Lakhan and Annette Kirchgessner, "The Emerging Role of Dietary Fructose in Obesity and Cognitive Decline," *Journal of Nutrition* 12, article no. 114 (August 2013), https://doi.org/10.1186/1475-2891-12-114.
9. Lakhan and Kirchgessner, "The Emerging Role of Dietary Fructose."
10. Eric Steen et al., "Impaired Insulin and Insulin-Like Growth Factor Expression and Signaling Mechanisms in Alzheimer's Disease—Is This Type 3 Diabetes?," *Journal*

of Alzheimer's Disease 7, no. 1 (2005): 63–80, https://doi.org/10.3233/JAD-2005 -7107.

11. Maria Stefania Spagnuolo, Susanna Iossa, and Luisa Cigliano, "Sweet but Bitter: Focus on Fructose Impact on Brain Function in Rodent Models," *Nutrients* 13, no. 1 (December 2020): 1, https://doi.org/10.3390/nu13010001.

12. Kathleen A. Page et al., "Effects of Fructose vs Glucose on Regional Cerebral Blood Flow in Brain Regions Involved with Appetite and Reward Pathways," *JAMA* 309, no. 1 (January 2013): 63–70, https://doi.org/10.1001/jama.2012.116975.

13. Pedro Cisternas et al., "Fructose Consumption Reduces Hippocampal Synaptic Plasticity Underlying Cognitive Performance," *Biochimica et Biophysica Acta* 1852, no. 11 (November 2015): 2379–90, https://doi.org/10.1016/j.bbadis.2015.08.016.

14. Karin van der Borght et al., "Reduced Neurogenesis in the Rat Hippocampus Following High Fructose Consumption," *Regulatory Peptides* 167, no. 1 (February 2011): 26–30, https://doi.org/10.1016/j.regpep.2010.11.002.

15. Rahul Agrawal et al., "Dietary Fructose Aggravates the Pathobiology of Traumatic Brain Injury by Influencing Energy Homeostasis and Plasticity," *Journal of Cerebral Blood Flow & Metabolism* 36, no. 5 (May 2016): 941–53, https://doi.org/10.1177 /0271678X15606719.

16. Matthew P. Pase et al., "Sugary Beverage Intake and Preclinical Alzheimer's Disease in the Community," *Alzheimer's & Dementia* 13, no. 9 (September 2017): 955–64, https://doi.org/10.1016/j.jalz.2017.01.024.

17. Richard J. Johnson et al., "Cerebral Fructose Metabolism as a Potential Mechanism Driving Alzheimer's Disease," *Frontiers in Aging Neuroscience* 12 (September 2012): 560865, https://doi.org/10.3389/fnagi.2020.560865. Also see Jonathan Q. Purnell et al., "Brain Functional Magnetic Resonance Imaging Response to Glucose and Fructose Infusions in Humans," *Diabetes, Obesity and Metabolism* 13, no. 3 (March 2011): 229–34, https://doi.org/10.1111/j.1463-1326.2010.01340.x.

18. Matthew C. L. Phillips et al., "Randomized Crossover Trial of a Modified Ketogenic Diet in Alzheimer's Disease," *Alzheimer's Research & Therapy* 13, article no. 51 (February 2021), https://doi.org/10.1186/s13195-021-00783-x.

19. Jasvinder A. Singh and John D. Cleveland, "Comparative Effectiveness of Allopurinol Versus Febuxostat for Preventing Incident Dementia in Older Adults: A Propensity-Matched Analysis," *Arthritis Research & Therapy* 20, article no. 167 (August 2018), https://doi.org/10.1186/s13075-018-1663-3.

20. Mumtaz Takir et al., "Lowering Uric Acid with Allopurinol Improves Insulin Resistance and Systemic Inflammation in Asymptomatic Hyperuricemia," *Journal of Investigative Medicine* 63, no. 8 (December 2015): 924–29, https://doi.org/10.1097 /JIM.0000000000000242.

21. Jane P. Gagliardi, "What Can We Learn from Studies Linking Gout with Dementia?," *American Journal of Geriatric Psychiatry* (February 2021): S1064-7481(21)00217-7, https://doi.org/10.1016/j.jagp.2021.02.044.

22. David J. Schretlen et al., "Serum Uric Acid and Cognitive Function in Community-Dwelling Older Adults," *Neuropsychology* 21, no. 1 (January 2007): 136–40, https://doi.org/10.1037/0894-4105.21.1.136.

Chapter 5: Acid Rain

1. William Osler, *The Principles and Practice of Medicine, Designed for the Use of Practitioners and Students of Medicine*, vol. 1 (n.p.: Andesite Press, 2015).
2. J. T. Scott, "Factors Inhibiting the Excretion of Uric Acid," *Journal of the Royal Society of Medicine* 59, no. 4 (April 1966): 310–13, https://doi.org/10.1177/003591576605900405.
3. For a general overview of the relationship between sleep and health, see National Institute of Neurological Disorders and Stroke, "Brain Basics: Understanding Sleep," https://www.ninds.nih.gov/Disorders/Patient-Caregiver-Education/Understanding-Sleep. Also refer to the works of Dr. Michael Breus, a noted authority on sleep medicine: http://www.thesleepdoctor.com/. Also see Matthew Walker, *Why We Sleep: Unlocking the Power of Sleep and Dreams* (New York: Scribner, 2017).
4. Karine Spiegel, Rachel Leproult, and Eve Van Cauter, "Impact of Sleep Debt on Metabolic and Endocrine Function," *The Lancet* 354, no. 9188 (October 1999): 1435–39, https://doi.org/10.1016/S0140-6736(99)01376-8.
5. For volumes of data about sleep and statistics about how much we get, refer to the National Sleep Foundation at https://sleepfoundation.org/.
6. Carla S. Möller-Levet et al., "Effects of Insufficient Sleep on Circadian Rhythmicity and Expression Amplitude of the Human Blood Transcriptome," *Proceedings of the National Academy of Sciences* USA 110, no. 12 (March 2013), E1132–41, https://doi.org/10.1073/pnas.1217154110.
7. Janet M. Mullington et al., "Sleep Loss and Inflammation," *Best Practice & Research Clinical Endocrinology & Metabolism* 24, no. 5 (October 2010): 775–84, https://doi.org/10.1016/j.beem.2010.08.014.
8. Michael R. Irwin, Richard Olmstead, and Judith E. Carroll, "Sleep Disturbance, Sleep Duration, and Inflammation: A Systematic Review and Meta-analysis of Cohort Studies and Experimental Sleep Deprivation," *Biological Psychiatry* 80, no. 1 (July 2016): 40–52, https://doi.org/10.1016/j.biopsych.2015.05.014.
9. Francesco P. Cappuccio et al., "Sleep Duration and All-Cause Mortality: A Systematic Review and Meta-analysis of Prospective Studies," *Sleep* 33, no. 5 (May 2010): 585–92, https://doi.org/10.1093/sleep/33.5.585.
10. Andrew J. Westwood et al., "Prolonged Sleep Duration as a Marker of Early Neurodegeneration Predicting Incident Dementia," *Neurology* 88, no. 12 (March 2017): 1172–79, https://doi.org/10.1212/WNL.0000000000003732.
11. Again, see the National Sleep Foundation website at https://sleepfoundation.org/.

12. Dorit Koren, Magdalena Dumin, and David Gozal, "Role of Sleep Quality in the Metabolic Syndrome," *Diabetes, Metabolic Syndrome and Obesity: Targets and Therapy* 9 (August 2016): 281–310, https://doi.org/10.2147/DMSO.S95120.

13. Francesco P. Cappuccio et al., "Meta-analysis of Short Sleep Duration and Obesity in Children and Adults," *Sleep* 31, no. 5 (May 2008): 619–26, https://doi.org/10.1093/sleep/31.5.619.

14. Chan-Won Kim et al., "Sleep Duration and Progression to Diabetes in People with Prediabetes Defined by HbA_{1c} Concentration," *Diabetic Medicine* 34, no. 11 (November 2017): 1591–98, https://doi.org/10.1111/dme.13432. Also see Karine Spiegel et al., "Effects of Poor and Short Sleep on Glucose Metabolism and Obesity Risk," *Nature Reviews Endocrinology* 5, no. 5 (May 2009): 253–61, https://doi.org/10.1038/nrendo.2009.23.

15. Christopher Papandreou et al., "Sleep Duration Is Inversely Associated with Serum Uric Acid Concentrations and Uric Acid to Creatinine Ratio in an Elderly Mediterranean Population at High Cardiovascular Risk," *Nutrients* 11, no. 4 (April 2019): 761, https://doi.org/10.3390/nu11040761.

16. Yu-Tsung Chou et al., "Association of Sleep Quality and Sleep Duration with Serum Uric Acid Levels in Adults," *PLOS ONE* 15, no. 9 (September 2020): e0239185, https://doi.org/10.1371/journal.pone.0239185.

17. Caiyu Zheng et al., "Serum Uric Acid Is Independently Associated with Risk of Obstructive Sleep Apnea-Hypopnea Syndrome in Chinese Patients with Type 2 Diabetes," *Disease Markers* 2019, article ID 4578327 (April 2019), https://doi.org/10.1155/2019/4578327.

18. Jeffrey J. Iliff et al, "A Paravascular Pathway Facilitates CSF Flow Through the Brain Parenchyma and the Clearance of Interstitial Solutes, Including Amyloid β," *Science Translational Medicine* 4, no. 147 (August 2012): 147ra111, https://doi.org/10.1126/scitranslmed.3003748.

19. Miguel A. Lanaspa et al., "High Salt Intake Causes Leptin Resistance and Obesity in Mice by Stimulating Endogenous Fructose Production and Metabolism," *Proceedings of the National Academy of Sciences* (USA) 115, no. 12 (March 2018): 3138–43, https://doi.org/10.1073/pnas.1713837115.

20. Lanaspa et al., "High Salt Intake." Also see Masanari Kuwabara et al., "Relationship Between Serum Uric Acid Levels and Hypertension Among Japanese Individuals Not Treated for Hyperuricemia and Hypertension," *Hypertension Research* 37, no. 8 (August 2014): 785–89, https://doi.org/10.1038/hr.2014.75; Yang Wang et al., "Effect of Salt Intake on Plasma and Urinary Uric Acid Levels in Chinese Adults: An Interventional Trial," *Scientific Reports* 8, article no. 1434 (January 2018), https://doi.org/10.1038/s41598-018-20048-2.

21. Susan J. Allison, "High Salt Intake as a Driver of Obesity," *Nature Reviews Nephrology* 14, no. 5 (May 2018): 285, https://doi.org/10.1038/nrneph.2018.23.

22. Giuseppe Faraco et al., "Dietary Salt Promotes Cognitive Impairment Through

Tau Phosphorylation," *Nature* 574, no. 7780 (October 2019): 686–90, https://doi .org/10.1038/s41586-019-1688-z.

23. Chaker Ben Salem, "Drug-Induced Hyperuricaemia and Gout," *Rheumatology* 56, no. 5 (May 2017): 679–88, https://doi.org/10.1093/rheumatology/kew293. Also see Mara A. McAdams DeMarco et al., "Diuretic Use, Increased Serum Urate Levels, and Risk of Incident Gout in a Population-Based Study of Adults with Hypertension: The Atherosclerosis Risk in Communities Cohort Study," *Arthritis & Rheumatology* 64, no. 1 (January 2012): 121–29, https://doi.org/10.1002/art.33315.

24. "Long-Term Use of PPIs Has Consequences for Gut Microbiome," Cleveland Clinic, https://consultqd.clevelandclinic.org/long-term-use-of-ppis-has-consequences-for -gut-microbiome/. Also see William B. Lehault and David M. Hughes, "Review of the Long-Term Effects of Proton Pump Inhibitors," *Federal Practitioner* 34, no. 2 (February 2017): 19–23.

25. Tuhina Neogi et al., "Alcohol Quantity and Type on Risk of Recurrent Gout Attacks: An Internet-Based Case-Crossover Study," *American Journal of Medicine* 127, no. 4 (April 2014): 311–18, https://doi.org/10.1016/j.amjmed.2013.12.019. Also see Hyon K. Choi and Gary Curhan, "Beer, Liquor, and Wine Consumption and Serum Uric Acid Level: The Third National Health and Nutrition Examination Survey," *Arthritis Care & Research* 51, no. 6 (December 2004): 1023–29, https://doi .org/10.1002/art.20821.

26. Rongrong Li, Kang Yu, and Chunwei Li, "Dietary Factors and Risk of Gout and Hyperuricemia: A Meta-analysis and Systematic Review," *Asia Pacific Journal of Clinical Nutrition* 27, no. 6 (2018): 1344–56, https://doi.org/10.6133/apjcn.201811 _27(6).0022.

27. Richard J. Johnson et al., "Umami: The Taste That Drives Purine Intake," *Journal of Rheumatology* 40, no. 11 (November 2013): 1794–96, https://doi.org/10.3899 /jrheum.130531.

28. Rene J. Hernández Bautista et al., "Obesity: Pathophysiology, Monosodium Glutamate–Induced Model and Anti-Obesity Medicinal Plants," *Biomedicine & Pharmacotherapy* 111 (March 2019): 503–16, https://doi.org/10.1016/j.biopha.2018.12.108.

29. Ka He et al., "Consumption of Monosodium Glutamate in Relation to Incidence of Overweight in Chinese Adults: China Health and Nutrition Survey (CHNS)," *American Journal of Clinical Nutrition* 93, no. 6 (June 2011): 1328–36, https://doi .org/10.3945/ajcn.110.008870.

30. Zumin Shi et al., "Monosodium Glutamate Is Related to a Higher Increase in Blood Pressure Over 5 Years: Findings from the Jiangsu Nutrition Study of Chinese Adults," *Journal of Hypertension* 29, no. 5 (May 2011): 846–53, https://doi .org/10.1097/HJH.0b013e328344da8e.

31. Kamal Niaz, Elizabeta Zaplatic, and Jonathan Spoor, "Extensive Use of Monosodium Glutamate: A Threat to Public Health?," *EXCLI Journal* 17 (March 2018): 273–78, https://doi.org/10.17179/excli2018-1092.

32. Ignacio Roa and Mariano del Sol, "Types I and III Parotid Collagen Variations and Serum Biochemical Parameters in Obese Rats Exposed to Monosodium Gluta-mate," *International Journal of Morphology* 38, no. 3 (June 2020), http://dx.doi .org/10.4067/S0717-95022020000300755.

33. Joseph F. Merola et al., "Psoriasis, Psoriatic Arthritis and Risk of Gout in US Men and Women," *Annals of the Rheumatic Diseases* 74, no. 8 (August 2015): 1495–1500, https://doi.org/10.1136/annrheumdis-2014-205212.

34. Renaud Felten et al., "At the Crossroads of Gout and Psoriatic Arthritis: 'Psout'," *Clinical Rheumatology* 39, no. 5 (May 2020): 1405–13, https://doi.org/10.1007 /s10067-020-04981-0.

35. Nicola Giordano et al., "Hyperuricemia and Gout in Thyroid Endocrine Disor-ders," *Clinical and Experimental Rheumatology* 19, no. 6 (November–December 2001): 661–65.

36. Eswar Krishnan, Bharathi Lingala, and Vivek Bhalla, "Low-Level Lead Exposure and the Prevalence of Gout: An Observational Study," *Annals of Internal Medicine* 157, no. 4 (August 2012): 233–41, https://doi.org/10.7326/0003-4819-157-4-20120 8210-00003.

37. J. Runcie and T. J. Thomson, "Total Fasting, Hyperuricaemia and Gout," *Postgrad-uate Medical Journal* 45, no. 522 (April 1969): 251–53, https://doi.org/10.1136 /pgmj.45.522.251.

38. Patrick H. Dessein et al., "Beneficial Effects of Weight Loss Associated with Mod-erate Calorie/Carbohydrate Restriction, and Increased Proportional Intake of Protein and Unsaturated Fat on Serum Urate and Lipoprotein Levels in Gout: A Pilot Study," *Annals of the Rheumatic Diseases* 59, no. 7 (July 2000): 539–43, https:// doi.org/10.1136/ard.59.7.539.

39. I-Min Lee et al., "Effect of Physical Inactivity on Major Non-Communicable Diseases Worldwide: An Analysis of Burden of Disease and Life Expectancy," *The Lancet* 380, no. 9838 (July 2012): 219–29, https://doi.org/10.1016/S0140-6736(12)61031-9.

40. World Health Organization, "Physical Inactivity a Leading Cause of Disease and Disability, Warns WHO," April 4, 2002, https://www.who.int/news/item/04-04-2002 -physical-inactivity-a-leading-cause-of-disease-and-disability-warns-who. Also see the World Health Organization's fact sheet on obesity and overweight at https:// www.who.int/news-room/fact-sheets/detail/obesity-and-overweight.

41. Aviroop Biswas et al., "Sedentary Time and Its Association with Risk for Disease Incidence, Mortality, and Hospitalization in Adults: A Systematic Review and Meta-analysis," *Annals of Internal Medicine* 162, no. 2 (January 2015): 123–32, https://doi.org/10.7326/M14-1651.

42. Srinivasan Beddhu et al., "Light-Intensity Physical Activities and Mortality in the United States General Population and CKD Subpopulation," *Clinical Journal of the American Society of Nephrology* 10, no. 7 (July 2015): 1145–53, https://doi.org /10.2215/CJN.08410814.

43. Doo Yong Park et al., "The Association Between Sedentary Behavior, Physical Activity and Hyperuricemia," *Vascular Health and Risk Management* 15 (August 2019): 291–99, https://doi.org/10.2147/VHRM.S200278.
44. Jun Zhou et al., "Physical Exercises and Weight Loss in Obese Patients Help to Improve Uric Acid," *Oncotarget* 8, no. 55 (October 2017): 94893–99, https://doi .org/10.18632/oncotarget.22046.

Chapter 6: New Habits to LUV

1. MRC London Institute of Medical Sciences, "Too Much Sugar Leads to Early Death, but Not Due to Obesity," *ScienceDaily*, March 19, 2020, www.sciencedaily .com/releases/2020/03/200319141024.htm and https://www.eurekalert.org/news-re leases/621703. Also see Esther van Dam et al., "Sugar-Induced Obesity and Insulin Resistance Are Uncoupled from Shortened Survival in *Drosophila*," *Cell Metabolism* 31, no. 4 (April 2020): 710–25, https://doi.org/10.1016/j.cmet.2020.02.016.
2. See Christoph Kaleta's papers at https://scholar.google.de/citations?user=qw172u QAAAAJ&hl=en.
3. Shijun Hao, Chunlei Zhang, and Haiyan Song, "Natural Products Improving Hyperuricemia with Hepatorenal Dual Effects," *Evidence-Based Complementary and Alternative Medicine* 2016, article ID 7390504 (2016), https://doi.org/10.1155 /2016/7390504. Also see Lin-Lin Jiang et al., "Bioactive Compounds from Plant-Based Functional Foods: A Promising Choice for the Prevention and Management of Hyperuricemia," *Foods* 9, no. 8 (July 2020): 973, https://doi.org/10.3390/foods 9080973.
4. Yuanlu Shi and Gary Williamson, "Quercetin Lowers Plasma Uric Acid in Pre-hyperuricaemic Males: A Randomised, Double-Blinded, Placebo-Controlled, Cross-Over Trial," *British Journal of Nutrition* 115, no. 5 (March 2016): 800–806, https://doi.org/10.1017/S0007114515005310. Also see Cen Zhang et al., "Mechanistic Insights into the Inhibition of Quercetin on Xanthine Oxidase," *International Journal of Biological Macromolecules* 112 (June 2018): 405–12, https://doi.org/10 .1016/j.ijbiomac.2018.01.190.
5. Maria-Corina Serban et al., "Effects of Quercetin on Blood Pressure: A Systematic Review and Meta-Analysis of Randomized Controlled Trials," *Journal of the American Heart Association* 5, no. 7 (July 2016): e002713, https://doi.org/10.1161/JAHA .115.002713.
6. Marina Hirano et al., "Luteolin-Rich Chrysanthemum Flower Extract Suppresses Baseline Serum Uric Acid in Japanese Subjects with Mild Hyperuricemia," *Integrative Molecular Medicine* 4, no. 2 (2017), https://doi.org/10.15761/IMM.1000275.
7. Muhammad Imran et al., "Luteolin, a Flavonoid, as an Anticancer Agent: A Review," *Biomedicine & Pharmacotherapy* 112 (April 2019): 108612, https://doi .org/10.1016/j.biopha.2019.108612.

8. Stuart Wolpert, "Fructose and Head Injuries Adversely Affect Hundreds of Brain Genes Linked to Human Diseases," UCLA *College*, https://www.college.ucla .edu/2017/07/11/fructose-and-head-injuries-adversely-affect-hundreds-of-brain -genes-linked-to-human-diseases/.

9. Janie Allaire et al., "A Randomized, Crossover, Head-to-Head Comparison of Eicosapentaenoic Acid and Docosahexaenoic Acid Supplementation to Reduce Inflammation Markers in Men and Women: The Comparing EPA to DHA (ComparED) Study," *American Journal of Clinical Nutrition* 104, no. 2 (August 2016): 280–87, https://doi.org/10.3945/ajcn.116.131896.

10. Stephen P. Juraschek, Edgar R. Miller III, and Allan C. Gelber, "Effect of Oral Vitamin C Supplementation on Serum Uric Acid: A Meta-analysis of Randomized Controlled Trials," *Arthritis Care & Research* 63, no. 9 (September 2011): 1295–306, https://doi.org/10.1002/acr.20519.

11. Hyon K. Choi, Xiang Gao, and Gary Curhan, "Vitamin C Intake and the Risk of Gout in Men: A Prospective Study," *Archives of Internal Medicine* 169, no. 5 (March 2009): 502–7, https://doi.org/10.1001/archinternmed.2008.606.

12. Juraschek, Miller, and Gelber, "Effect of Oral Vitamin C Supplementation on Serum Uric Acid."

13. Mehrangiz Ebrahimi-Mameghani et al., "Glucose Homeostasis, Insulin Resistance and Inflammatory Biomarkers in Patients with Non-alcoholic Fatty Liver Disease: Beneficial Effects of Supplementation with Microalgae *Chlorella vulgaris*: A Double-Blind Placebo-Controlled Randomized Clinical Trial," *Clinical Nutrition* 36, no. 4 (August 2017): 1001–6, https://doi.org/10.1016/j.clnu.2016.07.004.

14. Yunes Panahi et al., "A Randomized Controlled Trial of 6-week *Chlorella vulgaris* Supplementation in Patients with Major Depressive Disorder," *Complementary Therapies in Medicine* 23, no. 4 (August 2015): 598–602, https://doi.org/10.1016/j .ctim.2015.06.010.

15. Christopher J. L. Murray et al., "The State of US Health, 1990–2016: Burden of Diseases, Injuries, and Risk Factors Among US States," JAMA 319, no. 14 (2018): 1444–72, https://doi.org/10.1001/jama.2018.0158.

16. "Insulin Resistance & Prediabetes," National Institute of Diabetes, Digestive and Kidney Diseases at https://www.niddk.nih.gov/health-information/diabetes/over view/what-is-diabetes/prediabetes-insulin-resistance.

17. Amir Tirosh et al., "Normal Fasting Plasma Glucose Levels and Type 2 Diabetes in Young Men," *New England Journal of Medicine* 353, no. 14 (October 2005): 1454–62, https://doi.org/10.1056/NEJMoa050080.

18. Adam G. Tabák et al., "Prediabetes: A High-Risk State for Diabetes Development," *The Lancet* 379, no. 9833 (June 2012): 2279–90, https://doi.org/10.1016 /S0140-6736(12)60283-9.

19. To hear more from Dr. Casey Means and gain an introductory class on continuous glucose monitoring, I invite you to listen to my interview with her on my podcast,

accessible through my website at https://www.drperlmutter.com/continuous-glu
cose-monitoring-a-powerful-tool-for-metabolic-health/.

20. Heather Hall et al., "Glucotypes Reveal New Patterns of Glucose Dysregulation," *PLOS Biology* 16, no. 7 (July 2018): e2005143, https://doi.org/10.1371/journal.pbio.2005143.

21. Felicity Thomas et al., "Blood Glucose Levels of Subelite Athletes During 6 Days of Free Living," *Journal of Diabetes Science and Technology* 10, no. 6 (November 2016): 1335–43, https://doi.org/10.1177/1932296816648344.

22. Viral N. Shah et al., "Continuous Glucose Monitoring Profiles in Healthy Nondiabetic Participants: A Multicenter Prospective Study," *Journal of Clinical Endocrinology and Metabolism* 104, no. 10 (October 2019): 4356–64, https://doi.org/10.1210/jc.2018-02763.

23. Alexandra E. Butler et al., "β-Cell Deficit and Increased β-Cell Apoptosis in Humans with Type 2 Diabetes," *Diabetes* 52, no. 1 (January 2003): 102–10, https://doi.org/10.2337/diabetes.52.1.102.

24. Li Li et al., "Acute Psychological Stress Results in the Rapid Development of Insulin Resistance," *Journal of Endocrinology* 217, no. 2 (April 2013): 175–84, https://doi.org/10.1530/JOE-12-0559.

25. "Survey: Nutrition Information Abounds, but Many Doubt Food Choices," Food Insight, May 2017, https://foodinsight.org/survey-nutrition-information-abounds-but-many-doubt-food-choices/.

26. See my interview with Dr. Casey Means on my podcast of June 1, 2021, at https://www.drperlmutter.com/continuous-glucose-monitoring-a-powerful-tool-for-metabolic-health/.

27. Satchin Panda, *The Circadian Code: Lose Weight, Supercharge Your Energy, and Transform Your Health from Morning to Midnight* (New York: Rodale, 2018). For more about Dr. Panda and his research work, visit his lab's website at the Salk Institute: https://www.salk.edu/scientist/satchidananda-panda/.

28. Panda, *The Circadian Code*.

29. Emily N. Manoogian et al., "Time-Restricted Eating for the Prevention and Management of Metabolic Diseases," *Endocrine Reviews* (2021): bnab027, https://doi.org/10.1210/endrev/bnab027.

30. Endocrine Society, "Intermittent Fasting Can Help Manage Metabolic Disease: Popular Diet Trend Could Reduce the Risk of Diabetes and Heart Disease," *ScienceDaily*, www.sciencedaily.com/releases/2021/09/210922090909.htm (accessed October 7, 2021).

31. Malini Prasad et al., "A Smartphone Intervention to Promote Time Restricted Eating Reduces Body Weight and Blood Pressure in Adults with Overweight and Obesity: A Pilot Study," *Nutrients* 13, no. 7 (June 2021): 2148, https://doi.org/10.3390/nu13072148.

32. Nidhi Bansal and Ruth S. Weinstock, "Non-Diabetic Hypoglycemia," *Endotext*, May 20, 2020.

33. Fernanda Cerqueira, Bruno Chausse, and Alicia J. Kowaltowski, "Intermittent Fasting Effects on the Central Nervous System: How Hunger Modulates Brain Function," in *Handbook of Famine, Starvation, and Nutrient Deprivation: From Biology to Policy*, ed. Victor Preedy and Vanood B. Patel (Springer, Cham), https://doi.org/10.1007/978-3-319-40007-5_29-1.

34. Humaira Jamshed et al., "Early Time-Restricted Feeding Improves 24-Hour Glucose Levels and Affects Markers of the Circadian Clock, Aging, and Autophagy in Humans," *Nutrients* 11, no. 6 (May 2019): 1234, https://doi.org/10.3390/nu11061234.

PART II: U-Turn

1. Joana Araújo, Jianwen Cai, and June Stevens, "Prevalence of Optimal Metabolic Health in American Adults: National Health and Nutrition Examination Survey 2009–2016," *Metabolic Syndrome and Related Disorders* 17, no. 1 (February 2019): 46–52, https://doi.org/10.1089/met.2018.0105.

Chapter 7: Prelude to LUV

1. Adriano Bruci et al., "Very Low-Calorie Ketogenic Diet: A Safe and Effective Tool for Weight Loss in Patients with Obesity and Mild Kidney Failure," *Nutrients* 12, no. 2 (January 2020): 333, https://doi.org/10.3390/nu12020333.

Chapter 8: Dietary Edits to Lower Uric Values

1. "Health Effects of Dietary Risks in 195 Countries, 1990–2017: A Systematic Analysis for the Global Burden of Disease Study 2017," *The Lancet* 393, no. 10184 (April 2019): 1958–72, https://doi.org/10.1016/S0140-6736(19)30041-8. Also see Nita G. Forouhi and Nigel Unwin, "Global Diet and Health: Old Questions, Fresh Evidence, and New Horizons," *The Lancet* 393, no. 10184 (April 2019): 1916–18, https://doi.org/10.1016/S0140-6736(19)30500-8.

2. For everything you want to know about BDNF and brain health, including references to studies, see the updated edition of my book *Grain Brain: The Surprising Truth About Wheat, Carbs, and Sugar—Your Brain's Silent Killers* (New York: Little, Brown, 2018).

3. May A. Beydoun et al., "Dietary Factors Are Associated with Serum Uric Acid Trajectory Differentially by Race Among Urban Adults," *British Journal of Nutrition* 120, no. 8 (October 2018): 935–45, https://doi.org/10.1017/S0007114518002118. Also see Daisy Vedder et al., "Dietary Interventions for Gout and Effect on Cardiovascular Risk Factors: A Systematic Review," *Nutrients* 11, no. 12 (December 2019): 2955, https://doi.org/10.3390/nu11122955; M. A. Gromova, V. V. Tsurko, and A. S. Melekhina, "Rational Approach to Nutrition for Patients with Gout," *Clinician* 13,

nos. 3–4 (2019): 15–21, https://doi.org/10.17650/1818-8338-2019-13-3-4-15-21; Kiyoko Kaneko et al., "Total Purine and Purine Base Content of Common Foodstuffs for Facilitating Nutritional Therapy for Gout and Hyperuricemia," *Biological and Pharmaceutical Bulletin* 37, no. 5 (2014): 709–21, https://doi.org/10.1248/bpb.b13-00967.

4. Jotham Suez et al., "Artificial Sweeteners Induce Glucose Intolerance by Altering the Gut Microbiota," *Nature* 514, no. 7521 (October 2014): 181–86, https://doi.org/10.1038/nature13793.

5. Matthew P. Pase, et al., "Sugar- and Artificially Sweetened Beverages and the Risks of Incident Stroke and Dementia," *Stroke* 48, no. 5 (April 2017): 1139–1146, https://doi.org/10.1161/STROKEAHA.116.016027; Matthew P. Pase et al., "Sugary Beverage Intake and Preclinical Alzheimer's Disease in the Community," *Alzheimer's & Dementia* 13, no. 9 (September 2017): 955–64, https://doi.org/10.1016/j.jalz.2017.01.024.

6. Francesco Franchi et al., "Effects of D-allulose on Glucose Tolerance and Insulin Response to a Standard Oral Sucrose Load: Results of a Prospective, Randomized, Crossover Study," *BMJ Open Diabetes Research and Care* 9, no. 1 (February 2021): e001939, https://doi.org/10.1136/bmjdrc-2020-001939.

7. Here's a small collection of research on honey to get you started: Noori Al-Waili et al., "Honey and Cardiovascular Risk Factors, in Normal Individuals and in Patients with Diabetes Mellitus or Dyslipidemia," *Journal of Medicinal Food* 16, no. 12 (December 2013): 1063–78, https://doi.org/10.1089/jmf.2012.0285; Nur Zuliani Ramli et al., "A Review on the Protective Effects of Honey Against Metabolic Syndrome," *Nutrients* 10, no. 8 (August 2018): 1009, https://doi.org/10.3390/nu10081009; Omotayo O. Erejuwa, Siti A. Sulaiman, and Mohd S. Ab Wahab, "Honey—A Novel Antidiabetic Agent," *International Journal of Biological Sciences* 8, no. 6 (2012): 913–34, https://doi.org/10.7150/ijbs.3697.

8. Anand Mohan et al., "Effect of Honey in Improving the Gut Microbial Balance," *Food Quality and Safety* 1, no. 2 (May 2017): 107–15, https://doi.org/10.1093/fqsafe/fyx015.

9. Salma E. Nassar et al., "Effect of Inulin on Metabolic Changes Produced by Fructose Rich Diet," *Life Science Journal* 10, no. 2 (January 2013): 1807–14.

10. World Health Organization, "Global Strategy on Diet, Physical Activity and Health," https://www.who.int/dietphysicalactivity/strategy/eb11344/strategy_english_web.pdf.

11. Gabsik Yang et al., "Suppression of NLRP3 Inflammasome by Oral Treatment with Sulforaphane Alleviates Acute Gouty Inflammation," *Rheumatology* 57, no. 4 (April 2018): 727–36, https://doi.org/10.1093/rheumatology/kex499. Also see Christine A. Houghton, "Sulforaphane: Its 'Coming of Age' as a Clinically Relevant Nutraceutical in the Prevention and Treatment of Chronic Disease," *Oxidative Medicine and Cellular Longevity* 2019, article ID 2716870 (October 2019), https://doi.org/10.1155/2019/2716870.

12. Albena T. Dinkova-Kostova et al., "KEAP1 and Done? Targeting the NRF2 Pathway with Sulforaphane," *Trends in Food Science and Technology* 69, part B (November 2017): 257–69, https://doi.org/10.1016/j.tifs.2017.02.002.
13. Robert A. Jacob et al., "Consumption of Cherries Lowers Plasma Urate in Healthy Women," *Journal of Nutrition* 133, no. 6 (June 2003): 1826–29, https://doi.org/10.1093/jn/133.6.1826. Also see Keith R. Martin and Katie M. Coles, "Consumption of 100% Tart Cherry Juice Reduces Serum Urate in Overweight and Obese Adults," *Current Developments in Nutrition* 3, no. 5 (February 2019): nzz011, https://doi.org/10.1093/cdn/nzz011; Naomi Schlesinger, Ruth Rabinowitz, and Michael Schlesinger, "Pilot Studies of Cherry Juice Concentrate for Gout Flare Prophylaxis," *Journal of Arthritis* 1, no. 1 (2012): 101, https://doi.org/10.4172/2167-7921.1000101.
14. Jiahong Xie et al., "Delphinidin-3-O-Sambubioside: A Novel Xanthine Oxidase Inhibitor Identified from Natural Anthocyanins," *Food Quality and Safety* 5 (April 2021): fyaa038, https://doi.org/10.1093/fqsafe/fyaa038.
15. Marc J. Gunter et al., "Coffee Drinking and Mortality in 10 European Countries: A Multinational Cohort Study," *Annals of Internal Medicine* 167, no. 4 (August 2017): 236–47, https://doi.org/10.7326/M16-2945. Also see Hyon K. Choi and Gary Curhan, "Coffee, Tea, and Caffeine Consumption and Serum Uric Acid Level: The Third National Health and Nutrition Examination Survey," *Arthritis & Rheumatology* 57, no. 5 (June 2007): 816–21, https://doi.org/10.1002/art.22762.
16. Song-Yi Park et al., "Prospective Study of Coffee Consumption and Cancer Incidence in Non-white Populations," *Cancer Epidemiology, Biomarkers & Prevention* 27, no. 8 (August 2018): 928–35, https://doi.org/10.1158/1055-9965.EPI-18-0093.
17. Choi and Curhan, "Coffee, Tea, and Caffeine Consumption."
18. Yashi Mi et al., "EGCG Ameliorates High-Fat- and High-Fructose-Induced Cognitive Defects by Regulating the IRS/AKT and ERK/CREB/BDNF Signaling Pathways in the CNS," *FASEB Journal* 31, no. 11 (November 2017): 4998–5011, https://doi.org/10.1096/fj.201700400RR.
19. Hyon K. Choi et al., "Alcohol Intake and Risk of Incident Gout in Men: A Prospective Study," *The Lancet* 363 no. 9417 (April 2004): 1277–81, https://doi.org/10.1016/S0140-6736(04)16000-5.

Chapter 9: Companions to LUV

1. Scott Shannon et al., "Cannabidiol in Anxiety and Sleep: A Large Case Series," *Permanente Journal* 23 (2019), https://doi.org/10.7812/TPP/18-041.

Chapter 10: A Sweet Opportunity

1. Alpana P. Shukla et al., "Food Order Has a Significant Impact on Postprandial Glucose and Insulin Levels," *Diabetes Care* 38, no. 7 (July 2015): e98–99, https://doi.org/10.2337/dc15-0429.
2. Andrea R. Josse et al., "Almonds and Postprandial Glycemia — A Dose-Response Study," *Metabolism* 56, no. 3 (March 2007): 400–404, https://doi.org/10.1016/j.metabol.2006.10.024.
3. Austin Perlmutter, "The Coronavirus Took Advantage of Our Weaknesses," *Elemental*, October 21, 2020, https://elemental.medium.com/the-coronavirus-took-advantage-of-our-weaknesses-e7966ea48b75.
4. Goodarz Danaei et al., "The Preventable Causes of Death in the United States: Comparative Risk Assessment of Dietary, Lifestyle, and Metabolic Risk Factors," *PLOS Medicine* 6, no. 4 (April 2009): e1000058, https://doi.org/10.1371/journal.pmed.1000058.

Epilogue

1. Robert N. Proctor, *Golden Holocaust: Origins of the Cigarette Catastrophe and the Case for Abolition* (Berkeley: University of California Press, 2012).
2. Katherine Gourd, "Fritz Lickint," *Lancet Respiratory Medicine* 2, no. 5 (May 2014): 358–59, https://doi.org/10.1016/S2213-2600(14)70064-5.
3. Colin Grabow, "Candy-Coated Cartel: Time to Kill the U.S. Sugar Program," CATO Institute policy analysis no. 837, April 10, 2018, https://www.cato.org/policy-analysis/candy-coated-cartel-time-kill-us-sugar-program.
4. Yujin Lee et al., "Cost-Effectiveness of Financial Incentives for Improving Diet and Health through Medicare and Medicaid: A Microsimulation Study," *PLOS Medicine* 16, no. 3 (March 2019): e1002761, https://doi.org/10.1371/journal.pmed.1002761.
5. Sarah Downer et al., "Food Is Medicine: Actions to Integrate Food and Nutrition into Healthcare," *BMJ* 369 (June 2020): m2482, https://doi.org/10.1136/bmj.m2482.
6. Katie Riley et al., "Reducing Hospitalizations and Costs: A Home Health Nutrition-Focused Quality Improvement Program," *Journal of Parenteral and Enteral Nutrition* 44, no. 1 (January 2020): 58–68, https://doi.org/10.1002/jpen.1606.

Index

Note: Italic page numbers refer to illustrations.

adenine, 10
Adler, Isaac, 274
adolescents
    fructose consumption of, 93–94
    hypertension and uric acid levels, 28
    hyperuricemia in, 36
    metabolic syndrome and, 93–94
    obesity in, 37–38
    sleep and, 205
Aduhelm (aducanumab), 97–98, 99
advanced glycation end products (AGEs),
    139, 146
agave syrup, 76, 185
age-related macular degeneration, 34
aging
    AMPK and, 66, 156
    brain aging, 106–7
    cognitive decline and, 100, 101
    premature aging, 146, 229
    time-restricted eating and, 157
agricultural revolution, 52, 171
alcohol, 20, 26, 32, 79–80, 126–27, 195, 209
aldose reductase, 122
Alexander the Great, 7
allantoin, 56
allopurinol, 28, 108–9, 139, 162
allulose, 177, 182, 183–86
Alzheimer's disease
    abdominal fat and, 86
    as cause of death, 98–99
    cerebral fructose metabolism and, 40
    chronic inflammation and, 33
    C-reactive protein and, 34
    effects of fructose on brain, 87, 105
    fructose consumption and, 107
    long-term complications of COVID-19
        infection and, 41
    medical treatment for, 17, 97–99, 108, 110
    metabolic syndrome and, 39
    microbiome and, 69
    prevention of, 99, 102, 110
    sleep and, 121
    type 2 diabetes and, 39
    as type 3 diabetes, 102–11
    uric acid levels and, 4
American Diabetes Association, 78
American Heart Association, 78, 81
American Medical Association, 81
AMP (adenosine monophosphate), 67–68, 83, 127
AMPD2 (adenosine monophosphate
    deaminase 2), 67, 68
AMPK (adenosine monophosphate–activated
    protein kinase), 66–68, 156, 161, 211
Anne (queen of Great Britain), 7
anthocyanins, 189
appetite, 88–94, 113, 117, 123
Aristotle, 23
artificial sweeteners, 177, 182–83
asthma, 69, 125
astrobiology, 47
asymptomatic hyperuricemia, 7–8, 28, 32, 33,
    40, 109
ATP (adenosine triphosphate), 10–11, 59, 83,
    103, 127, 135, 145, 147
attention deficit hyperactivity disorder
    (ADHD), 92–93
Attia, Peter, 3–4
autism, 69
autoimmune diseases, 47
autophagy, 47, 133, 156–58

BDNF (brain-derived neurotrophic factor),
    140, 174
Beatles, 113

beer, 11, 126, 195
berberine, 67
beverage industry, 76, 278
beverages. *See also* drinks
  alcohol, 20, 26, 32, 79–80, 126–27, 195,
    209
  fructose-sweetened beverages, 43, 73, 77–78,
    86, 105–7, *106*, 122, 127
  water, 194–95
Biden, Joe, 94
Bidwell, Amy J., 85
bipolar disorder, 93
blood fats, 4, 21, 28, 32, 37, 61, 80
blood flow, 24, 25, 45
blood glucose levels
  asymptomatic hyperuricemia and, 8
  as biomarker, 43
  cognitive decline and, 40, 99
  continuous glucose monitor for, 36–37,
    149–52, 166–67, 203
  dementias and, 16
  diabetes and, 148
  diets and, 5
  drugs and lifestyle strategies for, 39
  fructose and, 80, 85
  lifestyle strategies for, 39
  management of, 9, 16, 74, 144–47, 159
  metabolic syndrome and, 38
  nature and, 215
  self-assessment of, 166
  time-restricted eating and, 157
blood pressure. *See also* hypertension
  as biomarker, 43
  as health marker, 54, 159
  human evolution and, 58–59
  management of, 9
bloodstream, uric acid building up in, 26
blue light, 206
BMI (body mass index), 54, 64, 65, *65*, 99
body fat
  asymptomatic hyperuricemia and, 8, 36
  health marker of, 54
  highs and lows of, 48
  human genome and, 51
  metabolic syndrome and, 38
body mass index (BMI), 54, 64, 65, *65*, 99
body weight, 43, 64. *See also* obesity; weight
    control
bone health markers, 54
bowel disorders, 69
brain damage, 34
brain-derived neurotrophic factor (BDNF),
    140, 174

brain function
  dopamine signaling and, 92
  fructose and, 87, 88, 96, 104
  hemoglobin A1c levels and, 16
  insulin resistance and, 103
  lifestyle strategies for, 99
  long-term complications of COVID-19
    infection and, 41
  neural resilience and, 104–5
  sugary beverages and, 105–7, *106*
  uric acid levels and, 100–101
Brain Maker (Perlmutter), 68, 168
Brain Wash (Perlmutter), 215
breads, 11, 176, 226
breakfast
  Recipes to LUV, 232–41
  staples for, 223–24
Bredesen, Dale, 203
Breus, Michael, 208
broccoli sprouts, 187–89

cancer
  chronic inflammation and, 33
  ketogenic diet and, 170
  microbiome and, 69
  uric acid levels and, 6, 24, 59
carbohydrates
  consumption of, 81–82, 85, 112, 115, 155,
    225–26
  glucose as product of breakdown of, 145
cardiopulmonary functionality, 54
cardiorenal disease, 30
cardiovascular disease
  in children, 36, 93
  chronic inflammation and, 33
  C-reactive protein and, 34, 35
  erectile dysfunction and, 46
  Framingham Heart Study, 26–27
  gout associated with, 6
  hyperuricemia and, 9, 35
  metabolic syndrome and, 39
  metabolism and, 4
  mortality and, 26
  triglyceride levels and, 85
  uric acid levels and, 6, 13, 20, 24, 27, 31, 35,
    37, 62
cells
  autophagy and, 47, 133, 156–58
  perpetual state of death and renewal, 26, 66
  purines in, 10
cerebral fructose metabolism, 40
Charlemagne, 7
cherries, 12, 189

children
    cardiovascular disease in, 36, 93
    obesity in, 36, 37–38, 101
    sleep and, 116
    uric acid levels of, 36
chlorella, 142–43, 168
cholesterol levels
    asymptomatic hyperuricemia and, 8
    C-reactive protein and, 34
    drugs and lifestyle strategies for, 39
    metabolic syndrome and, 38, 73
    ratio of good to bad cholesterol, 43
chronic degenerative diseases, 5, 8, 14, 89
chronic inflammatory conditions, 14, 33, 34
chronic kidney disease, 131
circadian rhythms, 117, 151, 153–54, 157,
    205–6, 210, 216
coenzymes, 11
coffee, 12, 128, 192–93
cognitive decline
    blood glucose levels and, 40, 99
    C-reactive protein and, 34
    fear of, 99
    fructose and, 87, 104
    metabolism and, 4
    obesity and, 99–100, 101
    sleep and, 116
    uric acid levels and, 21, 40, 88, 100, 108–9,
    110, 202
cognitive reserve, 104
Colbin, Annemarie, 230
Columbus, Christopher, 7
continuous glucose monitor (CGM), 36–37,
    149–52, 161
Corn Refiners Association, 74–75
coronary artery disease, 4, 33, 42, 46, 86
cortisol, 119, 215
COVID-19 infection, 16, 38, 40–42, 47,
    227
COVID-19 pandemic, 3, 36, 41–42, 212–13,
    221, 226–28, 276–77
C-reactive protein (CRP)
    cherries and, 189
    optimal range of, 165
    sleep and, 115
    systemic inflammation and, 8, 34–35, 73
    uric acid levels and, 34–35
CRISPR, 70
curiosity, 12
cytokines, 35, 115

dairy products, 53, 127–28, 176, 190
death. *See* mortality

dementias
    blood glucose levels and, 16
    C-reactive protein and, 34
    fructose and, 87, 102, 104, 107–8
    medical treatment of, 98–99
    metabolic syndrome and, 39
    obesity and, 99–100
    uric acid levels and, 4, 6, 24, 59, 100, 108, 109
depression
    chlorella and, 143
    C-reactive protein and, 34
    long-term complications of COVID-19
        infection and, 41
    microbiome and, 69
    sleep and, 115
    uric acid levels and, 6, 24
desserts, fructose in, 77
DHA (docosahexaenoic acid), 140–41, 167
diabetes. *See also* type 2 diabetes; type 3
        diabetes
    blood glucose levels and, 148
    in children, 36
    chronic inflammation and, 33, 146
    cognitive decline and, 99, 101
    COVID-19 infection and, 42
    C-reactive protein and, 34
    DNA and, 63
    hemoglobin A1c levels for diagnosis of, 16
    high-fructose corn syrup consumption and,
        81
    metabolic syndrome and, 39
    microbiome and, 69
    nonalcoholic fatty liver disease caused by,
        32
    prediabetes, 16, 72, 102, 117, 148, 150
    prevalence of, 37, 60
    salt consumption and, 90, 122
    sleep and, 115
    uric acid levels and, 4, 6, 9, 13, 30, 32, 45,
        62, 85
diets. *See also* LUV Diet
    ancient diets, 174
    crash diets, 16
    immune function and, 42
    ineffectiveness of, 5
    ketogenic diet, 107, 133–34, 167, 170–72
    low-purine diets, 11
    uric acid levels and, 12, 24
    uric acid-stimulating ingredients in, 4
dinner
    Recipes to LUV, 251–64
    sleep and, 209–10
    staples for, 224–25

dinosaurs, 50–51
DNA
  caloric load and, 49
  diabetes and, 63
  foods and, 174
  fructose and, 84
  purines and, 10, 25
  sleep and, 114
Doll, Richard, 274
dopamine signaling, 92
drinks, Recipes to LUV, 269–71
dysbiosis, 182–83
dyslipidemia, 32

eating behavior, 30
eating out, 195–96, 222–23
eggs, 176, 180, 190
Einstein, Albert, 24
endothelium, 11, 44, 45, 46, 123, 141
epigenetics, 20, 174
epilepsy, 6, 24, 170
erectile dysfunction (ED), 46
estrogen replacement therapy, 34
evolution
  blood pressure and, 58–59
  chronic inflammation and, 33–34
  evolutionary compromises, 29–30
  timeline of human evolution, 52
evolutionary/environmental mismatch, 51–59,
  61, 84
exercise
  amping it up, 212–13
  AMPK and, 67, 211
  excessive exercise, 16, 133, 136, 167, 214
  fat burning and, 66, 67
  frequency of, 134–36
  group exercise, 213
  health and, 19, 30
  immune function and, 42
  lifestyle strategy for, 211–14
  motionless days, 214
  removing barriers to, 212
  routines for, 211–12
  time-restricted eating and, 157–58
  timing of workouts, 37
  types of, 213–14
  uric acid levels and, 12, 14, 135–36, 167

Fanconi syndrome, 48
fast foods, 79, 93, 174
fasting, 16, 133, 153, 155, 169–70, 217
fasting glucose levels, 86, 148–49, 150, 165
fasting insulin concentrations, 54, 165

fat metabolism
  AMPK and, 66–68, 161
  fructose and, 30, 68, 84
  time-restricted eating and, 154, 157
fats, consumption of, 81–82, 141, 180
fat storage
  abdominal fat stores, 67, 86, 93, 146
  AMPD2 and, 67
  burning fat and, 66–68
  fructose and, 29–30, 58–59, 77, 79, 80, 83,
  84
  hyperuricemia and, 13, 20
  metabolic syndrome and, 39
  survival of the fattest, 28, 29, 52, 55–56, 58
fat switch, 29–30, 52, 53
fatty liver
  beer and, 126
  fructose and, 80, 91
  hibernation and, 67
  nonalcoholic fatty liver disease, 4, 20, 30,
  32–33, 36, 121, 122, 143
  salt and, 122
febuxostat, 108
fecal microbial transplants (FMT), 70
feedback potentiation, 83
fiber
  in ancient diets, 174
  food pairing and, 225–26
  in fruits, 77, 186–89
  in vegetables, 77, 186–89
fish, purines in, 127
flavonoids, 162, 189
flavonols, in fruits, 77
food access, 277–78
Food and Drug Administration (FDA), 75, 97,
  98, 169
food industry, 76, 278
Food Is Medicine Coalition, 277
"food is medicine" interventions, 190, 276
food scarcity, 13, 28, 29, 52, 55, 84
food systems, 277
Framingham Heart Study, 26–27, 105
Franklin, Benjamin, 7, 153
free radicals, 87, 107, 147, 149, 188
fructokinase, 83–84, 122
fructose. *See also* high-fructose corn syrup
  (HFCS)
  alcohol compared to, 79–80
  biological mechanisms of, 10
  cerebral fructose metabolism, 40
  consumption of, 61, 73, 77, 78, 81, 93–95,
  102
  DHA and, 140–41

effects in liver, 87
elevated uric acid levels and, 9–10, 30, 49, 77, 82–88, 95, 96, 103, 107, 112
endogenous fructose, 90, 122, 123
glucose distinguished from, 79, 82, 83, 86, 88–89, 90
glycemic index of, 60
in honey, 59, 76, 80, 184
hunger cues and, 80, 84, 88–94
insulin resistance and, 30, 61, 80, 84, 85, 86, 91, 103
marketing of, 9, 60, 79, 82–83, 85
metabolic effects of, 10, 58–59, 61, 68, 77, 79, 82–88, 103, 122
metabolic syndrome and, 43
metabolized by liver, 60–61, 83, 84–85, 86
mitochondria and, 59
as monosaccharides, 76
salt and, 90–91, 122, 123
as source of uric acid, 20, 29–30, 43, 68, 73–74, 77, 79, 85, 86, 87, 122
sources of, 9–10, 59–60, 64, 67, 76–81
sucrose distinguished from, 76–82
in whole, unprocessed foods, 76–77
fruit juice, 77, 78, 105–6
fruits
fiber in, 77, 186–89
flavonoids in, 162
fructose in, 77, 80, 95, 186
gout and, 112
purines in, 127
whole-fruit intake, 78
Yes list, 181

Gagliardi, Jane P., 109
Galen, 6, 23
Garrod, Alfred Baring, 132
gastroesophageal reflux disease (GERD), 125
gene expression, 147, 174, 187
genetically modified organisms (GMO), 168
genetic predispositions, 34
ghrelin, 88–89, 90, 117
glucokinase, 83
gluconeogenesis, 145
glucoraphanin, 188
glucose. *See also* blood glucose levels
cellular energy and, 82
fructose distinguished from, 79, 82, 83, 86, 88–89, 90
as monosaccharides, 76
sleep and, 113–14
glutamate, 129
gluten-free grains, 186

glycation, 135, 146
glycemic excursions, 149
glycemic variability, 149, 151, 226
glycogen, 44, 59, 145
glymphatic system, 121
Goldilocks zone, 47–48
gout
carbohydrates and, 112
cherries and, 189
fecal microbial transplants and, 70
gout-associated bacteria, 70
history of, 6–7
ketogenic diet and, 171, 172
lead poisoning and, 132
low-purine diets for, 11
as metabolic disease, 7
nighttime attacks of, 114, 119
prevalence of, 7, 59, 62–63, 64
psoriasis associated with, 130–31
risk with foods, 128
sugar-sweetened beverages and, 78
uric acid levels and, 3, 6, 7, 12–13, 17, 24, 32, 40, 109, 132
vitamin C and, 142
Grain Brain (Perlmutter), 94, 99, 176, 202
growth hormone, 156
guanine, 10
gut permeability, 69

habits
CGM technology, 149–52
maintenance of, 161
nature, 159, 161, 215–16
regular movement, 159, 161
rethinking, 16
sleep, 159, 161, 205
supplements, 138–43, 161, 167–69, 208
time-restricted eating, 153–58, 159, 161
tolerance for, 5
tweaks to daily habits, 20
uric acid levels and, 52
Hackethal, Veronica, 63
Haig, Alexander, 6, 8, 12, 24–25
HbA1c levels, 16, 135, 146, 165
health. *See also* metabolic health
factors influencing, 19
hyperuricemia associated with challenges to, 7, 9, 130–34
risks of COVID-19 infection to future health, 16
sleep and, 19, 30, 204
sugar as threat to, 4–5, 94, 96
health markers, 53–54

hedonic pathway, 80, 103
hemoglobin A1c levels, 16, 135, 146, 165
hemorrhagic stroke, 34
Hendrickson, Sue, 50n
Henry VIII (king of England), 7
hibernation, 67, 77, 84
high blood pressure. *See* hypertension
high-density lipoprotein (HDL) levels, 38, 159
high-fructose corn syrup (HFCS)
    ADHD and, 92
    consumption of, 52–53, 60, 81, 87, 95, 132
    dopamine signaling and, 92
    fructose combined with, 60–61
    marketing of, 74–76, 77
    sources of, 10, 73, 78–79
    type-2 diabetes and, 82
Hippocrates, 23
homeostasis, 205
hominoid family, 29
honey
    as added sugar, 60
    fructose in, 59, 76, 80, 184
    glucose metabolism and, 185
    In Moderation list, 181–82
hormonal signaling, sleep and, 113
human genome, 51–54, 57, 64, 134
human origin story, 58
humorism, as system of medicine, 6
hunger cues, 80, 84, 88–94, 103
hunter-gatherers, 51, 53–54, 84
hypertension
    asymptomatic hyperuricemia and, 8, 32
    as cardiovascular disease risk, 27
    in children, 36
    cognitive decline and, 99
    C-reactive protein and, 34
    drugs and lifestyle strategies for, 39
    fructose and, 80, 84, 91
    lifestyle strategies for, 39
    metabolic syndrome and, 38
    mortality and, 26
    nitric oxide and, 45
    nonalcoholic fatty liver disease and, 32
    rates of, 5
    salt and, 58, 90, 121
    uric acid levels and, 4, 6, 8, 13, 20–21, 24,
        27–28, 30, 32, 62, 91
hyperuricemia (elevated uric acid)
    asymptomatic hyperuricemia, 7–8, 28, 32,
        33, 40, 109
    cardiovascular disease and, 9, 35
    in children, 36
    chronic hyperuricemia, 145

consequences of, 11, 275
fat storage and, 13, 20
foods associated with, 128
fructose-induced hyperuricemia, 10, 88, 91
genetic mutations and, 13
health conditions associated with, 7, 9,
    130–34
intestinal barrier dysfunction and, 70
men and, 31
metabolic syndrome and, 43, 88, 91, 104
Pacific hyperuricemia, 64–65
pharmaceutical treatments for, 8
Polynesians and, 61–65
sedentary behavior and, 136
sugar consumption as cause of, 7
as survival mechanism, 8, 13, 59, 84
hypoglycemia, 156
hypopnea, 120
hypothalamus, 154
hypothyroidism, 131–32

immune dysfunction, 47, 70
immune function
    circadian rhythms and, 154
    COVID-19 pandemic and, 227–29
    microbiome and, 69
    obesity and, 42
    sleep and, 42, 115
independent risk factors
    for dementias, 100
    uric acid levels as, 9, 13–14, 204
Industrial Revolution, 52
inflammation levels
    abdominal fat and, 86
    blood glucose levels and, 146
    cognitive decline and, 99
    fructose and, 80, 84, 103
    gluten and, 176
    leptin and, 89
    microbiome and, 69
    obesity and, 89
    sleep and, 113
inflammatory markers
    C-reactive protein as, 34–35
    interleuken-6 as, 35
    sleep and, 115–16
    uric acid levels as, 28, 35
insomnia, 116
insulin
    as pro-inflammatory molecule, 89
    as trophic hormone, 103
insulin gene, expression of, 46
insulin-glucose correspondence, 44–45

insulin release, 60, 82, 85, 86, 145
insulin resistance
  abdominal fat and, 86
  Alzheimer's disease and, 102
  brain function and, 103
  in children, 36
  fructose and, 30, 61, 80, 84, 85, 86, 91, 103
  glucose and, 145
  nitric oxide levels and, 44–45, 103
  nonalcoholic fatty liver disease and, 32
  salt and, 121, 122
  sleep and, 117
  as survival mechanism, 28–29
  uric acid levels and, 4, 9, 44, 45, 107, 145–46
insulin sensitivity, 54, 133, 149, 154
insulin-signaling system, 46, 107, 117
interleuken-6 (IL-6), 35, 115
intermittent fasting. *See* time-restricted eating
intestinal barrier dysfunction, 69–70
inulin, 186–87

Jenner, Edward, 24
Johnson, Richard (Rick), 4, 25, 27–29
junk foods, 52, 93, 117

ketogenic diet, 107, 133–34, 167, 170–72
ketosis, 171–72
kidney disease
  chronic kidney disease, 131
  lead poisoning and, 132
  metabolic syndrome and, 39
  uric acid levels and, 30, 32, 40
kidney function, 27–28
kidney stones
  ketogenic diet and, 172
  low-purine diets for, 11
  uric acid levels and, 3, 6, 7, 12–13, 17, 32,
    109
Kooi, Earl R., 81

Lahtela, Petteri, 210
laws of nature, 23
LDL (low-density lipoprotein) levels, 43, 147
lead poisoning, 132–33
leaky gut, 69–70
legumes, purines in, 11
Leonardo da Vinci, 7, 204–5
leptin, 30, 54, 61, 88–90, 117, 131–32
leptin resistance, 89–91, 122
Lickint, Fritz, 274
lifestyle strategies
  for blood glucose levels, 39
  for brain function, 99

for cholesterol levels, 39
for COVID-19 infection, 42
for exercise, 211–14
for hypertension, 39
for sleep, 203–11
for time-restricted eating, 216–17
for uric acid levels, 8, 17, 33
light therapy, 206
lipogenesis, 84
liver
  daily cycles of, 154
  effects of fructose in, 87
  fructose metabolized by, 60–61, 83, 84–85,
    86
liver (organ meat), purines in, 26, 127
liver cells, production of fat in, 32, 67, 86
liver disease
  fructose and, 30
  uric acid levels and, 6
longevity
  factors influencing, 21, 134, 174
  limits of, 51
LPS (lipopolysaccharide), 69, 70
Ludwig, David, 34
lunch
  Recipes to LUV, 242–50
  staples for, 224–25
Lustig, Robert, 79
luteolin, 139–40, 167
LUV Diet. *See also* Recipes to LUV
  as acronym for lower uric values, 12, 159
  dietary principles of, 199–200
  drinks, 192–95
  fasting and, 169–70
  food journal for, 195–96, 220
  food pairing, 225–26
  GERD and, 125
  In Moderation list, 181–82
  No list, 169, 176–80
  protocol for, 175–76, 222, 278
  sample seven-day LUV meal plan, 196–99
  snacks, 191
  staples for, 223–25
  sugar substitutes, 182–86
  uric acid levels and, 109, 127, 133–34, 173
  Yes list, 180–81
LUV plan of action
  focal points of, 158, 159–62
  week 1, 161–62, 173–200
  week 2, 162, 201–17
  week 3, 162, 218–29
LUV program
  establishing rhythm, 219–22

LUV program (*cont.*)
flexibility and, 221–22
glycemic variability and, 149
goals of, 161, 175, 229
intentions for, 219–20, 229
lab tests for, 165–67
microbiome and, 68
opportunities of, 226–29
planning for, 220–21
prelude to, 163–72
tackling stress, 221

malaria, 63–64
Maori people, 62–63
margarine, 79, 177
market medicine, 190
Marshall, Richard O., 81
meal timing, 66. *See also* time-restricted eating
Means, Casey, 94–95, 150, 152, 203–4, 225
meats
consumption of, 165, 171
In Moderation list, 182
No list, 177–78
purines in, 11, 24, 26, 127, 171
medical advancements, 273
medications, uric acid levels and, 12, 14,
124–25, 209
memory
Aduhelm for, 97–98
body weight and, 101
episodic memory, 106–7
fructose and, 103–4
insulin resistance and, 102
nitric oxide and, 88, 108
sleep and, 113, 115, 121
uric acid levels and, 101, 107, 202
men
alcohol and, 127
coffee and, 128, 192, 193
gout and, 7, 31
uric acid levels of, 31, 165
menopause, 7, 165
metabolic dysregulation, 92
metabolic health
achievement of, 16, 161, 228
CGM technology and, 150
definition of, 159–60
markers of, 61
sleep and, 120, 204
time-restricted eating and, 154, 216, 217
triglyceride levels and, 159
uric acid and, 4
waist circumference and, 159–60

metabolic syndrome
adolescents and, 93–94
appetite and, 90
characteristics of, 38–39, 73
cognitive impairment and, 102
COVID-19 infection and, 38, 40–42
diagnosis of, 72–73
gut microbiome and, 70
hyperuricemia and, 43, 88, 91, 104
prevalence of, 7, 38
salt and, 121, 123
sleep and, 116
sleep apnea and, 120
uric acid levels and, 30, 43–47, 73–74, 91,
101
metabolism. *See also* fat metabolism
cerebral fructose metabolism, 40
low-purine diets and, 11
regulatory mechanisms of, 4
sleep and, 113, 114
thyroid hormones and, 73
uric acid as inert waste product of, 4, 6,
17, 131
uric acid levels affecting, 26
metformin, 66–67
MetS. *See* metabolic syndrome
microbiome
changes in, 53, 70
medications and, 125
physiological functions of, 68–69, 71
probiotics and, 168–69
uric acid levels and, 12, 68–71, 168
migraines, 6, 24, 130
migration, 55, 58, 84
Milton, John, 7
Miocene epoch, 54–59
mitochondria, 59, 157
mitochondrial dysfunction, 83–84, 147
modern age, 51–53, 61
monk fruit, 182, 185–86
monosodium glutamate (MSG), 129–30
mortality
Alzheimer's disease and, 98–99
cardiovascular disease and, 26
COVID-19 infection and metabolic
syndrome, 40–42
hazard ratio for all-cause mortality, 31
hypertension and, 26
metabolic syndrome and, 39
poor diet and, 173–74
premature death, 4, 32, 138
reducing risk of, 21
sedentary behavior and, 135

sleep and, 114, 116, 117
uric acid levels and, 4, 9, 31–32
motivation, 19, 160
movement, lack of regular movement, 134–36
multiple sclerosis, 69
muscle mass, 156
myrosinase, 188

native Hawaiians, 63
natural selection, 51
natural stevia, 182, 185
nature, lifestyle strategies for, 159, 161, 215–16
Neel, James, 51–52
negative feedback system, 84
neurodegenerative diseases, 69, 97, 170, 202
neuroenergetics, 103, 104, 105, 107
neurological disorders, 4, 41
Newton, Isaac, 7, 23
New Zealand, 62–63
nitric oxide (NO), 44–45, 45, 46, 87–88, 103, 107–8, 123
nitrogenous bases, 25
nocturnal hypoglycemia, 210
nonalcoholic fatty liver disease (NAFLD)
in children, 36
chlorella and, 143
as emerging driver of hypertension, 32
salt and, 121, 122
uric acid levels and, 4, 20, 30, 32–33
Nrf2 pathway, 187–88, 194
nucleotide base pairs, 25
nucleotides, 10, 126
nutrition, importance of, 276

obesity. *See also* metabolic syndrome
ADHD and, 92
in children, 36, 37–38, 101
cognitive decline and, 99–100, 101
COVID-19 infection and, 42
dietary sugars linked with, 10, 59
fructose consumption and, 61, 90, 91
genes associated with, 64
high-fructose corn syrup consumption and, 81
immune function and, 42
inflammation levels and, 89
insulin resistance and, 44
metabolic syndrome and, 38
microbiome and, 69
nonalcoholic fatty liver disease caused by, 32
obstructive sleep apnea and, 119–20
prevalence of, 7, 37, 53, 61, 81–82

salt consumption and, 90, 121
sleep and, 116–17
uric acid levels and, 4, 6, 8, 13, 20–21, 28, 30, 32, 37, 53, 65, 99–100
obstructive sleep apnea (OSA), 119–20, *120*, 204
Office of Disease Prevention and Health Promotion (ODPHP), 78
omega-3 fats, 81, 141
organic foods, 168
Osler, William, 24, 112
oxidative stress, 27, 45, 46, 84, 85, 147, 202

Paleolithic era, 52
Paleo movement, 57
pancreas
beta cells in, 139–40, 150
fructose and, 82, 85
gut microbiome and, 69
honey and, 185
inflammatory effect of uric acid and, 45
insulin release and, 60, 82, 85, 86, 145
MSG and, 129
time-restricted eating and, 154
Panda, Satchidananda (Satchin), 153–55
parasympathetic nervous system, 156, 215
Parkinson's disease, 34, 69, 107, 170
Pasteur, Louis, 23–24
Perlmutter, Austin, 227–28
Phillips, Matthew, 107
Plato, 23
Pollan, Michael, 79
Polynesians, 61–65
polyphenols, 192, 193–94, 195
polysomnogram, 121
postprandial hyperglycemia, 151
potassium, in fruits, 77
Prader-Willi syndrome, 64
prebiotics, 168, 187
prediabetes, 16, 72, 102, 117, 148, 150
premature death, 4, 32, 138
probiotics, 168–69, 194
processed foods, 53, 60, 62, 76–79, 95, 130, 145, 174, 176–77
produce prescription programs, 277–78
proteins
consumption of, 81
glycation of, 135, 146
In Moderation list, 181–82
Yes list, 181
proton-pump inhibitors (PPIs), 125
pseudogenes, 29
psoriasis, 130–31

purines
  ATP and, 10–11
  from damaged, dying, or dead cells, 10, 26
  endogenous purines, 26
  exogenous purines, 26
  in foods, 11, 20, 26, 64, 67, 127–30
  hyperuricemia linked with, 10
  purine pool, 26
  as source of uric acid, 20, 25–26
  umami foods and, 129
  xylitol and, 126
pyrimidines, 25

quercetin, 12, 138–39, 167, 189

Randolphus of Bocking, 6
reactive oxygen species, 147
Recipes to LUV
  breakfast, 232–41
  dinner, 251–64
  drinks, 269–71
  guidelines for, 230–31
  lunch, 242–50
  snacks, 265–68
renal insufficiency, 131
rheumatism, 6
rheumatoid arthritis, 34
Rippe, James M., 75
RNA, purines and, 10, 25

salt
  consumption of, 121–24, 231
  definition of, 58n
  fructose levels and, 90–91, 122, 123
  hunger cues and, 88
  hypertension and, 58, 90, 121
  retention of, 27–28
  uric acid production triggered by, 90
  water retention and, 58, 59
Samoan people, 63
SARS-CoV-2, 227–28
seafoods, purines in, 11, 26
sedentary behavior, 134–36
Semmelweis, Ignaz, 24
Shakespeare, William, 215
Shaw, Jonathan, 61–62
Shinrin-yoku (forest bathing), 215
sitting, 134–36, 214
sleep
  appetite and, 88–89, 113
  avoiding sleep aids, 207–8
  biochemical effects of, 113
  cycles of, 115, 207

destructive forces of sleep deprivation, 118
  fat burning and, 66
  health and, 19, 30, 204
  immune function and, 42, 115
  length of, 207
  leptin and, 89
  lifestyle strategy for, 203–11
  nature and, 215
  signals of, 205–6
  substances hostile to, 208–9
  technology and, 210–11
  temperature for, 207
  time-restricted eating and, 155, 157–58
  timing for dinner, 209–10
  uric acid levels and, 12, 14, 113–21, 204
sleep apnea, 116, 119–20, *120*, 204
smoking tobacco, 5, 34, 75, 228, 273–75, 278
snacks
  guidelines for, 191
  Recipes to LUV, 265–68
soy, 127–28, 178
starvation pathway, 80, 89
stress reduction
  blood glucose levels and, 151
  coping skills, 221
  health and, 19
  immune function and, 42
  nature and, 215
  sleep and, 113
stroke
  hemorrhagic stroke, 34
  ischemic stroke, 31
  long-term complications of COVID-19
    infection and, 41
  uric acid levels and, 4, 6, 24, 31, 100
sucrase, 76
sucrose
  as added sugar, 60
  as disaccharide, 76
  fructose distinguished from, 76–82
  research on, 67
sugar. *See also* fructose
  consumption of, 5, 7, 59–60, 74, 94–95,
    110–11, 137–38
  dietary sugars linked with obesity, 10, 59
  elevated uric acid levels and, 7, 9, 137–38
  Industrial Revolution and, 52
  names on food labels, 178–80
  refined-sugar overload, 89
  as source of fructose, 80–81
  sources of added sugar, 60, 76, 78
  substitutes for, 182–86
  as threat to health, 4–5, 94, 96

Index

sulforaphane, 187–89
supplements, 138–43, 161, 167–69, 208
suprachiasmatic nucleus, 206
sympathetic nervous system activation, 149, 156, 215
syndrome X. *See* metabolic syndrome
systemic inflammation
  asymptomatic hyperuricemia and, 8, 33
  controlled levels of, 16
  C-reactive protein and, 8, 34–35, 73
  fructose and, 85
  gut microbiome and, 70

tastes, five basic tastes, 128–129
tau protein, 123
tea, 193–94
Tennyson, Alfred, Lord, 7
thirst cues, 84
thrifty genes, 51–52, 53, 62–64
thyroid function, 15, 47, 73, 131–32
time-restricted eating
  AMPK and, 67, 156
  forms of, 155–56
  health and, 30
  lifestyle strategies for, 216–17
  practice of, 133, 153–58
TNF-alpha, 115
tobacco industry, 75, 79, 94
triceps skin-fold measurements, 54
triglyceride levels
  beer and, 126
  as biomarker, 43
  fructose and, 84–85, 86, 90
  leptin resistance and, 90
  metabolic health and, 159
  metabolic syndrome and, 38, 73, 91
Trump, Donald, 95
tumor lysis syndrome, 133–34
two-minute challenge, 135
type 2 diabetes
  abdominal fat and, 86
  in children, 36, 93
  C-reactive protein and, 34
  dementia risk and, 39
  genetic basis of, 51
  gut microbiome and, 70
  high-fructose corn syrup and, 82
  insulin resistance and, 44, 145
  prevalence of, 82
  uric acid levels and, 8, 9, 45
type 3 diabetes, Alzheimer's disease as, 102–11
tyrannosaur skeleton (Sue), 50–51, 50n

umami foods, 128–29
USDA dietary guidelines, 95
uric acid
  AMP production and, 67–68
  autophagy and, 47
  biological effects of, 4, 20
  BMI and, 65, 65
  as contributory causal factor, 43
  as inert waste product of metabolism, 4, 6, 17, 131
  intestines and, 70
  as master conductor, 30
  metabolic health and, 4
  nitric oxide activity and, 44–45, 45
  purines as source of, 20, 25–26
  research on, 19–20
  sources of, 20
  waist circumference and, 65, 65
uric acid levels. *See also* hyperuricemia (elevated uric acid)
  allopurinol lowering, 28
  as biomarker of health, 43
  blocking uric acid in high-fructose diet, 91
  brain function and, 100–101
  cognitive decline and, 21, 40, 88, 100, 108–9, 110, 202
  C-reactive protein and, 34–35
  dementias and, 4, 6, 24, 59, 100, 108, 109
  diabetes and, 4, 6, 9, 13, 30, 32, 45, 62, 85
  exercise and, 12, 14, 135–36, 167
  fat metabolism and, 67–68
  gout and, 3, 6, 7, 12–13, 17, 24, 32, 40, 109, 132
  habits and, 52
  hypertension and, 4, 6, 8, 13, 20–21, 24, 27–28, 30, 32, 62, 91
  as independent risk factor, 9, 13–14, 204
  kidney disease and, 30, 32, 40
  kidney function and, 27–28
  kidney stones and, 3, 6, 7, 12–13, 17, 32, 109
  lifestyle adjustments for, 8, 17, 33
  low-purine diets and, 11
  management of, 5, 9, 12, 16, 20, 159, 160, 228–29, 276
  medications and, 12, 14, 124–25, 209
  metabolic syndrome and, 30, 43–47, 73–74, 91, 101
  microbiome and, 12, 68–71, 168
  nonalcoholic fatty liver disease and, 4, 20, 30, 32–33
  obesity and, 4, 6, 8, 13, 20–21, 28, 30, 32, 37, 53, 65, 99–100

323

uric acid levels (*cont.*)
   optimal range of, 16, 31, 48–49, 100–101, 165–66
   self-assessment of, 14–16
   serum uric acid levels, 9, 11, 26, 31
   sleep and, 12, 14, 113–21, 204
   sugar-sweetened beverages and, 78
   supplements for lowering, 138–43, 161, 167–69, 208
   tests for, 7, 36–37, 166, 170
   time-restricted eating and, 154
   understanding UA values, 16
   vitamin C and, 12, 142, 168
uricase enzyme, 29, 50–51, 56–58, 56
urine
   color of, 194
   uric acid excreted from body in, 4, 26

Van Cauter, Eve, 114
vasodilation, 44
vasopressin, 58–59
vegetable oils, 52–53, 177, 222
vegetables
   fiber in, 77, 186–89
   flavonoids in, 162
   fructose in, 76–77, 186
   In Moderation list, 182
   purines in, 11, 127
   Yes list, 181
visceral adipose tissue, 67, 86, 93
visual acuity, 54

vitamin C
   in fruits, 77
   uric acid levels and, 12, 142, 168

waist circumference
   cognitive decline and, 99
   metabolic health and, 159–60
   uric acid and, 65, 65
waist-to-height ratio, 54
waist-to-hip ratio, 99
water, 194–95
weight control
   diets and, 5
   excessive eating and, 80
   high-fructose corn syrup and, 92
   ketogenic diet and, 171, 172
   management of, 9, 19
   time-restricted eating and, 154
Williams, Tricia, 230
wine, 126, 127, 195
Wolfe, Tom, 3
women
   alcohol and, 127
   coffee and, 128, 192, 193
   gout and, 7, 31
   uric acid levels of, 31, 165
World Health Organization, 61, 134, 187

xanthine oxidase, 139, 162, 189, 192
xylitol, 126–27, 177, 183

About the Author

David Perlmutter, MD, is a board-certified neurologist and Fellow of the American College of Nutrition. He is a frequent lecturer at symposia sponsored by institutions such as the World Bank, Columbia University, New York University, Yale, and Harvard and serves as an associate professor at the University of Miami Miller School of Medicine. He is the recipient of numerous awards, including the Linus Pauling Award, for his innovative approaches to neurological disorders; the National Nutritional Foods Association Clinician of the Year Award; and the Humanitarian of the Year Award from the American College of Nutrition. He maintains an active blog at DrPerlmutter.com and is the author of *Brain Wash, Grain Brain, Brain Maker, The Grain Brain Whole Life Plan, The Grain Brain Cookbook, Raise a Smarter Child by Kindergarten, The Better Brain Book,* and *Power Up Your Brain.*